Beijing Medical College

DICTIONARY OF TRADITIONAL CHINESE MEDICINE

中醫藥詞典

Edited by:

Xie Zhufan, *Associate Professor of Medicine*

Huang Xiaokai, *Associate Professor of English*

Written by:

Xie Zhufan

Huang Xiaokai

Lou Zhicen, *Ph.D.(Lond.) Professor of Pharmacognosy*

Li Shuncheng, *Associate Professor of Medicine*

Zhou Luling, *Lecturer of English*

Yuan Shuo, *Lecturer of Medicine*

Zhou Shijun, *Lecturer of Medicine*

Yang Zhendan, *Lecturer of English*

Tang Zijin, *Associate Professor of Medicine*

DICTIONARY
OF
TRADITIONAL
CHINESE
MEDICINE

中醫藥詞典

Edited by: Xie Zhufan, Huang Xiaokai

GEORGE ALLEN & UNWIN
Sydney London Boston

First published in 1985
GEORGE ALLEN & UNWIN AUSTRALIA PTY. LTD.
8 Napier Street, North Sydney NSW 2060

GEORGE ALLEN & UNWIN (PUBLISHERS) LTD.
18 Park Lane, Hemel Hempstead, Herts HP2
4TE England

National Library of Australia
Cataloguing in publication entry:

DICTIONARY OF TRADITIONAL CHINESE MEDICINE
  Bibliography.
  Includes Indexes.

  ISBN 0 86861 781 4
  1. Medicine – China – Dictionaries. i. Xie,
  Zhufan. ii. Huang, Xiaokai.

  610' 951

Printed by
C & C JOINT PRINTING CO., (H.K.) LTD.
75, Pau Chung Street, Kowloon, Hong Kong

Preface

Terms of traditional Chinese medicine may number ten thousand. Only those which are of practical use, i.e., those which are commonly used in clinical work and teaching today are listed in this dictionary. Besides the English equivalent of each entry in boldface, most of the entries are given explanations in addition to carry their meaning and implication into English more fully for better comprehension.

The terms are arranged into 12 chapters so that those which are closely related in nature and meaning are grouped together and the readers who know little about traditional Chinese medicine may find it easier to grasp their idea.

Most of the terms of traditional Chinese medicine have specific notions which defy any attempt to find appropriate English equivalents and a few terms still lack commonly accepted definitions. However, the authors have done their best in bringing out the closest, if not the only, meanings of them.

The dictionary is prepared under the guidance of the authorites of the Beijing Medical College. Acknowledgement is made to them and to Dr. Cheng Zhi-fan, head of the Section of Medical History, who checked the entries in Chapter 10, and Drs. Li Sheng-hua, Qin Bo and Zheng Jun-hua of the Department of Pharmacognosy for their help in preparing Chapter 8.

The Editors

Notes on the Use of the Dictionary

1. This dictionary lists 3,325 commonly-used terms of traditional Chinese medicine and pharmacy, arranged in 12 chapters, with an index appended at the end of it.

2. The terms are in general listed separately, with Chinese phonetic transcriptions, English translation (in boldface) and explanations. Terms easy to comprehend or with notions close to those of terms of modern medicine will have English translations only.

3. Synonymous terms are given in one entry to avoid repetition, but they are separated with semicolons, and provided with Chinese phonetic transcription each, and then followed by their common English translation and explanation. *e.g.,*

肝陰虛 [gānyīnxū]; 肝陰不足 [gānyīn bùzú]

deficiency of Yin (vital essence) of the liver, usually due to its being poorly nourished by the blood, marked by ......

Terms which are close in meaning but actually differ from each other are listed separately and marked with (cf...) to refer to related entries.

4. Derived terms of an entry are not listed separately if their meaning is already made clear in this entry. But they are listed separately in the index so that they may be easy to be looked up. *e.g.*

胃 [wèi]

the (orb of) stomach....... The cavity of the stomach is called 胃脘 [wèiwǎn];......

Here 胃脘 is not given as separate entry.

5. If a term has two or more meanings, the different meanings are given separately and marked with numerals to distinguish one from the other. *e.g.*

寒热 [hán rè]

(1) **cold or heat**—two of the Eight Principal Syndromes showing ......; (2) **chills and fever**

6. The English equivalents of the Chinese terms, if possible, are given in the same part of speech as that of the original. If the Chinese term can be used in different parts of speech, the most commonly used part of speech is adopted in the English translation. In general, the English translation of Chinese terms (except proper nouns or names of drugs) is not initiated with a capital letter, nor terminates with a period, unless it is a complete sentence.

7. Since terms of traditional Chinese medicine often have specific notions and few of them have exact English equivalents, great efforts have been made to make the English translations as close as can be to the original and explanations are given wherever necessary. The content and form of explanations are determined by what is needed and emphasis is laid on elucidation of the essentials. For instance, for terms of differentiation of symptom-complexes stress is put on the description of clinical manifestations; for terms of Chinese drugs and prescriptions, on their actions and indications; for distinguished Chinese physicians in history, on their medical theories and achievements.

8. Some terms of traditional Chinese medicine are widely used in modern medicine. Yet there exists much difference between the two. Though marked distinction is observed between Chinese medicine and Western medicine in describing the structure and functions of the internal organs, 心, 肝, 脾, etc., they are rendered into English as heart, liver, spleen, etc. In defining or explaining other terms, these terms are italicized to remind the readers that they should be comprehended according to traditional Chinese medicine and avoid confusing them with terms of modern medicine.

9. Both English and Latin translations are given to names of Chinese Materia Medica, with the latter italicized to distinguish themselves from the former. In explanations, especially in prescriptions names of drugs are generally given in Latin.

10. A lot of books on acupuncture and moxibustion have been published in Western languages. To economize space, we present the acupuncture points in tables instead of describing them separately, and after the fashion accepted internationally, we give their phonetic transcriptions and order numbers only, without any explanation.

CONTENTS

I   Theories of Yin-Yang and the Five Elements

陰陽 Yin and Yang

陰陽〔yīnyáng〕
Yin and Yang: the two fundamental principles or forces in the universe, ever opposing and complementing each other—an ancient philosophical concept used in traditional Chinese medicine to refer to various antitheses in anatomy, physiology, pathology, diagnosis and treatment, e.g., feminine, interior, cold and hypofunction being Yin while masculine, exterior, heat and hyperfunction are Yang.

陰〔yīn〕
Yin: the female or negative principle, the structive or material aspect of an effective position, e.g., of an internal organ

陽〔yáng〕
Yang: the male or positive principle, the active or functional aspect of an effective position, e.g., of an internal organ

陰中之陽, 陰中之陰〔yīn zhōng zhī yáng, yīn zhōng zhī yīn〕
Yang in Yin and Yin in Yin: Yin may be subdivided into Yang and Yin, the resultant Yang and Yin are called Yang in Yin and Yin in Yin respectively, e.g., the night is regarded as Yin in relation to the day, the period from nightfall to midnight is said to be Yang in Yin, and the period of small hours Yin in Yin

陽中之陽, 陽中之陰〔yǎng zhōng zhī yáng, yáng zhōng zhī yīn〕
Yang in Yang, Yin in Yang: Yang may be subdivided into Yang and Yin, the resultant Yang and Yin are said to be Yang in Yang and Yin in Yang respectively, e.g., the day is regarded as Yang in relation to the night, the early part of the day between dawn and noon is said to be Yang in Yang and the afternoon Yin in Yang

陰陽互根〔yīnyáng hùgēn〕

the interdependence of Yin and Yang, the existence of the one being the prerequisite of the existence of the other

陰陽消長 [yīnyáng xiāo zhǎng]

the relative **waxing and waning of Yin and Yang**, the two opposites of a single entity, increase or excess of the one means decrease or deficiency of the other, which is usually used in explaining pathological changes

陽生陰長 [yáng shēng yīn zhǎng]

Growth of Yin depends upon normal development of Yang, which illustrates the interdependence of Yin and Yang from the aspect of growing.

陰陽轉化 [yīnyáng zhuǎnhuà]

the **transformation of Yin and Yang into each other** under certain conditions, e.g., an illness of heat nature in the extreme may show symptoms and signs of cold nature

陽生於陰 [yáng shēng yú yīn]

Yang exists with Yin as its prerequisite, e.g., vital function (a Yang factor) relies on vital essence (a Yin factor) as its material basis.

陰生於陽 [yīn shēng yú yáng]

Yin exists with Yang as its prerequisite, e.g., the production of vital essence (a Yin factor) depends on the activity of vital function (a Yang factor).

陰平陽秘 [yīn píng yáng mì]

Yin is even and well while Yang is firm, hence a relative equilibrium is maintained and health is guaranteed.

陰陽調和 [yīnyáng tiáohé]

harmony of Yin and Yang by which good health is guaranteed

陰陽失調 [yīnyáng shītiáo]; 陰陽不和 [yīnyáng bùhé]; 陰陽乖戾 [yīnyáng guāilì]

breakdown of balanced equilibrium of Yin and Yang, which is believed to be the general pathogenesis of all diseases

陰陽自和 [yīnyáng zìhé]

restoration of relative equilibrium of Yin and Yang, indicating recovery of a person from illness

陰勝則陽病 [yīn shèng zé yáng bìng]

Yin in excess makes Yang suffer, e.g., if exogenous or endogenous cold (a Yin factor) prevails, the vital function (a Yang factor) of the internal organs would be impaired.

陽勝則陰病 [yáng shèng zé yīn bìng]
Yang in excess makes Yin suffer, e.g., excessive exogenous or endogenous heat (a Yang factor) would injure vital essence and body fluid (a Yin factor).

陰損及陽 [yīn sǔn jí yáng]
Impairment of Yin would impede the generation of Yang, e.g., deficiency of vital essence is often complicated by lowered vital function in advanced cases.

陽損及陰 [yáng sǔn jí yīn]
Impairment of Yang would impede generation of Yin, e.g., insufficiency of vital function is often complicated by deficiency of vital essence in advanced cases.

重陰必陽 [chóng yīn bì yáng]; 陰極反陽 [yīn jí fǎn yáng]
Yin in its extreme will give rise to Yang, e.g., a chronic debilitated case in its extreme may show symptoms and signs of Yang nature such as feeling hot and thirsty, moving restlessly.

重陽必陰 [chóng yáng bì yīn]; 陽極反陰 [yáng jí fǎn yīn]
Yang in its extreme will give rise to Yin, e.g., febrile disease with intense heat may bring on symptoms and signs of cold such as chills and cold limbs.

陰陽離決 [yīn yáng lí jué]
divorce of Yin and Yang, which means the end of one's life

陽常有餘, 陰常不足 [yáng cháng yǒu yú, yīn cháng bù zú]
Yang is usually redundant while Yin is ever deficient — a theory advocated by Zhu Dan-xi (1281—1358 A.D.), according to which the method of reinforcing Yin (vital essence) is recommended as a basic principle in treating diseases

五行
The Five Elements

五行 [wǔxíng]

3

the Five Evolutive Phases or the Five Elements: wood, fire, earth, metal and water with their characteristic properties—an ancient philosophical concept to explain the composition and phenomena of the physical universe and later used in traditional Chinese medicine to expound the unity of the human body and the natural world, and the physiological and pathological relationship between the internal organs

相生〔xiāngshēng〕

the interpromoting relation of the Five Evolutive Phases or Elements in the following sequence — wood, fire, earth, metal and water — in which each Evolutive Phase or Element is conceived to promote or produce the subsequent one, namely, wood produces fire, fire produces earth, earth produces metal, etc.

相克〔xiāngkè〕

the interacting(conquest or checking) relation of the Five Evolutive Phases or Elements in the following sequence—water, fire metal, wood and earth—in which each Evolutive Phase or Element is considered to check the subsequent one, namely, water checks fire, fire checks metal, metal checks wood, etc.

相乘〔xiāngchéng〕

encroachment — to check in the severest way, e.g., if wood is redundant in energy, it will encroach on the quality of earth instead of merely checking it, and will violate metal by which it should itself be checked

相侮〔xiāngwǔ〕; 反克〔fǎnkè〕

violation — to check instead of being checked as in the ordinary checking sequence of the Five Elements, e.g., fire checks (violates) water instead of being checked by water

制化〔zhìhuà〕

the promoting (producing) and counteracting (checking) relations of the Five Elements taken as a whole, which forms a self-limiting balanced process, e.g., wood checks earth which produces metal that will check wood in turn

運〔yùn〕

(1) circuit phase; (2) to transmit

運氣〔yùnqì〕

4

(1) the circulation of the Qi (vital energy); (2) abbreviation of "五運六氣", the circular movement of the Five Elements (Evolutive Phases) and the Six Atmospheric Influences

五運六氣 [wǔyùn liùqì]
the Five Circuit Phases and the Six Atmospheric Influences

五臟所屬 [wǔzàng suǒ shǔ]
the Evolutive Phases which the Five Viscera correspond to: the *liver, heart, spleen, lung* and *kidney* correspond to wood, fire, earth, metal and water respectively

木喜條達 [mù xǐ tiáodá]
Wood or tree likes to spread out freely — a figure of speech to explain the physiological properties of the *liver* (which corresponds to wood), since the main function of the *liver* is to smooth the flow of vital energy and blood, if it being depressed, symptoms of stagnancy would occur.

木鬱化火 [mù yù huà huǒ]
A depressed liver (corresponding to wood) may give rise to symptoms of fire, marked by headache, dizziness, flushed face, hematemesis, hemoptysis, or even mania.

木火刑金 [mùhuǒ xíng jīn]
Fire of the liver (corresponding to wood) makes the lung (corresponding to metal) suffer by impairing the latter's essence and fluid and brings on dry cough, chest pain, hemoptysis, etc.

木克土 [mù kè tǔ]
Earth is checked by wood, which denotes: (1) the physiological relationship between the *liver* (represented by wood) and the *spleen* and *stomach* (represented by earth); (2) the pathological condition of the *spleen* or *stomach* caused by dysfunction of the *liver*.

火性炎上 [huǒxìng yánshàng]
Fire tends to flare upwards, which figuratively states the fact that the symptoms caused by fire tend to appear on the upper part of the body, esp. on the head, such as headache, sore throat, bloodshot eye, gum bleeding, epistaxis, etc.

火盛刑金 [huǒ shèng xíng jīn], 火旺刑金 [huǒ wàng xíng jīn]

5

Excessive fire hurts metal, which denotes: (1) fire of the *liver* makes the *lung* (represented by metal) suffer; (2) fire in the *heart* or evil heat injures the *lung*.

火不生土 [huǒ bù shēng tǔ]

Fire fails to support earth; by which is meant that the Yang (functional activities) of the *kidney* or fire of the Vital Gate fails to warm the *spleen* and *stomach* (represented by earth) and bringing on symptoms of indigestion, diarrhea, edema, intolerance of cold, etc.

土生萬物 [tǔ shēng wànwù]

Earth produces everything. The *spleen* and *stomach* (corresponding to earth) provide the material foundation for the whole organism by digesting food and transporting nutrients.

土喜溫燥 [tǔ xǐ wēn zào]

Earth prefers warmth and dryness— an explanation of the physiological properties of the *spleen* (which corresponds to earth). The *spleen* functions well under warm and dry conditions and is liable to be rendered diseased by cold and dampness; a diseased *spleen* often leads to accumulation of dampness with symptoms such as diarrhea and edema.

土不制水 [tǔ bù zhì shuǐ]

Earth fails to control water, which figuratively denotes failure of the *spleen* (represented by earth) in guaranteeing normal water metabolism, as a result, loose stool, edema, profuse frothy sputum may occur.

金水相生 [jīn shuǐ xiāngshēng]

The lung and the kidney (corresponding to metal and water), **promote one another.** If one is diseased, the other is liable to be affected.

金實不鳴 [jīn shí bùmíng]

"A muffled gong does not sound" figuratively referring to sudden onset of hoarseness of voice when the *lung* (corresponding to metal) is attacked by various external pathogenic factors (such as wind and cold, wind and heat).

水性潤下 [shuǐxìng rùn xià]

Water tends to run downwards — a metaphor to explain the down-

6

ward tendency of pathological changes due to dampness such as diarrhea, heaviness and edema of the lower extremities.

水火相濟 〔shuǐ huǒ xiāngjì〕
Water and fire (referring to the *kidney* and *heart*) complement each other to maintain a balanced interacting — relationship physiologically.

水火不濟 〔shuǐ huǒ bùjì〕
Water and fire fail to complement each other, denoting the breakdown of a balanced interacting—relationship between the *kidney* and *heart* which correspond to water and fire respectively, hence irritability, insomnia, lumbago and nocturnal emission may occur.

水不涵木 〔shuǐ bù hán mù〕
Water fails to provide wood with proper nourishment, by which is meant that due to deficiency of Yin (vital essence), the *kidney* (represented by water) fails to nourish the *liver* (represented by wood), as a result, symptoms of internal wind may occur.

母 〔mǔ〕; 母氣 〔mǔqì〕
the "mother": in the producing sequence the evolutive phase that produces, e.g., wood is the "mother" of fire

子 〔zǐ〕; 子氣 〔zǐqì〕
the "child": in the producing sequence the evolutive phase that is produced, e.g., fire is the "child" of wood

子盜母氣 〔zǐ dào mǔqì〕
A "child" organ may "rob" the "mother" organ. According to the theory of the Five Evolutive Phases applied to pathology, a diseased "child" organ, e.g., the *lung*, may render its "mother" organ, the *spleen*, affected.

母病及子 〔mǔ bìng jí zǐ〕
A diseased "mother" viscus may get its "child" viscus involved, e.g., a diseased *kidney* may affect the *liver*.

子病及母 〔zǐ bìng jí mǔ〕
A diseased "child" viscus may get its "mother" viscus involved, e.g., a diseased *spleen* may affect the *heart*.

7

II Structure and Function of the Human Body

臟腑
Viscera and Bowels

臟腑 [zàngfǔ]
internal organs; viscera and bowels; functional orbs (in traditional Chinese medicine emphasis is laid on various physiological functions of an organ rather than on its anatomical structure)

五臟 [wǔzàng]
the Five Viscera; the Five Yin Orbs: *heart, liver, spleen, lung and kidney.*

六臟 [liùzàng]
the Six Viscera: (1) *heart, liver, spleen, lung, kidney* and *pericardium*; (2) *heart, liver, spleen, lung, kidney* and Vital Gate

六腑 [liùfǔ]
the Six Bowels; the Six Yang Orbs: *gallbladder, stomach, large intestine, small intestine, urinary bladder* and the Triple Burners

牡臟 [mǔzàng]
the male viscera, referred to the *heart* and the *liver*, distinguished for their preponderant Yang quality

牝臟 [pìnzàng]
the female viscera, referred to the *spleen*, the *lung* and the *kidney*, distinguished for their preponderant Yin quality

心 [xīn]
the heart; the cardial orb, which controls blood circulation and mental activities

肝 [gān]
the liver; the hepatic orb, which stores blood, smooths the flow of vital energy, controls functions of sinews, with its outward manifestation reflected in the eyes and nails

8

脾 [pí]

the spleen; the splenic orb, which is believed to share with the *stomach* the function of digesting food, transport and distribute nutrients and water, reinforce the vital energy, keep the blood flowing within the blood vessels

肺 [fèi]

the lung; the pulmonic orb, which is mainly in charge of vital energy, performs the function of respiration, disseminates the vital energy and keeps it flowing downwards, helps maintain normal water metabolism, controls the functions of the skin

肾 [shèn]

the kidney; the renal orb, which installs vital essence and takes charge of growth, development, reproduction, and urinary functions. It also has direct effect on the condition of the bone and marrow, activities of the brain, hearing of the ears, inspiratory function of the respiratory system, etc.

心包 [xīnbāo]; 心包络 [xīnbāoluò]

the pericardium; the pericardial orb, which, surrounding the *heart*, protects it against attack of exogenous pathogenic factors. "Affection of pericardium" is actually the same as that of the *heart*, people avoid mentioning the latter from the feudalistic point of view that during the invasion of exogenous evil factors the *pericardium* should bear the brunt and serve as a "scapegoat" for the "monarch" organ, the *heart.*

命门 [mìngmén]

(1) "Vital Gate" or "Gate of Life", which is believed to be closely related to the *kidney* both physiologically and pathologically, and is taken as the source of heat energy of the body. 命门之火 [mìngmén zhī huǒ] the fire of Vital Gate is actually the same as the Yang of the *kidney* (肾阳); (2) an acupuncture point on the Back Midline Channel —Du Channel

膽 [dǎn]

the (orb of) gallbladder; a hollow organ with refined content or 中精之腑 [zhōng jīng zhī fǔ] , i.e., containing bile which is also called refined juice or 精汁 [jīng zhī] . The function of this organ is also related to psychic and emotional activities.

胃 [wèi]

the (orb of) stomach. Its chief function is to receive and digest food. The cavity of the stomach is called 胃脘 [wèiwǎn]; the upper part of the stomach, 上脘 [shàngwǎn]; the middle part of the cavity of the stomach, 中脘 [zhōngwǎn]; the lower part or the fundus of the stomach, 下脘 [xiàwǎn]

大腸 [dàcháng]

the (orb of) large intestine: a hollow organ to pass the waste

小腸 [xiǎocháng]

the (orb of) small intestine: a hollow organ to receive food content from the stomach and further digest it, absorb the useful and excrete the waste

膀胱 [pángguāng]

the (orb of) urinary bladder which stores and discharges urine

三焦 [sānjiāo]

the Triple Burners (or Heaters); tricaloria; the three portions of the body cavity

上焦 [shàngjiāo]

the Upper Burner; the upper portion of the body cavity: the portion above the diaphragm of the body cavity housing the *heart* and the *lung*

中焦 [zhōngjiāo]

the Middle Burner; the middle portion of the body cavity: the portion between the diaphragm and umbilicus of the body cavity housing the *spleen* and the *stomach*

下焦 [xiàjiāo]

the Lower Burner; the lower portion of the body cavity: the portion below umbilicus of the body cavity housing the *kidney, urinary bladder, small* and *large intestines,* including the *liver* owing to its pathophysiological relation with the *kidney*

三焦有名無形 [sānjiāo yǒu míng wú xíng]

The Triple Burner is an unsubstantial name without any particular bodily shape, as believed by some ancient Chinese physicians.

奇恒之腑 [jīhéng zhī fǔ]

the Extraordinary organs: brain, medulla, bones, blood vessels, gallbladder and uterus. They are so called because their physiological properties are different both from ordinary viscera and from bowels.

脈 [mài]

(1) blood vessels; (2) conduits of blood and vital energy; (3) pulse

宗脈 [zōngmài]

(1) confluence of channels; (2) cardinal conduit of the Lung Channel

女子胞 [nǚzǐbāo]; 胞宮 [bāogōng]; 子臟 [zǐzàng]; 胞臟 [bāozàng]

the uterus; the womb; the child-bearing organ

四海 [sìhǎi]

the four seas or the four reservoirs: the reservoir of marrow (the brain), the reservoir of blood (the Conception Channel), the reservoir of Qi or vital energy (the pectoral region) and the reservoir of water and grain (the stomach)

氣海 [qìhǎi]

(1) the sea or reservoir of vital energy, referred to the central part of the chest. Some hold there are two in number, with the pectoral region as the upper one and the region just below the umbilicus as the lower one; (2) a point on the Ren (Front Middle) Channel, one and half cun 寸 (4—5cm) below the umbilicus

髓海 [suǐhǎi]

the sea or reservoir of marrow (chiefly the spinal marrow), referred to the brain

腦爲元神之府 [nǎo wéi yuánshén zhī fǔ]

The brain is the seat of mentality.

血海 [xuèhǎi]

the sea or reservoir of blood, referred to: (1) the Conception Channel (冲脈); (2) the *liver*; (3) a point on the Spleen Channel

水穀之海 [shuǐgǔ zhī hǎi]

the reservoir of water and grain, referred to the stomach

血室 [xuèshì]

the blood chamber, referred to: (1) the uterus; (2) the *liver;* (3) the Conception Channel (冲脈)

11

臟象 [zàngxiàng]

organ picture: visceral outward manifestations through which physiological functions as well as pathological changes can be detected and state of health judged

五臟爲實, 藏而不洩 [wǔzàng wéi shí, cáng ér bú xiè]

The Five Viscera are solid, installing but not discharging (essence, energy, blood or body fluid).

六腑爲空, 洩而不藏 [liùfǔ wéi kōng, xiè ér bù cáng]

The Six Bowels are hollow, discharging their content but not installing it. Main functions of the Bowels are supposed to receive and digest food, supply the Viscera with food essence but not to keep it for themselves, and discharge the waste from the body.

五臟藏精氣而不洩 [wǔ zàng cáng jīngqì ér bú xiè]

The Five Viscera install and not eliminate essence and energy.

六腑傳化物而不藏 [liùfǔ chuán huàwù ér bù cáng]

The Six Bowels transform food into essence but not store it.

六腑以通爲用 [liùfǔ yǐ tōng wéi yòng]

The Six Bowels function well when they are unobstructed.

五臟所惡 [wǔzàng suǒ wù]

intolerance of the Five Viscera. The *heart, lung, liver, spleen* and *kidney* are said to be intolerant of heat, cold, wind, dampness and dryness respectively.

五臟所主 [wǔzàng suǒ zhǔ]

the charges of the Five Viscera. The *heart, lung, liver, spleen* and *kidney* are said to be in charge of the pulse, skin, tendons, muscles and bones respectively

五味所入 [wǔwèi suǒ rù]

accessibility of the Five Sapors (Flavors). The sour, bitter, sweet, pungent and salty are accessible to the Five Viscera: the *liver, heart, spleen, lung* and *kidney* respectively.

五志 [wǔzhì]

the Five Emotions: (1) joy, anger, anxiety, sorrow, and fear assigned to the *heart, liver, spleen, lung* and *kidney* respectively; (2) various emotional changes at large

臟腑相合 [zàngfǔ xiānghé]

12

connexion between the Viscera and the Bowels, which are inter-related and mutually influenced and are connected by the Channels

臟行氣於腑 [zàng xíng qì yú fǔ]

The Five Viscera provide the Bowels with energy for their proper functioning.

腑輸精於臟 [fǔ shū jīng yú zàng]

The Bowels supply the Viscera with nutrients.

臟氣 [zàngqì]

the Qi (functional activities) of the internal organs

心氣 [xīnqì]

the Qi (functional activities) of the heart, including mental activities

心屬火 [xīn shǔ huǒ]

The heart corresponds to fire according to the theory of the Five Evolutive Phases.

心血 [xīnxuè]

the blood controlled by the heart; blood in the heart, which nourishes various parts of the body and serves as the material basis of mental activities (hence deficiency of blood in the *heart* usually leads to mental disturbances)

心陰 [xīnyīn]

the Yin (vital essence) of the heart, especially the fluid in the *heart*

心陽 [xīnyáng]

the Yang (vital function) of the heart, especially the function of the cardiovascular system in general

心主血脈 [xīn zhǔ xuèmài]

The heart controls blood circulation.

心主神明 [xīn zhǔ shénmíng]

The heart is in charge of mental activities, including consciousness and thinking, and dysfunction of the *heart* may result in insomnia, amnesia, impairment of consciousness, psychosis, etc.

心，其華在面 [xīn, qí huá zài miàn]

The heart has its outward manifestation in the face or complexion, since the heart controls blood circulation, and the face is abundant in blood vessels.

舌爲心之苗 [shé wéi xīn zhī miáo]
The tongue is the body opening of the heart.

心開竅於舌 [xīn kāi qiào yú shé]
The heart has its specific opening in the tongue, i.e., the condition
of the *heart* is bound to be reflected in the tongue proper, e.g.,
dark purple of the tongue indicats blood stasis of the *heart*, pallor of the
tongue reveals blood deficiency of the *heart*, ulcer on the tongue
tells of excessive fire of the *heart*.

心腎相交 [xīn shèn xiāngjiāo]; 水火相濟 [shuǐ huǒ xiāngjì]
the mutual helping and checking relationship between the heart
and the kidney. The *heart* controls the fire, and the *kidney* the water.
Normally, the fire of the *heart* comes down to warm the *kidney* and
the water of the *kidney* goes up to irrigate the *heart*. If this balanced
relationship breaks down, especially when the water is insufficient
to check the fire, a series of fire symptoms of the *heart* such as fidget,
palpitation, insomnia may occur.

心合小腸 [xīn hé xiǎocháng]
The heart is connected with the small intestine functionally, e.g.,
pathologic heat of the *heart* may be transmitted to the *small intestine*,
resulting in urodynia and hematuria, and drugs to dispel heat from the
heart are effectual in treating these urinary symptoms which are said
to be caused by dysfunction of the *small intestine*.

心與小腸相表裏 [xīn yǔ xiǎocháng xiāng biǎolǐ]
The heart and small intestine are interior-exteriorly related, owing
to the connection of their channels and coordination in some of their
functions.

小腸主受盛 [xiǎocháng zhǔ shòuchèng]
The small intestine receives food content from the stomach.

小腸化食, 泌別清濁 [xiǎocháng huà shí, mìbié qīng zhuó]
The small intestine further digests food, separates the useful
from the waste and absorbs the useful, excretes the waste through the
large intestine and the *urinary bladder* (hence some urinary abnormalit-
ies are alleged to dysfunction of the *small intestine*).

肝氣 [gānqì]

14

the Qi (vital energy) of the liver; either in its physiological state or in pathological condition, particularly referred to a disturbance due to perverted functioning of the *liver*, marked by fullness of the chest, pain in the costal region with symptoms of indigestion or menoxenia

肝血 [gānxuè]

the blood stored in the liver

肝陰 [gānyīn]

the Yin (vital essence) of the liver

肝屬木 [gān shǔ mù]

The liver corresponds to wood, according to the theory of the Five Evolutive Phases.

肝陽 [gānyáng]

the Yang (vital function) of the liver

肝藏血 [gān cáng xuè]

The liver stores blood, serving as a reservoir of blood to regulate the circulating blood volume.

肝主疏洩 [gān zhǔ shūxiè]

The liver has the function of smoothing and regulating the flow of vital energy and blood. Either insufficiency of this function or its excessiveness is pathological.

肝主筋 [gān zhǔ jīn]

The condition of the liver determines the condition of the sinews; the *liver* supplies the sinews with nutrients to develop physical strength, if this function is impaired, numbness, tremor or spasm of the muscles and sluggishness of joint movement may occur.

肝，其華在爪 [gān, qí huá zài zhǎo]

The outward manifestation of the liver is reflected in the nails, lustrous nails signifying a sound *liver.*

肝開竅於目 [gān kāi qiào yú mù]

The liver has its specific body opening in the eyes, normal eyesight depends upon proper functioning of the *liver.*

爪爲筋之餘 [zhǎo wéi jīn zhī yú]

The nails are the odds and ends of tendon and so it reflects the condition of the *liver* which supplies the tendon with blood and nutrients.

肝藏魂 [gān cáng hún]
The liver stores the soul, i.e., it is believed to be the seat of one's soul, for patients with *liver* disease often complain of dreadful dreams and restlessness.

肝主怒 [gān zhǔ nù]
Irritability is one of the chief symptoms of liver diseases.

怒傷肝 [nù shāng gān]
The liver is easily affected by anger.

肝惡風 [gān wù fēng]
The liver is intolerant of wind, for the wind symptoms such as vertigo, tremor, convulsion are usually seen in diseases of the *liver*.

肝爲風木之臟 [gān wéi fēng mù zhī zàng]
The liver is a viscus of "wind and wood", because it smooths the flow of vital energy and blood like the tree to branch out freely and, if diseased, it gives rise to symptoms of wind such as vertigo, tremor, or even convulsion.

肝爲血海 [gān wéi xuèhǎi]
The liver is a reservoir of blood.

髮爲血之餘 [fà wéi xuè zhī yú]
Hair is the odds and ends of blood. It is nourished by blood; gray hair of the aged is alleged to insufficient blood stored in the *liver* and lowered function of the *kidney*.

肝爲剛臟 [gān wéi gāng zàng]
The liver is "a viscus of temperament"; if diseased, it will make one liverish, i.e., easily to become excited, fiery, and hard to be put under control or restraint.

肝爲牡臟 [gān wéi mǔzàng]
The liver is called a male organ as it is preponderantly of an active effective position, in contrast with the *spleen* and the *lung* (e.g., it checks the function of the *spleen*, its fire can make the *lung* suffer).

肝體陰而用陽 [gān tǐ yīn ér yòng yáng]
The liver is substantially Yin but functionally Yang, because it stores the blood (Yin factor) and, on the other hand, its physiological functions and pathological manifestations (e.g., normal and abnormal motility) are of Yang nature.

16

肝腎同源 [gān shèn tóng yuán]
The liver and the kidney have a common source, because (1) the *liver* and the *kidney* store blood and vital essence respectively and blood and vital essence have a common source; (2) the essence of the *liver* and *kidney* can reinforce each other, deficiency of the one will result in deficiency of the other.

肝合膽 [gān hé dǎn]
The liver communicates with the gallbladder.

肝與膽相表裏 [gān yǔ dǎn xiāng biǎolǐ]
The liver and gallbladder are interior-exteriorly related and can influence each other if diseased, owing to the connection of their channels and coordination in some of their functions.

膽主決斷 [dǎn zhǔ juéduàn]
The gallbladder has something to do with one's courage in making decisions, i.e., the *gallbladder* also has some function in connection with the central nervous system.

脾屬土 [pí shǔ tǔ]
The spleen corresponds to earth, according to the theory of the Five Evolutive Phases.

脾氣 [píqì]
Qi (functional activities) of the spleen, including digestion of food, assimilation, transportation and distribution of nutrients and water, and the function to keep the blood flowing within the blood vessels

脾陽 [píyáng]
the Yang of the spleen, referring to the vital function of the *spleen* and to the heat energy required for its functioning as well. Thus, when Yang of the *spleen* is insufficient, besides the manifestations of its hypofunction, symptoms of internal cold are bound to appear.

脾陰 [píyīn]
the Yin (vital essence) of the spleen

脾主運化 [pí zhǔ yùnhuà]
The spleen has the function of digestion and transportation, i.e., digesting food, transporting; distributing and transforming nut-

17

rients, and promoting water metabolism.

脾藏营 [pí cáng yíng]
The spleen has the function of storing nutrients (constructive energy).

脾主升清 [pí zhǔ shēng qīng]; 脾氣主升 [píqì zhǔ shēng]
The spleen has the function of sending clarity (food essence) upward (to the *lung*); the spleen keeps Qi (vital energy) going upward. If this function is impeded, diarrhea or ptosis of viscera may occur.

脾统血 [pí tǒng xuè]
The spleen has the function of keeping the blood flowing within the blood vessels. Its impairment usually leads to chronic hemorrhagic diseases.

脾主肌肉 [pí zhǔ jīròu]
The spleen has the function of nourishing the flesh. One with a healthy *spleen* usually has a full figure, and a diseased *spleen* makes one lose flesh.

脾主四肢 [pí zhǔ sìzhī]
The spleen has the function of nourishing the limbs. Strength of the limbs depends upon the nourishment guaranteed by the normal functioning of the *spleen*. A diseased *spleen* usually causes weakness of the limbs.

脾, 其華在唇 [pí, qí huá zài chún]
The spleen has its outward manifestation in the lips, red and lustrous lips signifying normal functioning of the *spleen*.

脾開竅於口 [pí kāi qiào yú kǒu]
The spleen has its specific body opening in the mouth, normal sensation of taste depends upon proper functioning of the *spleen*.

脾惡濕 [pí wù shī]
The spleen is intolerant of dampness which is apt to impair the transporting and transforming function of the *spleen*, leading to diarrhea, lassitude, edema, etc.

脾爲生化之源 [pí wéi shēnghuà zhī yuán]
The spleen is the source of nutrients for growth and development, since it has the function of digestion, assimilation, transportation and distribution of nutrients.

18

脾主後天 [pí zhǔ hòutiān]
The spleen determines the acquired constitution.

脾胃爲後天之本 [píwèi wéi hòutiān zhī běn]
The spleen and stomach provide the material basis of the acquired constitution.

脾胃爲倉廩之官 [píwèi wéi cānglǐn zhī guān]
The spleen and the stomach are "barn" organs, which store and supply nutrients for the whole body.

脾合胃 [pí hé wèi]
The spleen is closely related with the stomach.

脾與胃相表裏 [pí yǔ wèi xiāng biǎolǐ]
The spleen and the stomach are interior-exteriorly related, which is demonstrated by connection of their channels and functioning in coordination.

胃氣 [wèiqì]
the Qi (functional activities) of the stomach (and the intestines): (1) denoting the digestive function; (2) referred to the material basis of normal pulse.

胃陽 [wèiyáng]
the Yang (vital function) of the stomach

胃陰 [wèiyīn]; 胃津 [wèijīn]
the Yin (vital essence and fluid) of the stomach, also referred to the body fluid as a whole.

胃主受納 [wèi zhǔ shòunà]
The stomach has the function of receiving water and food.

胃爲水穀之海 [wèi wéi shuǐgǔ zhī hǎi]
The stomach serves as the reservoir of water and grains (food).

胃主腐熟 [wèi zhǔ fǔshú]
The main function of the stomach is to digest and transform food into chyme.

胃主降濁 [wèi zhǔ jiàngzhuó]; 胃氣主降 [wèiqì zhǔ jiàng]
The stomach has the function of sending down preliminarily digested food content, if this function is impeded, vomiting may occur.

肺屬金 [fèi shǔ jīn]

19

The lung corresponds to metal, according to the theory of the Five Evolutive Phases.

肺氣 [fèiqì]

the Qi (functional activities) of the lung, including the respiratory function

肺陰 [fèiyīn]; 肺津 [fèijīn]

the Yin (vital essence) of the lung, especially the fluid nourishing and moistening it

肺主氣，司呼吸 [fèi zhǔ qì, sī hūxī]

The lung is in charge of vital energy and performs the function of respiration.

肺主宣發 [fèi zhǔ xuān fā]

The lung keeps the pathway of air unobstructed and disseminates vital energy throughout. If this function is impeded, obstruction of nose, cough, dyspnea and fullness of the chest may occur.

肺主肅降 [fèi zhǔ sùjiàng]

The lung cleanses the inspired air and keeps it and the vital energy flowing downward. If this function is impeded, coughing, asthma, oliguria, edema may occur.

肺朝百脈 [fèi cháo bǎimài]

All blood vessels lead to the lungs, i.e., all blood within the body must pass through the *lung*.

肺主行水 [fèi zhǔ xíng shuǐ]; 肺主通調水道 [fèi zhǔ tōng tiáo shuǐdào]

The lung helps maintain normal water metabolism; the lung regulates the water course. If this function is impeded, oliguria and edema may occur.

肺爲水之上源 [fèi wéi shuǐ zhī shàngyuán]

The lung is the upper source of water circulation: Normal water circulation in the body, especially its flow into the urinary bladder, is guaranteed by the downward drive of the vital energy of the *lung*.

肺合皮毛 [fèi hé pímáo]

The lung is associated with the skin surface (especially the pores and sweat glands), supplying the skin with nutrient and defensive energy, dysfunction of the *lung* makes one liable to perspire spon-

20

taneously and vulnerable to the attack of colds.

肺主一身之表 [fèi zhǔ yīshēn zhī biǎo]

The lung is in charge of superficial resistance.

肺主聲 [fèi zhǔ shēng]

The lung is associated with one's voice, the volume of which is determined by the condition of the *lung.*

肺開竅於鼻 [fèi kāi qiào yú bí]

The lung has its specific body opening in the nose. Stuffed nose, nasal discharge and impairment of smelling are common symptoms when the *lung* is attacked by wind and cold.

肺爲華蓋 [fèi wéi huágài]

The lung is compared to a canopy, which, being the uppermost organ, shelters and protects all other internal organs.

肺爲嬌臟 [fèi wéi jiāozàng]

The lung is a delicate organ, vulnerable to the attack of atmospheric influences.

肺合大腸 [fèi hé dàcháng];肺與大腸相表裏 [fèi yǔ dàcháng xiāng biǎolǐ]

The lung and the large intestine are closely related; the lung and the large intestine are interior—exteriorly related, owing to the connection of their channels and coordination in some of their functions. Thus, purgation of the *large intestine* is beneficial in treating cough and asthma due to excessive heat in the *lung,* while replenishing the vital energy of the *lung* cures constipation in debilitated patients.

大腸主傳導 [dàcháng zhǔ chuándǎo]

The function of the large intestine is to pass its content on and finally eliminate the waste. Disturbance of its function usually gives rise to diarrhea or constipation.

腎屬水 [shèn shǔ shuǐ]

The kidney corresponds to water, according to the theory of the Five Evolutive Phases.

腎陰 [shènyīn]

the Yin (vital essence or vital sap) of the kidney, also called 元陰 [yuányīn]"the original essence", 眞陰 [zhēnyīn] "the genuine essence", 腎水 [shènshuǐ] "the kidney fluid", 眞水 [zhēnshuǐ] "the

21

genuine fluid", being the material basis of vital function of the *kidney*

腎陽 [shènyáng]

the Yang (vital function) of the kidney, which is believed to be the source of heat energy of the body. It is also called 元陽 [yuányáng] "the original vital function", 眞陽 [zhēnyáng] "the genuine vital function", 眞火 [zhēnhuǒ] "the genuine fire", 命門之火 [mìngmén zhī huǒ] "the fire of the Vital Gate", 先天之火 [xiāntiān zhī huǒ] "the fire inherited".

腎藏精 [shèn cáng jīng]

(1) The kidney stores the essence of life either congenital or acquired (i.e., derived from food); (2) The kidney stores the reproductive essence.

腎主水 [shèn zhǔ shuǐ]

The kidney regulates water circulation, including its conservation and excretion by "opening and closing the sluice-gate" 腎關開闔 [shènguān kāi hé] and its distribution by the dynamic of the fire of Vital Gate (vital function of the *kidney*), therefore the *kidney* plays the leading role in maintenance of fluid balance of the body.

腎爲水臟 [shèn wéi shuǐzàng]

The kidney is an organ of water; it corresponds to the Evolutive Phase "Water" and regulates water circulation.

腎其充在骨, 腎充則髓實 [shèn qí chōng zài gǔ, shèn chōng zé suǐ shí]

The kidney supplies the bone with marrow, and the bone marrow is full if the kidney is in good condition.

腎主骨 [shèn zhǔ gǔ]

The condition of the kidney determines the condition of the bone, as the bone is filled and nourished with marrow which is believed to be derived from the vital essence of the *kidney*.

齒爲骨之餘 [chǐ wéi gǔ zhī yú]

The teeth are the odds and ends of the bone, the condition of which is determined by the condition of the *kidney*.

腎主命門之火 [shèn zhǔ mìngmén zhī huǒ]

The kidney controls the fire of the Vital Gate, which is the source of heat energy of the body, serving as the dynamic force of functional activities of viscera, and also plays an important role in development, growth and sexual potency (fire of the Vital Gate concerning the sexual potency is also called 相火 [xiàng huǒ] or Ministerial Fire).

肾主纳气 [shèn zhǔ nàqì]

The kidney has the function of controlling and promoting inspiration, so tonifying the *kidney* is a therapy for relieving dyspnea.

肾主生殖 [shèn zhǔ shēngzhí]

The kidney is in charge of reproduction.

肾为先天之本 [shèn wéi xiāntiān zhī běn]

The kidney is the foundation of the native (inborn) constitution because growth, development and reproduction are attributed to the *kidney*.

腰为肾之府 [yāo wéi shèn zhī fǔ]

The loin or lumbus is the seat of the kidney, thus patients with *kidney* diseases often complain of lumbago.

肾藏志 [shèn cáng zhì]

The kidney has the function of concentration and remembrance, since inability to concentrate one's attention and forgetfulness are common symptoms in case of insufficient *kidney* function.

恐伤肾 [kǒng shāng shèn]

Fright affects the kidney, impairing its essence and leading to weakness, seminal emission, incontinence of urine, etc.

肾恶燥 [shèn wù zào]

The kidney is intolerant of dryness, for the latter may impair its vital essence.

肾，其华在发 [shèn, qí huá zài fà]

The kidney has its manifestation in the hair of the head, i.e., the function of the *kidney* reflects in the thickness and glossiness of hair.

肾开窍于耳 [shèn kāi qiào yú ěr]; 肾气通于耳 [shènqì tōng yú ěr]

The kidney has its specific body opening in the ears; the kidney is associated with the ear (healthy *kidney* ensures sharp hearing, and presbyterian deafness is believed to be caused by deficiency of vital essence of the *kidney*).

肾開竅於二陰 [shèn kāi qiào yú èryīn]

The ·kidney has its specific opening in the urino-genital orifice and the anus, i.e., *the kidney* is associated with the urinogenital orifice and the anus (chronic diarrhea, incontinence of urine and premature ejaculation should be treated by tonifying the *kidney*).

肾合膀胱 [shèn hé pángguāng]

The kidney and the urinary bladder are connected and closely related.

肾與膀胱相表裏 [shèn yǔ pángguāng xiāng biǎolǐ]

The kidney and the urinary bladder are interior-exteriorly related, owing to the connection of their channels and coordination in some of their functions such as urination.

膀胱藏津液 [pángguāng cáng jīnyè]

The urinary bladder stores urine.

膀胱爲州都之官 [pángguāng wéi zhōudū zhī guān]

The urinary bladder serves as a reservoir of urine.

三焦爲决瀆之官 [sānjiāo wéi juédú zhī guān]

The Triple Burners or the three portions of the body cavity may be compared to water communications. It is the foundation and controller of the circulation of body fluids.

三焦爲營衛之源 [sānjiāo wéi yíng wèi zhī yuán]

The Triple Burners or the three portions of body cavity are the source of both the constructive energy and the defensive energy.

上焦主納 [shàngjiāo zhǔ nà]

The Upper Burner or the upper portion of the body cavity has the function of taking in (air, water and food).

中焦主化 [zhōngjiāo zhǔ huà]

The Middle Burner or the middle portion of the body cavity is in charge of transforming, i.e., digesting food and transforming it into nutrients.

下焦主出 [xiàjiāo zhǔ chū]

The Lower Burner or the lower portion of the body cavity has the function of eliminating (waste and superfluous water).

上焦如霧 [shàngjiāo rú wù]

The Upper Burner or the upper portion of the body cavity is like a sprayer, for the *heart* and the *lung* being housed in it, have the function to spread nutrients and vital energy throughout the whole body.

中焦如漚 [zhōngjiāo rú òu]

The Middle Burner or the middle portion of the body cavity works like a fermentation tun, for the *stomach* and the *spleen* being housed in it are responsible for digesting food.

下焦如瀆 [xiàjiāo rú dú]

The Lower Burner or the lower portion of the body cavity works like gutters, for the *kidney, urinary bladder* and *large intestine* being housed in it have the function to filter and drain off waste and surplus water.

三焦氣化 [sānjiāo qìhuà]

the combined functional activities of the Triple Burners (referring to the *lung, spleen* and *kidney*) such as regulating water metabolism, production and transformation of food essence, etc.

心包絡合三焦 [xīnbāoluò hé sānjiāo]; 心包絡與三焦相表裏 [xīnbāoluò yǔ sānjiāo xiāng biǎolǐ]

The pericardium and the Triple Burners are interior-exteriorly related, which is referred to the inter-relationship of the corresponding channels.

其他組織、器官和體表部位
Other Tissues, Organs and Regions of the Body Surface

五官 [wǔguān]

the five sense organs: the nose, eyes, lips, tongue and ears connected by channels with the five viscera: the *lung, liver, spleen, heart* and *kidney*.

七竅 [qīqiào]

the seven orifices on the head: the ears, eyes, nostrils and mouth.

九竅 [jiǔqiào]

the nine body orifices or openings, consisting of (1) eyes, ears, nostrils, mouth, plus urethral orifice and anus; or (2) eyes, ears, nostrils, mouth plus the tongue and throat (according to 難經 or "the

Classic on Medical Problems")

上竅 [shàngqiào]
the upper orifices, referring to the orifices on the head

下竅 [xiàqiào]
the lower orifices, referring to urethral opening and anus

苗竅 [miáoqiào]
body opening reflecting the condition of an internal organ, e.g., the nose is the body opening of the *lung*

唇 [chún]
the lips, also called 飛門 [fēimén] the "Flying Door", the colour of which reflects the condition of the *spleen*

齒 [chǐ]
the teeth

眞牙 [zhēnyá]
the wisdom tooth

舌本 [shéběn]
the root of the tongue

舌質 [shézhì]
the tongue substance; the tongue proper

咽門 [yānmén]
the opening of the pharynx, through which food passes into the esophagus

咽喉 [yānhóu]
pharynx and larynx, the potential cavity at the back of the root of the tongue, which connects with the mouth, trachea and esophagus and through which many channels run

懸雍垂 [xuányōngchuí]; 小舌 [xiǎoshé]
uvula, also called "the small tongue"

喉核 [hóuhé]
the tonsils

喉關 [hóuguān]
the throat pass, formed by the tonsils, uvula and the back of the tongue

會厭 [huìyàn]
epiglottis.

26

七衝門 [qī chōngmén]

the seven important passes along the alimentary tract: the lips (飛門, "flying door"), teeth (戶門, "house door"), epiglottis (吸門, "inhalation door"), cardia (賁門), pylorus (幽門), the ileocecal conjunction (闌門) and the anus (魄門)

賁門 [bēnmén]

cardia, the esophageal orifice of the stomach

幽門 [yōumén]

pylorus, the distal (duodenal) aperture of the stomach

皮毛 [pímáo]

skin with hairs, referring to the body surface which is closely related to the *lung* functionally

毫毛 [háomáo]

down; fine hair of the skin

腠理 [còulǐ]

texture and interspace of the skin, muscle, etc. including the sweat pore

肌腠 [jīcòu]

texture and interspace of muscles, referring to the superficial layers of the human body

玄府 [xuánfǔ]; 元府 [yuánfǔ]

the sweat pore, also known as the 氣門 [qìmén] "portal of energy" or the 鬼門 [guǐmén] "devil's portal"

膈(膈) [gé]

diaphragm

筋 [jīn]

tendon or sinew, the function of which is believed to be controlled by the *liver*

募原 [mùyuán]; 膜原 [móyuán]

space between the pleura and the diaphragm; also referring to the part between the interior and exterior of the body in the diagnosis of febrile diseases

膏肓 [gāohuāng]

(1) space below the heart and above the diaphragm: the innermost part of the body (lesion in this part is said to be beyond cure); (2)

a point on the Urinary Bladder Channel

丹田 [dāntián]

elixir field, referring to: (1) the region three inches below the umbilicus, believed by the Taoists to be the seat of womb of the female and seminal vesicle of the male; (2) regions in the body to which one's will is focused while practising breathing exercise: the lower elixir field (region below the umbilicus), the middle elixir field (the pectoral region) and the upper elixir field (region between the eyebrows)

形 [xíng]

physical appearance

巔頂 [diāndǐng]; 巔 [diān]

the top of the head

顖 [xìn]; 顖門 [xìnmén]

fontanel

髮際 [fàjì]

hairline

前髮際 [qiánfàjì]

anterior hairline (above the forehead)

後髮際 [hòufàjì]

posterior hairline (above the neck)

天庭 [tiāntíng]

the central part of the forehead

闕 [què]; 闕中 [quèzhōng]; 印堂 [yìntáng]

the part or point between the eyebrows, inspection of which was thought to be a guide to diagnosing diseases of the lung in ancient times

闕上 [quèshàng]

the lower part of the forehead just above the eyebrows, inspection of which was thought to give informations on diagnosing diseases of the throat in ancient times

內眦 [nèizì]

the inner canthus

耳廓 [ěrkuò]

auricula

耳輪 [ěrlún]
helix
耳門 [ěrmén]
(1) **tragus:** the cartilaginous projection before the external meatus of the ear; (2) a point on the Triple Burners Channel; when mouth is open, the point is in the depression in front of the tragus and slightly superior to the condyloid process of the mandible

頰車 [jiáchē]
(1) **mandible;** the jaw bone; (2) a point on the Stomach Channel, anterior and superior to the angle of jaw at the prominence of the masseter muscle when the jaw is shut tight

人中 [rénzhōng]; 水溝 [shuǐgōu]
(1) **philtrum:** the vertical groove on the midline of the upper lip; (2) an acupuncture point on the Back Midline Channel located at the junction of the upper third and lower two thirds of the midline of the upper lip

承漿 [chéngjiāng]
(1) **the depression in the middle of the mental labial groove;** (2) a point on the Ren (Front Midline) Channel, located at the middle of the mental labial groove

吻 [wěn]
corner of the mouth where the upper and lower lips meet

缺盆 [quēpén]
(1) **supraclavicular fossa:** the depression on either side of the neck behind the clavicle; (2) a point on the Stomach Channel in the center of the supraclavicular fossa

膻中 [dànzhōng]
(1) **the central part of the chest,** between the two nipples; (2) a point on the Ren (Front Middle) Channel, at the very center of the above-mentioned spot

鳩尾 [jiūwěi]
(1) **xyphoid process;** (2) a point on the Ren (Front Middle) Channel half an inch below the xyphoid process

脅 [xié]
the costal region: the upper part of the side of the human body

季肋 [jìlèi]
the lower costal regions
大腹 [dàfù]
the upper part of the abdomen above the umbilicus
小腹 [xiǎofù]
the lower part of the abdomen below the umbilicus
少腹 [shàofù]
(1) lower abdomen; (2) lateral regions of the lower abdomen
神闕 [shénquè]
(1) umbilicus; (2) a point on the Ren (Front Middle) Channel
at the center of the umbilicus
橫骨 [hénggǔ]
(1) the pubic bone; (2) a point on the Kidney Channel located
in the lower abdomen on the superior border of the pubic symphysis
曲骨 [qūgǔ]
(1) the pubic symphysis; (2) a point on the Ren (Front Middle)
Channel, located on the superior border of the pubic symphysis
會陰 [huìyīn]
(1) perineum; (2) a point on the Ren (Front Middle) Channel, just
in the center of perineum
毛際 [máojì]
margin of the hairy part above the external genitalia
氣街 [qìjiē]
path of vital energy: (1) femoral artery at the groins; (2) the path
through which the Qi (vital energy) circulates
前陰 [qiányīn]
the front private parts— external genitalia including extenal orifice
of the urethra
後陰 [hòuyīn]
the back private parts—the anus
二陰 [èryīn]
the two (front and back) private parts — the external genitalia,
external urethral orifice and the anus
產門 [chǎnmén]; (陰户) [yīnhù]
the external viginal orifice

子門 [zǐmén]
external (vaginal) orifice of the uterus
廷孔 [tíngkǒng]
the external urethral orifice of the female
陰器 [yīnqì]
the private parts; external genitalis
睾 [gāo]
testicle; testis
莖 [jīng]
penis
腰 [yāo]
the lumbus; the loins
股 [gǔ]
the thigh
百骸 [bǎihái]
skeleton: the bones of the body collectively
高骨 [gāogǔ]
the eminent head of the radius at the wrist, proximal to the inner side of the thumb, where the tip of the physician's middle finger is placed on pulse-taking
輔骨 [fǔgǔ]
radius
髀 [bì]
thigh, esp. its anterior superior part
髀骨 [bìgǔ]
thigh—bone, i.e., femur
髀樞 [bìshū]
trochanteric region: the part over the major trochanter of the femur
尾骶 [wěidǐ]
sacrococcygeal region
尾骶骨 [wěidǐgǔ]
sacrococcyx
尾閭 [wěilǘ]
coccyx

31

尻 [kāo]
sacral region
尻骨 [kāogǔ]
sacrum
外輔骨 [wàifǔgǔ]
fibula
百節 [bǎijié]
the joints of the body on the whole
十二節 [shíèrjié]
the twelve joints, referring to the joints of the shoulder girdle, the elbow and the wrist on the upper limbs and the joints of the thigh, knee and ankle on the lower limbs
大節 [dàjié]
the large joints, referring to: (1) large joints of the human skeleton; (2) proximal joints of the fingers and toes
八豁 [bāxī]
the eight joints: joints at the elbow, wrist, knee and ankle
本節 [běnjié]
the eminences over the digitometacarpal and digitometatarsal joints seen at the back of the hands and feet
虎口 [hǔkǒu]
"the tiger's mouth": area between the thumb and the index finger. It is so called because it looks like an opening mouth of a tiger.
赤白肉際 [chìbáiròujì]
the junction of the "red and white" skin, such as that bordering the skin of the back and palm of a hand

III Material Basis of Vital Activities of the Human Body

氣 [qì]

(1) vital energy; (2) functional activities. Conception of Qi represents the naive cognition of the natural phenomena in the ancient times, in which Qi is believed to be the basic element which constitutes the cosmos and produces everything in the world through its movement and changes. Thus, Qi corresponds to or can be comprehended as configurative energy. In the field of medicine, Qi is referred to the basic element or energy which makes up the human body and supports its vital activities, such as 水谷之氣, i.e., food energy, 呼吸之氣, i.e., the breathed air. Since the existence of Qi in the human body can only be perceived through its resultant activities of organs and tissues, it is more frequently used with the meaning of functional activities, such as 臟腑之氣, i.e., the functional activities of viscera and bowels.

穀氣 [gǔqì]; 水穀之氣 [shuǐgǔ zhī qì]

food energy

水穀 [shuǐgǔ]

water and grains; food; diet

大氣 [dàqì]

cosmic energy—air, especially the air which is breathed

原氣 [yuánqì]; 元氣 [yuánqì]

original vital energy, as the dynamic of all visceral functions; vitality.

正氣 [zhèngqì]

(1) genuine energy (cf.眞氣); **(2) body resistance,** opposed to pathogenic factors; **(3) normal weather conditions** of the four seasons

眞氣 [zhēnqì]

vitality; genuine energy: the combination of the inborn original vital energy, the acquired energy derived from food and the air, serving as the dynamic force of all vital functions

宗氣 [zōngqì]

pectoral energy; food energy plus the air, stored in the chest, serving as the dynamic force of respiration and voice, and also related to the blood circulation and body metabolism

血氣 [xuèqì]

blood and vital energy

先天之氣 [xiāntiān zhī qì]

inborn vital energy; inborn configurative energy, also called 原氣 or the original energy, which originates in the *kidney* by transformation from the innate essence (先天之精) and combines with the acquired configurative energy (後天之氣) to form the genuine energy (眞氣)

後天之氣 [hòutiān zhī qì]

acquired vital energy; acquired configurative energy, which is formed from the food energy obtained by digestion in the *spleen* and *stomach* in combination with the fresh air inhaled in the *lung*

精氣 [jīngqì]

(1) **vital substance**, chiefly referred to that derived from food essence; (2) **vital essence and vital energy** as material basis of visceral functioning. The vital essence and energy stored in the *kidney* are closely related to sexual activity and reproduction.

臟氣 [zàngqì]

(1) **functional activities of a viscus**; (2) **visceral energy**

營氣 [yíngqì]

constructive energy, which moves through the conduits and nourishes all the organs

衛氣 [wèiqì]

defensive energy, which moves outside the conduits, permeating the surface of the body and warding off exogenous pathogens; superficial resistance of the body

清氣 [qīngqì]

(1) **fresh air**, usually referred to the air inspired in the *lungs*; (2) **food energy** or **nutrient**, esp. the clarified thin part of food essence; (3) **clear up the evil heat from the Qi system**: a method in treating febrile diseases

濁氣 [zhuóqì]

(1) dense part of food essence; (2) waste gas, e.g., the air expired or flactus discharged

經氣 〔jīnqqì〕

vital energy in the conduits, denoting: (1) the vital energy moving in the conduits; (2) all energy integrated into a physiological cycle; (3) vital function of the Channels of the body

衛氣營血 〔wèi qì yíng xuè〕

(1) defensive energy, vital energy, nutrients and blood— the chief substances and energy required for maintaining vital activities of human life; (2) the Wei (superficial defensive) system, the Qi (secondary defensive) system, the Ying (nutrient) system and the Xue (blood) system, denoting the four portions or strata of the body from the superficial to the deep to show the location and seriousness or stages of a febrile disease as a guide to diagnosis

衛分 〔wèifēn〕

the Wei (superficial defensive) system, often abbreviated as 衛 or the Wei

氣分 〔qìfēn〕

the Qi (secondary defensive) system, including functioning of the *lung*, the *spleen*, the *stomach*, the *gallbladder*, the *large intestine* etc., often abbreviated as 氣 or the Qi

營分 〔yíngfēn〕

the Ying (nutrient) system, closely related to the Xue (blood) system, often abbreviated as 營 or the Ying

血分 〔xuèfēn〕

the Xue (blood) system, often abbreviated as 血 or the Xue

氣機 〔qìjī〕

mechanism of the Qi (vital energy), referring either to functional expression of vital energy at large, or the flow of visceral vital energy in particular

氣化 〔qìhuà〕

activity of the Qi (vital energy), including vital function of the viscera, circulation and distribution of vital energy and blood, etc. In a narrow sense, it refers only to the functional activities of the Triple Burners, e.g., the regulation of water circulation

雜氣 [záqì]; 異氣 [yìqì]

impure, noxious atmospheric influences as exogenous pathogenic factors causing epidemic diseases

逆氣 [nìqì]

vital energy on adverse flow; vital energy running counter to normal movement or circulation

厥氣 [juéqì]

vital energy on perverted flow, usually giving rise to manifestations of syncope

中氣 [zhōngqì]

vital energy or function of the Middle Burner (of the *spleen* and the *stomach*)

血 [xuè]

blood—the red fluid circulating through the blood vessels and nourishing the body tissues. It is derived by transformation of the food essence and nutrients produced in the *spleen* and *stomach* and vital essence stored in the *kidney*. It is stored in the *liver* and distributed throughout the body in accordance with demand. Its circulation is promoted by the *heart* with the help of the *lung* and controlled by the *spleen*. Hence, dysfunction of any of the above viscera may lead to blood deficiency or abnormal blood flow, such as stasis due to insufficient activities of the *heart*, hemorrhage caused by functional deficiency of the *spleen*.

精血 [jīngxuè]

essence and blood

營血 [yíngxuè]

nutrients and blood, an equivalent for blood

血脈 [xuèmài]

(1) blood vessels; (2) conduits of blood and vital energy

精血同源 [jīngxuè tóng yuán]

Essence and blood have a common source; both constitute the material basis of the human body, blood comes from congenital essence and is nourished by acquired food essence.

津血同源 [jīnxuè tóng yuán]

Body fluid and blood are derived from a common source (i.e., from water and food), so they are closely related physiologically and pathologically.

氣為血帥 [qì wéi xuè shuài]

Qi (vital energy) is the "commander" of blood, for it serves as the dynamic force of blood flow, keeps the blood circulating within the vessels, and promotes the blood regeneration. Hence, stagnancy of Qi is apt to cause blood stasis, and deficiency of Qi may lead to chronic bleeding or deficiency of blood.

血為氣母 [xuè wéi qì mǔ]

Blood is the "mother" of vital energy for being the latter's material basis. Hence deficiency of blood usually causes insufficient vital energy, and massive loss of blood may lead to collapse (prostration of vital energy).

精 [jīng]

(1) essence of life: the fundamental substance which builds up the physical structure and maintains the body function; (2) semen

生殖之精 [shēngzhí zhī jīng]

reproductive essence

水穀之精 [shuǐgǔ zhī jīng]; 水穀精微 [shuǐ gǔ jīng wēi]

food essence: the essential substance derived from food, which is required for maintenance of vital activities and metabolism of the human body

先天之精 [xiāntiān zhī jīng]

congenital or innate essence, i.e. reproductive essence, the original substance which is essential for construction of the body

後天之精 [hòutiān zhī jīng]

acquired essence: the fundamental substance derived from food to maintain the body function and replenish the physical construction.

津液 [jīnyè]

(1) body fluid; a general term for all fluids in the body, including secretions such as saliva, tear, sweat, urine, etc. (2) liquid nutrients

津 [jīn]

(1) active thin body fluid which circulates with Qi (vital energy) and blood. It is mainly distributed over the exterior part of the body and can be secreted as tears, saliva, sweat, etc. (2) saliva

液［yè］

structive thick or mucous body fluid which does not circulate together with Qi (vital energy) and blood, but is stored in body cavities such as articular and cranial cavities

陰液［yīnyè］

Yin fluids: all kinds of nutrient fluid in the body, especially that of the viscera

清濁［qīng zhuó］

clarity and turbidity, often referred to essence and waste of digested food

五液［wǔyè］

five kinds of fluid: a classification of body fluid according to its origin in connection with viscera. They are: sweat (汗), tears (淚), snivel (涕), slobber (涎) and spittle (唾)

淚爲肝液［lèi wéi gānyè］

The tears are the fluid of the liver. The tears come from the eyes which reflect the condition of the *liver* as its specific opening. Lack of tears with dry eyes is a common symptom indicating deficiency of essence and blood of the *liver*.

汗爲心液［hàn wéi xīnyè］

The sweat is the fluid of the heart, for sweat comes from blood which, in turn, is regulated by the *heart*. Clinically, spontaneous sweating is commonly seen when Yang (vital function) of the *heart* is insufficient, while night sweating usually suggests deficiency of Yin (vital essence) of the *heart*.

涎爲脾液［xián wéi píyè］

The slobber is the fluid of the spleen, for the *spleen* has its specific body opening in the mouth. Clinically, dry mouth is frequently seen in cases of inadequacy of fluid in the *spleen* and *stomach* and dysfunction of the *spleen* in sending up the fluid.

涕爲肺液［tì wéi fèiyè］

The snivel is the fluid of the lung, for the nose is the specific body opening of the *lung*. Clinically, a dry nose is usually due to heat or dryness in the *lung*, while patients with the function of the *lung* impeded often have a running nose.

唾爲腎液 [tuò wéi shènyè]

The spittle is the fluid of the kidney, for the Kidney Channel runs through the sublingual area. Clinically, excessive spittle can be cured by tonifying the *kidney*.

神 [shén]

(1) mental faculties, which are believed to be functions of the *heart*; (2) expression: outward expression of the mental state

精神 [jīngshén]

spirit; mood; manifestation of the configurative force

志 [zhì]

(1) emotion or psychic reaction; (2) memory or faculty of memory

形體 [xíng tǐ]

configuration and constitution

IV Causes and Mechanisms of Diseases

三因 [sānyīn]

three categories of pathogeny: exogenous, endogenous and non-exo-endogenous—an ancient classification of etiology

外因 [wàiyīn]

exogenous causes of disease, referring chiefly to the six excessive and untimely atmospheric influences

内因 [nèiyīn]

endogenous causes of disease, referring chiefly to the excessive emotional changes

不内不外因 [bùnèi bùwài yīn]

non-exo-endogenous causes of disease: causes related neither to external nor to internal influences, such as intemperance in eating, drinking and sexual life, overwork, tumbling, animal bite, etc.

邪氣 [xiéqì]；邪 [xié]

pathogenic factors

外邪 [wàixié]

exogenous pathogenic factors, including the six excessive or untimely atmospheric influences and various infectious factors

時邪 [shíxié]

seasonal pathogenic factors, a general designation for the pathogenic factors causing seasonal diseases

六氣 [liùqì]

(1) six atmospheric influences: wind, cold, summer heat, dampness, dryness and fire; **(2) the six basic substances that maintain human life:** sperm, Qi (vital energy), nutrient sap, body fluid, blood and vessels

六淫 [liùyín]

the six excessive or untimely atmospheric influences as exogenous pathogenic factors: wind, cold, summer heat, dampness, dryness and fire

淫氣 [yínqì]

(1) **fullness of Qi** (vital energy), which keeps one healthy; (2) **excess of Qi** referring to excessive atmospheric influences and exuberance of Yin or Yang of the body which causes disease

四時不正之氣 [sìshí bùzhèng zhī qì]
abnormal weather changes of the four seasons, which are unfavourable to the normal growth and development of living beings and often cause diseases

戾氣 [lìqì]; 疫癘之氣 [yìlì zhī qì]
epidemic noxious factors

時行戾氣 [shíxíng lìqì]
prevalent epidemic pathogenic factors

客邪 [kèxié]
foreign pathogenic factor, i.e., any pathogenic factor which attacks a person from without

賊風 [zéifēng]
evil wind: (1) wind as a pathogenic factor; (2) abnormal weather changes harmful to one's health

陰邪 [yīnxié]
(1) **exogenous pathogenic factors of Yin nature**, i.e., cold and dampness, which tend to impede and injure Yang (vital function): (2) **pathogenic factors attacking the Yin channels**

陽邪 [yángxié]
(1) **pathogenic factors of Yang nature**, i.e., wind, summer heat, dryness and fire, which tend to take the form of heat and injure Yin (the vital essence and body fluid); (2) **pathogenic factors attacking the Yang channels**

伏氣 [fúqì]
(1) **latent noxious factors**, usually concealed in channels; (2) an abbreviation of 伏氣溫病 [fúqì wēnbìng] , i.e., febrile diseases caused by latent noxious factors

風 [fēng]
wind: (1) one of the six exogenous pathogenic factors; (2) name of a syndrome marked by dizziness, fainting, convulsion, tremor, numbness, etc.

風為百病之長 [fēng wéi bǎibìng zhī zhǎng]

Wind is the first and foremost factor to cause various diseases because it is the commonest factor seen in diseases caused by exogenous factors, and other factors often attack the human body in combination with wind, such as wind and cold, wind and heat, wind and dampness, etc.

内风 [nèifēng]

internal or endogenous wind, a pathological change due to excessive heat or deficiency of blood or vital essence marked by dizziness, fainting, convulsion, tremor, numbness, facial paralysis, etc.

外风 [wàifēng]

external or exogenous wind as pathogenic factor

伤风 [shāngfēng]

(1) illness due to attack of exogenous wind on the body surface; (2) common cold

寒 [hán]

cold – one of the six pathogenic factors

外寒 [wàihán]

external cold: (1) cold as an exogenous factor, bringing on such symptoms as chillness, headache, general aching, hypohidrosis, floating and tense pulse; (2) a morbid condition caused by deficiency of Yang (vital function), marked by intolerance of cold or liability to catch cold

内寒 [nèihán]

internal cold, due to lowered vital function of the internal organs, especially of the *kidney* and *spleen*, marked by watery diarrhea, abdominal pain,cold limbs,intolerance of cold,and slow and deep pulse

中寒 [zhōnghán]

cold in the middle portion of the body cavity due to lowered vital function of the *spleen* and *stomach* with symptoms such as abdominal pain which may be relieved by warmth, intolerance of cold, cold limbs, loss of appetite, loose bowel, etc.

中寒 [zhònghán]

direct attack of cold on the *stomach* and intestine, marked by abdominal pain, borborygmi, diarrhea, accompanied with chills or cold limbs

暑 [shǔ]

summer heat—one of the six exogenous pathogenic factors, bringing on symptoms such as fever, headache, thirst, fidget, sweating, rapid gigantic pulse

濕 [shī]

dampness: (1) one of the six pathogenic factors, attacking the organism from without and disturbing the normal flow of Qi and normal functioning of the *spleen* and *stomach*; (2) water retention due to impaired water circulation and distribution, often referred to as endogenous dampness (cf. 內濕)

外濕 [wàishī]

exogenous dampness: a pathogenic factor attacking a victim living and working in damp places, bringing on symptoms such as headache as if the head were tightly bound, lassitude, heaviness in the limbs, fullness in the chest, joint pains and swelling with sensation of heaviness, etc.

內濕 [nèishī]

endogenous dampness: stagnancy of water within the body caused by deficiency of Yang (vital function) of the *spleen* and *kidney*, manifested by loss of appetite, diarrhea, abdominal fullness, scanty urine, sallow face, edema of the lower limbs

水氣 [shuǐqì]

(1) **water retention** due to dysfunction of the *spleen* and *kidney*; (2) edema, as cited in "Synopsis of Prescriptions of the Gold Chamber" by Zhang Zhong-jing

濕毒 [shīdú]

noxious dampness: stagnated dampness as a noxious factor, which, if occurring in the intestines, may cause hematochezia, if occurring in the muscles and skin of the lower limbs, may cause ulcer on the shank

燥 [zào]

dryness: (1) one of the six pathogenic factors, which prevails in autumn and impairs visceral essence and body fluid, bringing on red eye, dryness of the nasal cavity, parched lips, dry cough, constipation, etc.; (2) symptoms of dryness caused by impairment of Yin (vital essence and body fluid)

内燥 [nèizào]

internal or endogenous dryness; symptoms of dryness such as fidget and thirst, parched lips, dry skin, etc., usually appearing at a late stage of febrile disease or after excessive vomiting, diarrhea, sweating or hemorrhage

火 [huǒ]

fire: (1) one of the Five Elements; (2) physiological energy of life; (3) one of the six pathogenic factors; (4) pathological manifestation of intense heat such as flushed face, bloodshot eyes, acute local inflammation, etc. resulting from excessive functional activities, immoderate emotional influences or affection by various pathogenic factors

火邪 [huǒxié]

pathogenic fire; fire as a pathogenic factor

温热 [wēnrè]

(1) **warmth and heat** as pathogenic factors causing febrile diseases. In the strict sense, the pathogenic warmth(温邪) attacks insidiously, causes milder disease and prevails in winter and spring, while the pathogenic heat (热邪) causes severe disease with sudden onset and prevails in summer; (2) **diseases caused by warmth and heat,** referred to acute febrile diseases at large or the febrile disease caused by heat exclusively, not in combination with dampness

火毒 [huǒdú]

noxious fire: (1) fire accumulated to be noxious, causing boils, ulcers and other purulent inflammations; (2) infection caused by burns and scalds

风寒 [fēnghán]

wind and cold: (1) wind and cold in combination as a pathogenic factor; (2) illness due to attack of wind and cold combined

风热 [fēngrè]

wind and heat: (1) wind and heat in combination as a pathogenic factor; (2) illness caused by attack of wind and heat

风湿 [fēngshī]

wind and dampness: (1) wind and dampness combined as a pathogenic factor; (2) illness caused by wind and dampness, such as rheumatism

44

風寒濕 [fēnghánshī]

wind, cold and dampness combined as a pathogenic factor, causing diseases such as rheumatic and rheumatoid arthritis

寒濕 [hánshī]

cold-dampness: (1) disease due to attack of dampness on the *spleen* leading to lowered vital function of this organ or due to insufficient vital function of the *spleen* and *kidney* with accumulation of dampness, marked by intolerance of cold, cold limbs, abdominal distension, diarrhea and edema; (2) cold and dampness combined as a pathogenic factor causing muscle pains, arthralgia, etc.

濕熱 [shīrè]

dampness and heat: (1) two pathogenic factors in combination; (2) febrile disease caused by dampness and heat, marked by fever, headache, anorexia, abdominal distension, yellow greasy fur of the tongue; (3) attack of dampness and heat on internal organs, e.g., on *large intestine* as seen in acute dysentery, on *urinary bladder* as seen in acute urinary infection, on *liver* and *gallbladder* as seen in acute icteric hepatitis

風燥 [fēngzào]

wind and dryness: (1) combined as a pathogenic factor, generally prevailing in autumn; (2) illness caused by wind and dryness, marked by fever and chilliness, headache, absence of perspiration, dry throat, dry cough, dry skin, etc.

燥熱 [zàorè] ；燥火 [zàohuǒ]

dryness and heat, or dryness and fire: symptoms of heat or fire brought on by dryness, such as sore throat, redness of the eye, dry cough and coughing blood, etc.

六鬱 [liùyù]

six kinds of stagnancy, i.e., stagnancy of Qi (vital energy), blood, dampness, fire, phlegm (mucus) and food, the first two being the most important

七情 [qīqíng]

the seven emotional factors: joy(喜), anger(怒), melancholy(憂), anxiety (思), sorrow (悲), fear (恐) and fright (驚), considered to be endogenous factors causing diseases if in excess

45

五志過極 [wǔzhì guòjí]

five emotions in excess: excessive joy (喜), anger(怒), melancholy (憂), anxiety (思) and fear (恐) may influence the normal circulation of Qi (vital energy) and blood of the internal organs, causing morbid condition

五志化火 [wǔzhì huàhuǒ]

transformation of the five emotions into fire: the uncontrolled overflow of the five emotions (joy, anger, melancholy, anxiety and fear) may disturb the natural flow of Qi and injure the genuine Yin (vital essence), giving rise to symptoms of fire, such as irritability, insomnia, bitterness in the mouth, chest pain, hemoptysis, etc.

邪火 [xiéhuǒ]

evil fire: pathogenic or pathological fire as opposed to the physiological fire (cf. 火)

勞倦 [láojuàn]

overfatigue and overstrain, which may cause chronic or wasting diseases

房勞 [fángláo];房室傷 [fángshìshāng]

exhaustion caused by intemperance in sexual life

蟲獸傷 [chóngshòushāng]

insect, reptile or animal bite as a pathogenic factor

膏粱厚味 [gāoliáng hòuwèi]

rich, greasy food, overfeeding on which may bring on endogenous heat, ulcers and carbuncles

五味偏嗜 [wǔwèi piānshì]

partiality for a particular kind of food or taste, which may give rise to disease, e.g., partiality for pungent taste often induces constipation, ulceration in the mouth, and hemorrhoids; partiality for sweets causes acid regurgitation

癖嗜 [pǐshì]

addiction as a pathogenic factor, such as smoking and drinking

勞復 [láofù]

relapse of disease due to fatigue, such as overwork, mental stress, intemperance in sexual life, etc.

燙火傷 [tànghuǒshāng]

burns and scalds

瘀血 [yūxuè]

stagnated blood, including extravasated blood and the blood moving sluggishly in circulation or congested in a viscus

痰 [tán]

phlegm: (1) pathologic secretions of the diseased respiratory organs, also called "phlegm visible"(有形之痰) since it is visible when spat; (2) a pathologic product of diseased internal organs, especially the *spleen*, which in turn, may cause various troubles, e.g., nausea and vomiting when the stomach being affected by it, palpitation, impairment of consciousness or even mania when the *heart* being invaded by it, scrofula when it accumulating subcutaneously. These troubles are thought to be caused by "phlegm invisible" (無形之痰) chiefly because they can be cured by similar therapeutic methods as cases with "visible phlegm"

濕痰 [shītán]; 痰濕 [tánshī]; 痰濁 [tánzhuó]

wet phlegm or phlegm-dampness, produced by long standing retention of dampness due to deficiency of vital energy of the *spleen*, bringing on symptoms such as profuse frothy sputum, nausea, fullness in the chest, cough and dyspnea, plump tongue with slippery or greasy coat

頑痰 [wántán]

persistent phlegm, e.g., a lingering case of asthma with repeated attacks is believed to be due to persistent phlegm lingering in the pleurodiphragmatic quarters

中毒 [zhòngdú]

poisoning

中惡 [zhòngè]

illness due to attack of noxious factors, usually with sudden onset of syncope or mental disorder

水土不服 [shuǐtǔ bù fú]

climatic sickness, illness due to temporary inadaptability of a person to the climate of a new dwelling place, with symptoms such as loss of appetite, abdominal distension, diarrhea, menstrual complaints in women, etc.

胎毒 [tāidú]
noxious heat got at the fetus stage, which is believed to be the cause of boils, and skin eruptions of the newborns

諸蟲 [zhū chóng]
parasites, especially of the intestines, which cause diseases

山嵐瘴氣 [shānlán zhàngqì]; 瘴毒 [zhàngdú]
miasma; swamp vapour; noxious pathogenic vapour in woody mountainous regions, a term usually referring to malaria

病機 [bìngjī]
pathological mechanism; pathogenesis

病機十九條 [bìngjī shíjiǔ tiáo]
nineteen guiding-rules of pathological mechanism given in Su Wen "Plain Questions" of Nei Jing " Canon of Medicine"

諸風掉眩，皆屬於肝 [zhū fēng diàoxuàn jiē shǔyú gān]
Endogenous winds marked by vertigo, spasm and convulsion are pathological changes related to the liver.

諸寒收引，皆屬於腎 [zhū hán shōuyǐn, jiē shǔyú shèn]
Endogenous colds marked by contraction are pathological changes related to the kidney.

諸氣膹鬱，皆屬於肺 [zhū qì fèn yù, jiē shǔyú fèi]
Respiratory disorders such as dyspnea and stuffiness of the chest are pathological changes related to the lung.

諸濕腫滿，皆屬於脾，[zhū shī zhǒngmǎn, jiē shǔyú pí]
Endogenous dampness marked by water retention and edema are pathological changes related to the spleen.

諸熱瞀瘛，皆屬於火 [zhū rè mào qì, jiē shǔyú huǒ]
High fevers with impaired consciousness and convulsion are related to the symptom-complex of fire.

諸痛癢瘡，皆屬於心 [zhū tòng yǎng chuāng, jiē shǔyú xīn]
Skin abscesses or sores with pain and itching are pathological changes related to the heart.

諸厥固洩，皆屬於下 [zhū jué gù xiè, jiē shǔyú xià]
Disorders such as constipation, diarrhea and cold extremities are related to the lower portion of the body cavity.

諸痿喘嘔,皆屬於上 [zhū wěi chuǎn ǒu, jiē shǔyú shàng]

Illnesses marked by consumption, dyspnea and vomiting are related to the upper portion of the body cavity, i.e. to the *lung* and the *stomach.*

諸禁鼓慄, 如喪神守, 皆屬於火 [zhū jìn gǔlì, rú sàng shén shǒu, jiē shǔyú huǒ]
Febrile illnesses with trismus, shivering chills and delirium are related to symptom-complex of fire

諸痙項強, 皆屬於濕 [zhū jìng xiàngjiāng, jiē shǔyú shī]
Rigidity such as stiff neck and other locomotive restrictions are pathological changes due to dampness.

諸逆衝上, 皆屬於火 [zhū nì chòngshàng, jiē shǔyú huǒ]
Disorders with upward perverted flow of gas or liquid such as cough and spouting vomiting are related to symptom-complex of fire.

諸脹腹大, 皆屬於熱 [zhū zhàng fùdà, jiē shǔyú rè]
Abdominal distension and swelling are related to symptom-complex of heat.

諸躁狂越, 皆屬於火 [zhū zào kuángyuè, jiē shǔyú huǒ]
Restlessness and mania are related to symptom-complex of fire.

諸暴強直, 皆屬於風 [zhū bào jiāngzhí, jiē shǔyú fēng]
Sudden onset of muscular spasm and rigidity is related to symptom-complex of wind.

諸病有聲, 鼓之如鼓, 皆屬於熱 [zhū bìng yǒu shēng, gǔ zhī rú gǔ, jiē shǔyú rè]
Abdominal distension like a drum with borborygmi is related to symptom-complex of heat.

諸病胕腫, 疼酸驚駭, 皆屬於火 [zhū bìng fùzhǒng, téng suān jīnghài, jiē shǔyú huǒ]
Illnesses with swelling and aching of back of the feet and nervous tension are related to symptom-complex of fire.

諸轉反戾, 水液混濁, 皆屬於熱 [zhū zhuǎn fǎnlì, shuǐyè hūnzhuó, jiē shǔyú rè]
Spasm, rigidity and opisthotonus with turbid urine is related to symptom-complex of heat.

諸病水液, 澄澈清冷, 皆屬於寒 [zhū bìng shuǐyè, chéng chè qīnglěng, jiē shǔyú hán]

Thin, clear and watery discharge of the body is related to symptom-complex of cold.

諸嘔吐酸, 暴注下迫, 皆屬於熱 〔zhū ǒu tǔsuān, bàozhù xiàpò, jiē shǔyú ré〕

Vomiting with sour vomitus or spouting diarrhea with tenesmus is related to symptom-complex of heat.

天人相應 〔tiān rén xiāngyìng〕

the relevant adaptation of the human body to natural environment —one of the basic theories in traditional Chinese medicine, according to which the physical structure and physiological phenomena of human body as well as the pathological changes are in adaptative confirmity with the variations of the natural environment, and hence in diagnosis and treatment the influences of environmental factors such as climatic conditions, geographical localities, etc., should be considered

正邪相爭 〔zhèng xié xiāngzhēng〕

confrontation between vital energy of the human body and pathogenic factors, which is the process of all diseases and, in a narrow sense, denotes the mechanism of intermittent chills and fever occurring in febrile diseases

正虚邪實 〔zhèngxū xiéshí〕

vital energy undermined while pathogenic factors are prevailing, denoting the patient is in an unfavorable state with lowered resistance

邪氣盛則實 〔xiéqì shèng zé shí〕

Symptom-complexes of excessiveness occur when pathogenic factors are in abundance while the body resistance is sufficient to give corresponding reactions with increased functional activities. Hence the symptom-complex of excessiveness may have two groups of clinical manifestations: one including those showing the presence of abundant pathogenic factors such as retained water and dampness, indigested food, stagnant blood, etc.; the other including those showing increased functional activities such as high fever, restlessness, forceful pulse, etc.

精氣奪則虚 〔jīngqì duó zé xū〕

Symptom-complexes of insufficiency occur when the patient's vital essence and energy are severely damaged. Hence the chief clinical manifestations are those showing lowered body resistance and insuf-

50

ficiency of functions such as pallor, fatigue, palpitation, shortness of
breath, spontaneous and night sweats, feeble pulse, general debility,
etc.

思則氣結 [sī zé qì jié]
Mental anxiety makes the Qi (vital energy) of the spleen depressed,
causing indigestion.

怒則氣上 [nù zé qì shàng]
Anger causes the Qi (vital energy) of the liver to go perversely
upward, as a result, stuffiness in the chest, headache and redness of the
eye may occur.

恐則氣下 [kǒng zé qì xià]
Fear causes the Qi (vital energy) of the kidney to sink, as a result,
incontinence of urine and stool and seminal discharge may occur.

勞則氣耗 [láo zé qì hào]
Overwork renders the vital energy consumed, and hence results in
lassitude and listlessness.

陽虛陰盛 [yáng xū yīn shèng]
Deficiency of Yang leads to preponderance of Yin, i.e., lowered
vital function of the *kidney* and *spleen* being unable to warm up and
nourish all other internal organs, brings on symptoms of endogenous
cold (such as intolerance of cold, cold limbs) and symptoms showing
the presence of pathological factors of Yin nature (such as diarrhea and
edema showing the presence of excessive fluid within the intestines
and in the tissue spaces of the body)

陰盛陽衰 [yīn shèng yáng shuāi]
Preponderance of Yin renders Yang impaired, i.e., excessive endogenous cold renders the vital function damaged, mostly due to predominance of dampness (a pathogenic factor of Yin nature) of being
overdosed with medicines of cold nature

陽盛 [yángshèng]
exuberance of Yang (vital function), usually indicating presence
of excessive pathogenic heat, manifested by high fever, irritability,
thirst, etc.

陰盛 [yīnshèng]
predominance of Yin, usually with manifestations of endogenous

cold (such as intolerance of cold, cold limbs) and/or symptoms showing the presence of other pathological factors of Yin nature (such as diarrhea with watery stool)

陰虛陽亢 [yīnxū yángkàng]
exuberance of Yang due to deficiency of Yin. Deficiency of vital essence, blood or body fluid may lead to breakdown of the equilibrium between Yin and Yang, resulting in exuberance of the latter with symptoms such as headache, dizziness, malar flush, heat sensation in the chest, palms and soles, afternoon fever, night sweat, hemoptysis, irritability, insomnia, hyperaphrodisia, nocturnal emission, etc.

陰虛火旺 [yīnxū huǒwàng]
deficiency of Yin (vital essence) accompanied with flaming up of evil fire, with symptoms such as flushed cheeks, irritability, hyperaphrodisia, hemoptysis, etc. (cf.陰虛陽亢)

陽盛格陰 [yáng shèng gé yīn]
predominating Yang screened by Yin, a case of high fever with symptoms of pseudo-cold as Yang (heat) is being prevented from coming out. The patient may have symptoms such as cold extremities and a deep pulse, and yet with no intention of putting on more clothes.

陰盛格陽 [yīn shèng gé yáng]
predominating Yin screened by Yang, a case of excessive endogenous cold with pseudo-febrile symptoms. The patient may feel hot, yet likes to keep warm; he may feel thirsty, yet drinks very little, his pulse being full yet feeble.

陰盛則寒 [yīn shèng zé hán]
Preponderance of Yin gives rise to endogenous cold due to hypofunction of the organism.

陽盛則熱 [yáng shèng zé rè]
Preponderance of Yang leads to heat manifestations due to hyperfunction of the organism

陽虛則外寒 [yáng xū zé wài hán]
Deficiency of Yang (functional activities) brings on symptoms of external cold, such as intolerance of cold, cold limbs, etc.

陰虛則內熱 [yīn xū zé nèi rè]
Deficiency of Yin (vital essence) leads to internal heat, with symp-

toms such as afternoon fever, irritability, heat sensation in the chest, palms and soles, night sweats, thirst, red tongue, and fine and rapid pulse.

陰陽兩虛 [yīn yáng liǎngxū]
deficiency of both Yin and Yang seen usually at the advanced stage of a disease

脫陰 [tuōyīn]
exhaustion of Yin (vital essence) of the viscera, especially of the *liver* and *kidney*, leading to sudden deterioration of eye sight, usually seen at late stage of febrile diseases, malnutrition, postpartum weakness, etc.

脫陽 [tuōyáng]
exhaustion of Yang: (1) prostration due to exhaustion of Yang, bringing on preponderance of Yin factor internally, with symptoms of illusion, etc.; (2) prostration of the male due to exhaustion after sexual intercourse

虛陽上浮 [xūyáng shàng fú]; 孤陽上越 [gūyáng shàng yuè]
upward floating of desolate Yang due to lowered vital function of the *kidney*, a case of endogenous cold with superficial pseudo-heat manifestation

表氣不固 [biǎoqì bù gù]; 衛氣不固 [wèiqì bù gù]
lowered superficial resistance; unconsolidated defensive energy, which makes one susceptible to exogenous pathogenic factors, especially cold, and liable to perspire spontaneously

逆傳心包 [nì chuán xīnbāo]
adverse attack on the pericardium: pathogenic factor of an epidemic fever directly attacks the central nervous system (instead of the vital energy system as in an ordinary transmission of febrile diseases) soon after the onset of disease, causing impairment of consciousness or coma

陽虛水泛 [yángxū shuǐfàn];
generalized edema due to lowered vital function of the spleen and kidney, more marked in the loins and lower extremities, with scanty urine, ascites, loose bowels, pale tongue and white smooth fur, deep and fine pulse, seen usually in nephrotic syndrome, cardiac edema, etc.

營衛不和 [yíng wèi bù hé]

derangement of the constructive energy and defensive energy (the latter being the consolidating force of the body surface that regulates the excretion of sweat while the former related to the formation of sweat), resulting in spontaneous sweating in cases of exterior symptom-complexes. There are two kinds of derangement: (1) 衛弱營强 [wèi ruò yíng qiáng] —the defensive energy is weakened while the constructive energy is relatively strong, which leads to spontaneous sweating without fever; (2) 衛强營弱 [wèi qiáng yíng ruò] —the defensive energy being relatively strong while the constructive energy is weakened, which results in sweating only during the fever.

衛氣同病 [wèi qì tóng bìng]
symptom-complex showing both the Wei (the superficial defensive) system and Qi (secondary defensive) system are involved in epidemic fevers, marked by high fever, thirst, irritability together with intolerançe of cold and wind, general pains, etc.

營衛同病 [yíng wèi tóng bìng]
symptom-complex showing both Wei (the superficial defensive) system and Ying (the nutrient) system are involved, in which symptoms such as high fever, delirium are observed together with chills, headache, general aching, etc.

氣營兩燔 [qì yíng liǎng fán]
blazing of evil heat in both the Qi (the secondary defensive) and Ying (the nutrient) systems, marked hy high fever, thirst, mental irritability, delirium, barely visible skin eruption, etc.

氣血兩燔 [qì xuè liǎng fán]
blazing of evil heat in both the Qi (the secondary defensive) and the blood systems, marked by high fever, delirium, hemoptysis rhinorrhagia, skin eruptions, convulsion, etc.

熱入心包 [rè rù xīnbāo]
penetration of evil heat into the pericardium, causing high fever with delirium or even coma

熱入血分 [rè rù xuèfēn]
invasion of the blood system by evil heat— the late and severest stage of febrile disease, with fever, restlessness, delirium, skin eruption, bleeding (hematemesis, epistaxis, hematochezia), etc.

血分热毒 [xuèfēn rèdú]

noxious heat in the blood system: (1) penetration of heat into the blood system in epidemic febrile disease, marked by high fever, delirium, skin eruption, hematuria, etc.; (2) the common mechanism of acute pyogenic infections marked by recurrent local inflammation or boil formation

热入血室 [rè rù xuèshì]

attack of evil heat on the blood chamber (uterus), symptoms of which are abdominal distension, menstruous disturbances, alternate fever and chills, delirium at night, etc.

瘀热 [yūrè]

stagnant heat: (1) a febrile case due to heat and phlegm-dampness accumulating in the interior of the body; (2) heat produced by stagnated blood

伏热在裏 [fúrè zài lǐ]

evil heat collected within the stomach and intestines, manifested by dry throat, foul breath, red tongue, constipation, scanty yellow urine, etc.

血分瘀热 [xuèfèn yū rè]

stagnant heat in the blood system: (1) pathological heat accumulated in the blood system; the last stage of febrile disease with deep penetration of pathogenic factor into internal organs including the *heart, liver* and *kidney*; (2) heat produced by stagnated blood

热盛风动 [rè shèng fēng dòng]; 热极生风 [rè jí shēng fēng]

symptoms of wind produced by extreme heat, referred to convulsion or opisthotonus in high fever

风胜则动 [fēng shèng zé dòng]

Prevailing of endogenous wind produces involuntary movement, such as vertigo, giddiness, convulsion, tremor, spasm, etc.

血虚生风 [xuèxū shēng fēng]

internal wind due to deficiency of blood resulting from persisting anemia or profuse bleeding, marked by dizziness, twitching, tremor, etc.

风湿相搏 [fēng shī xiāngbó]

wind and dampness in contest: pathological changes caused by contending pathogenic factors wind and dampness after gaining access to the patient's muscles and joints, with muscle aching, joint pain and stiffness as main symptoms

濕熱內蘊[shīrè nèi yùn]
gathering and brewing of dampness and heat in the body, especially in the *stomach, spleen, liver* and *gallbladder,* manifested by persistent fever, heaviness feeling of the body, lassitude, loss of appetite, abdominal distension, or jaundice, seen usually in icteric hepatitis, typhoid fever, etc.

濕熱下注 [shīrè xià zhù]; 下焦濕熱 [xiàjiāo shīrè]
downward drive of dampness and heat into the Lower Burner or the lower portion of the body cavity, seen in acute entero-colitis, dysentery, infection of urinary tract, leukorrhea, etc.

濕毒流注 [shīdú liúzhù]
lingering of noxious dampness in muscles and skin, causing ulcer or fester on the shank

寒熱錯雜 [hán rè cuòzá]
coexistence and interlocking of cold and heat, a complicated pathological condition such as heat in the upper part with cold in the lower part of the body or cold in the exterior and heat in the interior of the body

寒極生熱, 熱極生寒 [hán jí shēng rè, rè jí shēng hán]
Extreme cold may bring on heat and vice versa, which denotes: (1) the change of weather in the four seasons of a year; (2) pathologic changes, e.g., a disease of cold nature in its extreme may show symptoms of pseudo-heat.

久熱傷陰 [jiǔrè shāng yīn]
Long-standing pathologic heat injures Yin (vital essence) of internal organs, and hence in the late stage of febrile disease the nutrient fluid of the *lung* and *stomach* may be impaired, with symptoms such as thirst, dry cough, reddened and dry tongue, fine and rapid pulse, and in severe cases the vital essence of the *liver* and *kidney* may also be injured, resulting in symptom-complex of wind, such as tremors of extremities and tongue.

虛火上炎 [xūhuǒ shàng yán]

56

flaring up of the asthenic fire caused by deficiency of vital essence of the *kidney*, marked by dry and sore throat, dizziness, restlessness, red eye, oral ulcers, etc.

壮火食氣 [zhuànghuǒ shí qì]
Hyperactivity consumes vital energy.

化热 [huàrè]
heat-transformation: pathological changes resulting from the heat produced in the process of transmission of external pathogenic factors, such as wind, cold, dryness, etc., into the interior of the body, manifested by intolerance of heat, thirst, irritability, reddened tongue with yellow fur, rapid pulse, etc.

化火 [huàhuǒ]
fire-transformation: pathological changes resulting from the fire produced when pathologic heat goes to extreme in the course of a disease. Many factors, exogenous and endogenous, may also transform into fire under certain conditions. Manifestations are varied, including persistent thirst, blood-shot eyes and flushed face, parched lips, dry and sore throat, hemoptysis, epistaxis, hematuria, and in severe cases impairment of consciousness or raving madness

胃热化火 [wèirè huà huǒ]
flaring up of heat in the stomach, characterized by inflammation and ulceration of the mouth in addition to the symptoms of heat in the *stomach*

化風 [huàfēng]
wind-transformation: pathologic changes in the course of febrile disease or due to severe damage to the blood and essence, with symptoms such as giddiness, convulsion, tremor, etc.

化燥 [huàzào]
dryness-transformation: pathological changes resulting from impairment of body fluid caused by heat factors or loss of blood, symptoms of which include thirst, dry throat and lips, constipation, dry cough, etc.

氣機不利 [qìjī bù lì]
obstruction of the vital energy flow, which is referred to dysfunction of the internal organs at large, especially functional der-

angement in sending things up or down, as manifested by hiccup, stuffiness feeling in the chest, abdominal distension, diarrhea, etc.

升降失常 [shēngjiàng shícháng]

disturbance in upward and downward functional activities: e.g., disturbance of the function of the *spleen* in sending food essence and water up and of the stomach in sending food contents down, causing abdominal distension, anorexia, diarrhea, vomiting, regurgitation, etc.

下陷 [xiàxiàn]

sinking due to deficiency of vital energy, usually of the *spleen*

内陷 [nèixiàn]

penetration of pathogenic factors into the interior of the body when the body's vital energy is weakened, which aggravates the patient's condition

肺氣不利 [fèiqì bù lì]

disturbance of the functional activities of the lung, especially referred to its function in maintaining normal water metabolism, giving rise to oliguria and edema together with respiratory symptoms

肺氣不宣 [fèiqì bù xuān]

impediment of the functional activities of the lung, usually referred to the exterior symptom-complex caused by exogenous pathogenic factors, with chills, fever and upper respiratory symptoms such as stuffed nose with nasal discharge, cough, etc.

肺津不布 [fèijīn bù bù]

failure of the lung's normal function in distributing nutrient essence and fluid, leading to production of sputum and causing cough and asthma

肺失清肅 [fèi shī qīngsù]

impairment of the normal function of the lung in clarifying the passage and sending down the air and vital energy—one of the common mechanisms seen in *lung* diseases, giving rise to cough, dyspnea, expectoration of sputum, fullness of the chest, etc.

肺氣上逆 [fèiqì shàngnì]

upward perversion in the functioning of the lung — an advanced case of impaired sending-down function of the *lung,* marked by cough and asthma

胃氣不降 [wèiqì bù jiàng]; 胃失和降 [wèi shī héjiàng]
dysfunction of the stomach in sending down food content, with symptoms such as anorexia, nausea, vomiting, belching, stuffiness feeling over the gastric region, etc.

胃氣上逆 [wèiqì shàngnì]
upward perversion in the functioning of the stomach, with belching, hiccup and vomiting as main symptoms

氣化不利 [qìhuà bù lì]
(1) disturbance in metabolic functions in a broad sense, denoting metabolic disorders of all sorts of vital essence and energy; (2) in a narrow sense, disturbance in urine excretion due to dysfunction of the *kidney* and the *urinary bladder*—one of the causes of edema and difficulty in urination

寒凝氣滯 [hánníng qìzhì]
stagnancy of the flow of Qi (vital energy) due to accumulated cold, often causing spasms and pains

氣滯血瘀 [qìzhì xuèyū]
stagnation of vital energy and stasis of blood. Various pathogenic factors such as emotional depression, improper diet, infection and injury can impede the normal circulation of vital energy and result in its stagnation with stuffiness and pain as main symptoms. Long standing or severe stagnation of vital energy may lead to blood stasis, marked by aggravation of local pain with tenderness, or even mass formation.

氣虛則寒 [qì xū zé hán]
Deficiency of Qi (vital energy) brings on cold with symptoms such as intolerance of cold, cold limbs, loose bowels, etc.

氣虛不攝 [qìxū bù shè]
Qi (vital energy) of the spleen being insufficient to keep the blood circulating within the vessels, which usually leads to chronic bleeding

氣虛中滿 [qìxū zhōngmǎn]
abdominal distension due to deficiency of Qi (vital energy) of the spleen, usually accompanied by loss of appetite, loose bowels, etc.

氣陰兩虛 [qì yīn liǎng xū]
deficiency of both Qi (vital energy) and Yin (vital essence, including blood and fluid) seen in chronic consumptive cases and in the late

stage of febrile diseases

氣有餘便是火 [qì yǒu yú biàn shì huǒ]

Excess of Qi (vital energy) gives rise to manifestations of fire : a hypothesis propounded by Zhu Zhen-heng for explanation of various kinds of fire syndromes, e.g., in cases with deficiency of vital essence, fire symptoms may be caused by the preponderance of vital function, and in cases with uncontrolled overflow of emotions, fire symptoms may be brought on by stagnancy and smouldering of vital energy.

氣血失調 [qì xuè shītiáo]

derangement of Qi (vital energy) and blood, which may bring on pathological changes such as menstruous complaints, chronic hemorrhage, persistent pain, etc.

血虛 [xuèxū]

deficiency of blood, with symptoms such as pallor, dizziness, palpitation, insomnia, etc., usually resulting from profuse bleeding or chronic hemorrhage, or impaired blood production due to diminished function of the internal organs, especially of the *spleen*

血脱氣脱 [xuè tuō qì tuō]; 氣隨血脱 [qì suí xuè tuō]

prostration of Qi (vital energy) after great loss of blood, marked by pale complexion, cold extremities, profuse sweating, thready and barely perceptible pulse, as seen in shock.

血不歸經 [xuè bù guī jīng]; 血不循經 [xuè bù xún jīng]

escape of blood from vessels instead of flowing within them (such as hemoptysis, epistaxis, uterine bleeding, ecchymoses, etc.) which may be caused by various factors, e.g., deficiency of perverted flow of vital energy, intense heat and fire

冲任損傷 [chōng rèn sǔnshāng]

damage of the Chong (Vital) and Ren (Conception) Channels, usually caused by infection, intemperance in sexual life, or frequent pregnancy, resulting in dysmenorrhea, pain in the lower abdomen and loins, uterine bleeding, abortion, etc.

冲任不固 [chōng rèn bú gù]

weakness of the Chong (Vital) and Ren (Conception) Channels—a pathological change seen in the damage of these channels (cf. 衝任損傷), leading to uterine bleeding or abortion

60

V Method of Diagnosis

诊法 [zhěnfǎ]; 四诊 [sìzhěn]
(the four) methods of diagnosis: inspection, auscultation and olfaction, interrogation (history taking), and pulse feeling and palpation

望诊 [wàngzhěn]
inspection; examination by the eye—one of the four methods of diagnosis, including inspection of complexion, facial expression, behaviour, body surface, tongue, excreta and secretions

望神 [wàng shén]
observation of the patient's expression, esp. facial expression and lustre of the eye (the outward manifestation of one's vitality) to judge his general condition and body resistance

得神 [déshén]
being full of spirit. A patient full of spirit is apt to recover from his illness and usually has a good prognosis.

失神 [shīshén]
lack of vitality with skinny figure, lack-lustre eyes or even impaired consciousness, indicating a poor prognosis.

假神 [jiǎshén]
false manifestation of vitality: momentary spurt of activity just before death

望色 [wàng sè]
observation of the patient's complexion, especially the natural colour, appearance, etc. of the face as a reference for diagnosis

气色 [qìsè]
complexion; outward manifestation of vital energy

病容 [bìngróng]
sickly appearance and complexion

五色 [wǔsè]
the five colours: blue, red, yellow, white and black. According to the doctrine of Five Evolutive Phases or theory of Five Elements, they

correspond to the *liver* (wood), *heart* (fire), *spleen* (earth), *lung* (metal) and *kidney* (water) respectively.

青色 [qīngsè]

bluish discoloration (cyanosis) of the skin or complexion, usually caused by stagnancy or obstruction of vital energy and blood, indicating presence of cold, pains, blood stasis, convulsion or illness of the *liver*.

黄色 [huángsè]

yellow discoloration of the skin or complexion, seen in cases of dysfunction of the *spleen* or in icteric patients, indicating presence of dampness and heat

萎黄 [wěihuáng]

sallow skin or complexion, usually caused by dysfunction of the *spleen* or deficiency of blood

赤色 [chìsè]

redness of the skin or complexion caused by excessive filling of skin capillaries, indicating presence of heat

白色 [báisè]

white colour (pallor) of the skin or complexion, usually indicating presence of cold or deficiency of blood and vital energy

黑色 [hēisè]

dark colour of the skin or complexion seen usually in severe and chronic cases of blood stasis, cold, pains, and lowered vital function of the *kidney*

五色主病 [wǔsè zhǔ bìng]

diagnostic significance of the five colours. The five colours reveal illness in corresponding viscera, i.e. blue, red, yellow, white, and black suggest disease in the *liver, heart, spleen, lung* and *kidney* respectively. This theory has been developed in later ages and may be given as follows: the blue colour suggests disease of wind, cold, pains, convulsion, or blood stasis; the red colour hints disease of heat; the yellow colour reveals dampness or blood deficiency; the white colour indicates debility and symptom-complex of cold; and the balck colour suggests cold, pain, exhaustion or blood stasis

望形態 [wàng xíngtài]

inspection of the patient's physical build: musculature, skeleton, posture, gait, etc, to judge his constitution, development and nutrition, severity of the illness, location of the injury, etc.

审苗窍 [shěn miáoqiào]
inspection of the body opening to judge the condition of its corresponding internal organ, e.g., the condition of the *heart* is revealed on the tongue proper

望目 [wàng mù]; 察目 [chá mù]
inspection of the eye, the lustre, expressiveness and acuity of vision may reveal the vital function of the viscera, especially that of the *liver*

舌诊 [shézhěn]
inspection of the tongue, its size, form, colour and smoothness (moisture) of both the tongue proper and its fur as one of the findings for diagnosis

舌的部位 [shé de bùwèi]; 舌的分部 [shé de fēnbù]
parts of the tongue. Different parts of the tongue reflect the condition of various internal organs: the tip, middle, root and the borders of the tongue reveal pathologic changes of the *heart*, the *spleen* and *stomach*, the *kidney*, the *liver* and the *gallbladder* respectively.

舌质 [shézhì]
the tongue substance or the tongue proper. In diagnosis the size, form, colour, motility and moisture of the tongue may reveal the condition of blood circulation, body fluid and vital function of the internal organs.

舌色 [shésè]
colour of the tongue as a criterion of semeiology

舌淡白 [shédànbái]
whitish tongue, that is, paler than normal, indicating deficiency of vital energy and blood

舌红 [shéhóng]
reddened tongue, that is, redder than normal, indicating presence of heat

舌绛 [shéjiàng]
deep redness of the tongue proper, indicating intense heat, usually

seen in febrile disease when the Ying (nutrient) system is involved

舌青紫[shéqīngzǐ]
blue and purple (cyanosis) of the tongue, indicating blood stasis

舌有瘀點 [shé yǒu yūdiǎn]；舌有瘀斑[shé yǒu yūbān]
purple dots or spots on the tongue—a sign of blood stasis

舌老嫩 [shélǎonèn]
solid, dark-coloured tongue or soft, light-coloured tongue, the former indicating symptom—complex of excessiveness while the latter indicates symptom-complex of insufficiency

舌胖 [shépàng]；舌體胖大 [shétǐ pàngdà]
plump tongue, often with teeth prints at the lower borders, brought on in most cases by deficiency of vital function of the *spleen* and *kidney*

齒痕舌 [chǐhénshé]；舌有齒痕 [shé yǒu chǐhén]
the tongue with teeth prints at its borders, indicating hypofunction of the *spleen* if the tongue is plump as well

芒刺舌 [mángcìshé]
prickly tongue, resulting from proliferation and hypertrophy of taste buds, indicating intense heat of the viscera

舌裂 [shéliè]
fissured tongue, a sign showing impairment of the essence, usually seen in protracted or exhausted case

舌腫 [shézhǒng]
swollen tongue with pains, usually due to toxic fire in the blood (hyperemia and inflammation) of the Heart Channel

重舌 [chóngshé]
double tongue: a togue-like swelling of the sublingual veins due to blood stagnancy, which may be brought on by accumulated heat in *heart* and *spleen* or exposal to wind after heavy drinking

舌瘦癟 [shéshòubiě]
thin and shrunken tongue. A thin and light-coloured tongue usually suggests deficiency of vital energy and blood, while a deep red, shrunken tongue indicates intense heat with impairment of body fluid.

舌强 [shéjiàng]

stiffness of the tongue, usually seen in cases of apoplexy or acute
febrile disease (the central nervous system is always involved)

舌謇 [shéjiǎn]
sluggish tongue, usually curled and stiff, seen in cases of apoplexy,
encephalitis and their sequelae

舌戰 [shézhàn]
tremor of the tongue, often seen in cases of debility or disease
due to endogenous wind (which is marked by tremors)

舌痿 [shéwěi]
paralysis of the tongue; inability to move the tongue—a sign
of debility and exhaustion'(especially of vital essence)

舌歪 [shéwāi]
wry tongue, turning to one side while stuck out, usually seen in
apoplexy

舌短 [shéduǎn] 舌體短縮 [shétí duǎnsuō]
shortened or contracted tongue, seen in cases of severe cold with
whitish tongue or febrile disease with reddened tongue due to deficiency of body fluid, also in apoplexy, being a sign of critical condition if accompanied with loss of consciousness

舌卷囊縮 [shéjuǎn náng suō]
curled tongue and retracted testicles, seen in critical stage of
febrile diseases and apoplexy

木舌 [mùshé]
swollen and hardened tongue, due to excessive fire of the *heart*
or accumulated heat in the *heart* and *spleen*

伸舌 [shēnshé]
sticking the tongue out frequently to lick the lips, which reveals
internal dryness of the *spleen* and *stomach* and deficiency of fluid

吐弄舌 [tǔnòngshé]
playing with the tongue: sticking the tongue out to lick the lips
and drawing it back frequently, seen in children with defective development of the brain, and also in febrile disease especially when the
central nervous system is involved

舌苔 [shétāi]
fur; coat of the tongue

苔色 [tāisè]

colour of the fur of the tongue, as a criterion of semeiology

白苔 [báitāi]

white coat of the tongue, usually indicating cold factor or disease with the surface of the body involved only

黄苔 [huángtāi]

yellow coat of the tongue, indicating illness with heat

灰黑苔 [huīhēitāi]

ashy black coat of the tongue, indicating severe condition of the patient. A pale tongue with moistened and ashy black coat is often seen in cases of endogenous cold or cold-dampness and a red tongue with dry and black-ashy coat is usually seen in cases of intense heat with impairment of the body essence.

染苔 [rǎntāi]

staining of the fur by food or medicine, which should be distinguished from its natural colour on inspection of the tongue

苔的厚薄 [tāi de hòubó]

thickness of the fur of the tongue. A thin coat usually indicates a mild case or only the body surface is being attacked by exogenous pathogenic factors while a thick coat indicates inward penetration of pathogenic factors or presence of stagnancy of food or phlegm.

苔的润燥 [tāi de rùnzào]

moist or dry coat of the tongue. Moist coat indicates that the body fluid is not impaired or the disease is caused by dampness, while dry coat is a sign of impairment of body fluid.

腐苔 [fǔtāi]

spongy curdy coat of the tongue, capable of being wiped off, reflecting retention of food in the *stomach*

腻苔 [nìtāi]

slimy and greasy coat of the tongue hard to wipe off, indicating presence of excessive phlegm and dampness or stagnancy of food

滑苔 [huátāi]

smooth, slippery coat of the tongue, indicating presence of dampness

剥苔 [bōtāi]; 剥脱苔 [bōtuōtāi]

66

shedding of the tongue fur. Map-like shedding indicates parasitosis, a furless mirror-like tongue suggests severe case with impoverished essence of the *liver* and *kidney*.

光剥苔 [guāngbōtāi]
sudden disappearance of the fur on tongue, usually indicating deficiency of vital energy and essence of the *stomach*

舌面如镜 [shémiàn rú jìng]   镜面舌 [jìngmiànshé]
a furless, smooth, mirror-like tongue, redder than normal, seen usually in patients with deficiency of essence of the *liver* and *kidney*

唇腫 [chúnzhǒng]
swollen lips, seen in cases of accumulated heat in the *spleen* and *stomach* or food poisoning

唇裂 [chúnliè]
cracked lips due to dryness or impairment of fluid by febrile diseases

望齒 [wàng chǐ]
inspection of the teeth, including the gum, not only for diagnosis of local illness, but also for finding clues to detecting diseases of internal organs, e.g., luxated teeth suggesting hypofunction of the *kidney*, red swollen and tender gum often indicating excessive heat in the *stomach*

望痰 [wàng tán]
inspection of the sputum: clear, thin whitish foamy sputum indicating cold; scanty sticky sputum indicating dryness; profuse whitish sputum, easy to expectorate, indicating dampness; condensed, yellow and sticky sputum indicating heat; sputum with blood streaks or stains, indicating fire due to deficiency of essence of the *lung* and *kidney;* purulent and bloody sputum suggesting presence of pulmonary abscess

望指紋 [wàng zhǐwén]
inspection of superficial veins of the finger — a pediatric diagnosing method for children under three years old. The extending and colour of these veins on the palmar side of the index finger are taken as reference for diagnosis; e.g., red veins with yellowish tint, faintly visible, not extending beyond the proximal segment of the finger indicate health; deep red veins suggest presence of heat; dark veins suggest blood

stagnation; purple and blue veins are usually seen in convulsion and pains.

三關 [sānguān]

the Three Passes: on examining the superficial veins of the index finger of a child, the three segments of the finger are named 風關 [fēngguān]or Wind Pass (the proximal segment), 氣關 [qìguān] or Vital Energy Pass (the middle segment), and 命關 [mìngguān]or Life Pass (the distal segment). The veins only visible at Wind Pass usually indicate mild disease. The farther the veins extend, the more serious is the case.

通關射甲 [tōngguān shèjiǎ]   透關射甲 [tòuguān shè jiǎ]

extending of the superficial veins through the Three Passes toward the tip of the index finger, often indicating the child is dangerously ill

望皮膚 [wàng pífū]

inspection of the skin

腫脹 [zhǒngzhàng]

edema and distension. The former may take place at any part of the body, while the latter is usually referred to the abdomen only.

斑疹 [bānzhěn]

macula and papula

白痦 [báipéi];   晶痦 [jīngpéi]

miliaria alba; sudamina crystallina − skin eruption of crystalline vesicles appearing on the neck and then spreading to other parts of the body in the course of acute febrile disease

聞診 [wénzhěn]

ausculation and olfaction − one of the four methods of diagnosis

聞聲音 [wén shēngyīn]

auscultation, to listen to the patient's voice, sounds of breath and cough, etc.

語聲 [yǔshēng]

voice, which may give a clue to judging the patient's general condition, e.g., a debilitated patient usually speaks in a feeble voice

譫語 [zhānyǔ]

delirious speech, usually occurring during high fever, especially when the pericardium (which is refered to the central nervous system)

68

is attacked by evil heat

失音 [shīyīn]; 喑 [yīn]; 瘖 [yīn]

aphonia; loss of voice. An acute case with sudden onset of aphonia, 暴瘖 [bàoyīn], is usually due to affection of exogenous pathogenic factors while a chronic case is more likely caused by deficieny of essence in the *lung* and *kidney*.

痰鳴 [tánmíng]

wheezing due to excessive phlegm

太息 [tàixī]

sighing — deep breathing with prolonged expiration (with a ratio to pulse of 1:5). Frequent sighing is considered as a symptom of stagnancy of vital energy of the *liver* and the *gallbladder* or disharmonious flow of the vital energy of the *lung*

嗅氣味 [xiù qìwèi]

smelling the odour of the patient, his or her compartment and bodily discharge as a reference for diagnosis, e.g., purulent fetid odour suggests presence of ulceration

腥臭氣 [xīngchòuqì]

stink — horrid and offensive smell as given off from stools in steatorrhea or from cancerous discharges

口氣 [kǒuqì]

odour in the mouth. A normal person does not give any bad smell from the mouth while talking. Foul breath (口氣臭穢 [kǒuqì. chòuhuì]) usually indicates presence of heat in the *lung* or *stomach*. Sour smell in the mouth (口氣酸臭 [kǒuqì suān chòu]) is a sign of indigestion.

十問 [shíwèn]

the Ten Questions: ten questions recommended by Zhang Jie-bin 張介賓 (1553—1640), for a physician to ask of his patient while making diagnosis: (1) chills and fever; (2) perspiration; (3) headache and general pains; (4) urination and defecation; (5) appetite; (6) feeling in the chest and abdomen; (7) hearing; (8) thirst; (9) pulse taking and observation; (10) auscultation and smelling. Chen Xiu-yuan 陳修園 (1753-1823) made some alterations and additions. According to Chen, the 9th and 10th questions are about the patient's past disease and the cause of the present illness respectively. And in addition, inquiry should be made into the efficacy of medicine taken, about menstruation for women patients and history of smallpox and measles for children.

脈息 [màixī]
the tempo of pulse beat

脈象 [màixiàng]
pulse condition, generally including its rate, rhythm, volume, tension, etc., as felt by the finger tips of the physician

脈學 [màixué]
pulse lore, theory of the pulse by which the relationship between different kinds of pulse-beat and physiopathological changes is explained

切診 [qièzhěn]
pulse feeling and palpation—one of the four methods of diagnosis

脈診 [màizhěn]
pulse feeling manual study of the pulse

切脈 [qièmài]
feeling the pulse, the art of feeling the patient's pulse by the physician with the index, middle and ring fingers

寸、關、尺 [cùn、guān、chǐ]
inch, bar and cubit — three places on the wrist over the radial artery to feel the pulse. The bar is just over the eminent head of the radius at the wrist, where the tip of the physician's middle finger is placed, the inch is next to it on the distal side, where the tip of the physician's index finger rests, the cubit is on the proximal side where the tip of the physician's ring finger is placed. The inch, bar and cubit on the left represent the pulse of the *heart, liver* and *kidney* respectively while those on the right represent the pulse of the *lung, spleen* and Vital Gate

舉、按、尋 [jǔ、àn、xún]
lifting, pressing and searching (manipulations used in pulse-taking). By lifting is meant to rest the fingers on the wrist very lightly, by pressing is meant to feel the pulse with proper force, and by searching is meant to vary the force or move the fingers to get a more distinct pulse-

70

reading

平息 [píngxī]

normal, even respiration (with a ratio to pulse of 1:4 normally) which a physician should assume while examining a patient and use it as a reference for judging the frequency of the latter's pulse

三部九侯 [sānbù jiǔhòu]

three-portion and nine-position pulse taking method: (1) to take pulse on the three portions of the body: the head, the upper and the lower limbs, in each portion pulses of three arteries examined (temporal art. at point Taiyang (太陽) for the state of the head, auricular art. at point Ermen (耳門) for ears, art. buccinatoria at points Dicang (地倉) and Daying (大迎) for mouth and teeth, radial art. at *inch* for the *lung*, ulnar art. at point Shenmen (神門) for the *heart*, pulse at point Hegu (合谷) for the chest, pulse at points Wuli (五里) and Taichong (太冲) for the *liver*, pulse at points Qimen (期門) and Chongyang (冲陽) for the *spleen* and *stomach*, pulse at point Taixi (太谿) for the *kidney* — a method of general examination adopted in the ancient times; (2) three areas over the radial art. on the wrist for pulse feeling, designated as *inch*, *bar* and *cubit*, each area felt with light, moderate and strong force to study superficial, medium and deep pulse

寸口 [cùnkǒu]; 氣口 [qìkǒu];脈口 [màikǒu]

entrance of pulse, the place on the wrist over the radial artery where pulse is felt. It is called *cunkou* because it is one inch (*cun*) proximal to the point Yuji (魚際). (Yuji is located at the junction of the "red and white" skin of the hand corresponding to the midpoint of the first metacarpal bone.)

寸口脈 [cùnkǒumài]

the radial artery on the wrist where the pulse is routinely taken for diagnosis

趺陽脈 [fúyángmài]

arteria dorsalis pedis where pulsation is easily felt

人迎脈 [rényíngmài]

arteria carotis communis, the pulsation of which is easily felt beside Adam's apple

病脈 [bìngmài]

71

abnormal pulse, indicating pathological changes

二十八脉 [èrshíbāmài]

(1) twenty-eight kinds of pulses: floating, sinking (deep), slow, rapid, smooth, hesitant, feeble, forceful, long, short, full, faint, tense, relaxed, taut, hollow, hard and hollow, firm, soft, weak, scattered, fine, hidden, tremulous, running, slow and uneven, intermittent, gigantic; (2) the twenty eight channels in acupuncture

浮脉 [fúmài]

floating pulse, which can be felt by light touch and grows faint on hard pressure, seen usually in the initial stage of diseases caused by exogenous factors, indicating the exterior of the body being affected. Debilitated patients may show floating and feeble pulse.

沉脉 [chénmài]

deep or sinking pulse, which can only be felt while pressing hard, showing that disease is located in the interior of the body

伏脉 [fúmài]

hidden pulse, as if embedded in muscles, only felt on strong pressure, seen in cases of syncope, shock, severe pain, etc.

数脉 [shuòmài]

rapid or frequent pulse, a pulse with more than 5 beats to one cycle of the physician's respiration or more than 90 beats per minute, indicating presence of heat

迟脉 [chímài]

slow or retarded pulse, a pulse with less than four beats to one cycle of respiration, or less than 60 beats per minute, usually indicating presence of cold or obstruction or deficiency of the Yang function. It may be observed normally in some athletes

缓脉 [huǎnmài]

(1) moderate pulse, four beats to one cycle of respiration, with even rhythm and moderate tension, indicating a normal condition; (2) relaxed or loose pulse, a pulse with diminished tension and moderate frequency, seen in cases with dampness and dysfunction of the spleen

虚脉 [xūmài]

feeble pulse, a pulse felt feeble and void to the physician's finger, seen in cases of debility

实脉 [shímài]

replete or forceful pulse, a pulse felt forceful on both light and heavy pressure, seen in excessiveness symptom-complexes with undamaged body resistance

洪脉 [hóngmài]

full pulse, a pulse beating like dashing waves with forceful rising and gradual decline, seen usually in cases with excessive evil heat

细脉 [xìmài]

fine or thready pulse, a pulse as thin as a silk thread, feeble yet always perceptible on hard pressure, indicating exhaustion of vital essence, blood and body fluid

微脉 [wēimài]

faint pulse, thready and soft, scarcely perceptible, showing exhaustion to the extreme

弱脉 [ruòmài]

weak pulse, usually deep and soft, seen in cases of general debility

濡脉 [rúmài]

soft pulse, superficial and fine, like thread floating on water, which can be felt on light pressure but grows faint on hard pressure, seen in cases with deficiency of blood and vital essence or collection of dampness

滑脉 [huámài]

smooth or slippery pulse, pulse beating like beads rolling on a plate, seen in patients with phlegm and dampness or stagnation of food, and also in pregnant women and normal persons

涩脉 [sèmài]

hesitant pulse, with small, fine, slow joggling tempo like scraping bamboo with knife, indicating sluggishness of blood circulation caused by deficiency of blood and essence or stagnancy of vital energy and blood

革脉 [gémài]

hard and hollow pulse, large and taut yet as hollow as touching the surface of a drum, indicating loss of blood and semen

牢脉 [láomài]

firm pulse, a forceful and taut pulse, felt only by hard pressure, usually seen in cases with accumulation of cold factor such as formation of firm masses

長脈 [chángmài]

long pulse, a pulse with large extent and prolonged stroke. Long pulse with moderate tension may be found in normal persons, but long and taut pulse is observed in cases where confrontation between the body resistance and the invading factors is going on hard.

短脈 [duǎnmài]

short pulse, a pulse with short extent, easily to be felt at the bar part yet not obviously, no volume, while felt at the inch and cubit parts. It strikes the finger (mainly the middle finger) sharply and leaves it quickly, showing stagnancy or deficiency of vital energy.

疾脈 [jímài]

swift pulse, over 7-8 beats to one cycle of respiration or 120-140 beats per minute, seen in febrile diseases with high fever or advanced cases of consumption

促脈 [cùmài]

running pulse, rapid with irregular intermittence, seen usually in cases with excessive heat and stagnation of vital energy, blood and phlegm

代脈 [dàimài]

intermittent pulse pausing at regular intervals, indicating the feeble condition of the viscera, seen in patients with heart disease, severe trauma or being seized with terror

結脈 [jiémài]

slow and uneven pulse, pausing at irregular intervals, seen usually in stagnation of vital energy and blood

緊脈 [jǐnmài]

tense pulse, felt like a tightly stretched cord, seen usually in cases with exterior or interior cold

散脈 [sǎnmài]

scattered pulse, a pulse diffusing on light touch and faint on hard pressure, seen in critical cases

弦脈 [xiánmài]

taut pulse, string tight pulse, a pulse beating like a tremulous music string, seen usually in cases with *liver* troubles or severe pains

芤脈 [kōumài]

hollow pulse, floating, large and empty inside, felt like a scallion stalk, seen in cases with massive loss of blood

大脈 [dàmài]

large or gigantic pulse, with a high pulse wave which lifts the finger to a greater height than normal, either forceful (seen in cases with undamaged body resistance and excessive heat) or weak (seen in cases with general debility)

動脈 [dòngmài]

(1) tremulous pulse, quick and jerky, which can be felt like a dancing pea, seen in cases with pain or being frightened or in pregnant women; (2) arterial pulsation that can be felt anywhere on the human body

七怪脈 [qīguàimài]; 七絕脈 [qījuémài]

seven kinds of pulses indicating impending death

雀啄脈 [quèzhuómài]

pecking pulse, an abrupt, quick, arrythmic pulse resembling the pecking of a bird-one of the seven kinds of pulses indicating impending death

魚翔脈 [yúxiángmài]

fish-swimming pulse, an extremely short pulse resembling a swimming fish with only its tail wagging—one of the seven pulses indicating impending death

蝦游脈 [xiāyóumài]

shrimp—darting pulse, a nearly imperceptible pulse with occasional darting beats—one of the seven pulses indicating impending death

釜沸脈 [fǔfèimài]

boiling pulse, an extremely floating and rapid pulse like bubbles rising to the surface in boiling water—one of the seven pulses indicating impending death

屋漏脈 [wūlòumài]

dripping pulse, an extremely retarded pulse resembling water dripping from a roof crack—one of the seven pulses indicating impending death

彈石脈 [tánshímài]

flicking pulse, a deep and solid pulse resembling flicking stones with finger tips—one of the seven pulses indicating impending death

解索脈 [jiěsuǒmài]

snapping pulse, a rhythmless pulse resembling the snapping of a cord—one of the seven pulses indicating impending death

喜脈 [xǐmài]

pulse indicating pregnancy

單一脈象 [dānyī màixiàng]

single-feature pulse—pulse with only one distinct feature, such as slow pulse, full pulse, etc.

相兼脈象 [xiāngjiān màixiàng]

multi-feature pulse—pulse with two or more than two distinct features, such as floating and tense pulse, deep, fine and rapid pulse, etc.

反關脈 [fǎnguānmài]

dorsally located radial artery, an anatomic anomaly of the radial artery which makes the pulse beat felt on the dorsal of the wrist

斜飛脈 [xiéfēimài]

slantly located radial artery, an anatomic anomaly of the radial artery which makes the pulse beat felt running from the *cubit* outwardly and slantly to the back of the hand

脈合四時 [mài hé sìshí]

The pulse changes in response to the change of the four seasons, e.g., the normal pulse may be slightly taut in spring, full in summer, floating in autumn, and sinking in winter.

四診合參 [sìzhěn hé cān]

an overall analytical study of the data gained by the four methods of diagnosis

脈證合參 [mài zhèng hé cān]

making a diagnosis in the light of pulse condition and symptoms observed, taking into account their agreements and disagreements, penetrating phenomena and grasping the reality

舍脈從證 [shě mài cóng zhèng]

making a diagnosis rather on the basis of symptoms and signs than on the basis of pulse condition if there exists disagreement between the two, especially in acute and complicated cases when the pulse is unable to furnish accurate information on the essential nature of the disease

舍證從脈 [shě zhèng cóng mài]

making a diagnosis rather on the basis of pulse condition than on symptoms and signs in case of contradiction between the two, so doing usually in chronic and complicated cases

按診 [ànzhěn]; 觸診 [chùzhěn]

palpation, feeling or pressing the skin, the collateral channels and points, the chest, the abdomen or any other part of the body surface to check the temperature, hardness, tenderness and other qualities

按尺膚 [àn chǐfū]; 診尺膚 [zhěn chǐfū]

palpation of the forearm (from the elbow to the wrist) to examine texture of the skin, development of the muscles, temperature of the extremities, etc.

按胸腹 [àn xiōngfù]; 診胸腹 [zhěn xiōngfù]

palpation of the chest and abdomen to determine the location and extent of the affected area, its temperature, presence of tenderness, lumps or accumulation of fluid, and to see if the pain is relieved by pressure

VI Differentiation of Symptom-Complexes

辨證 [biànzhèng]

differentiation of symptom-complexes on the basis of an overall analysis of symptoms and signs, including the cause, nature and location of the illness and the patient's physical condition

證 [zhèng]

(1) **symptom-complex or syndrome**, including the cause, mechanism, location and nature of the disease as well as the condition of the struggle between the invading pathogenic factors and body resistance; (2) **evidences of illness**

證候 [zhènghòu]

symptoms and signs

八綱 [bāgāng]

Eight Principal Syndromes, i.e., Yin and Yang, exterior and interior, heat and cold, insufficiency (or deficiency) and excessiveness

八綱辨證 [bāgāng biàn zhèng]

analysing and differentiating pathological conditions in accordance with the Eight Principal Syndromes

陰陽 [yīn yáng]

Yin and Yang —two comprehensive categories of Eight Principal Syndromes serving as a guidance in differential diagnosis

陰證 [yīnzhèng]

Yin symptom-complex, in which manifestations of debility, depression, hypofunction, decreased metabolism, etc., especially in chronic diseases are observed. Syndromes of interior, cold, and insufficiency generally belong to this category.

陽證 [yángzhèng]

Yang symptom-complex, in which manifestations of hyperactivity, excitability, hyper-function, increased metabolism, etc., especially in acute diseases, are observed. Syndromes of exterior, heat, and excessiveness generally belong to this catagory.

表裏 [biǎo lǐ]
exterior and interior of the body—two of the Eight Principal Syndromes showing the relative location and severity of illnesses

表證 [biǎozhèng]
exterior symptom-complex, marked by fever and chills, headache, joint pains or general aches, stuffy nose or cough, floating pulse, etc., indicating that the external part of the human body is affected or attacked by exogenous pathogenic factors

裏證 [lǐzhèng]
interior symptom-complex, indicating that the internal organ or the interior of the body is affected

寒熱 [hán rè]
(1) cold or heat—two of the Eight Principal Syndromes showing two main features of illnesses; (2) chills and fever

寒證 [hánzhèng]
cold symptom-complex, caused by cold factor or diminished vital function, marked by intolerance of cold, fondness of warmth, loose bowels, pallor, pale tongue with white fur, etc.

熱證 [rèzhèng]
heat symptom-complex, caused by pathogenic heat or excessive vital function, marked by feverishness, flushed face, thirst, craving for cold drink, constipation, red tongue with yellow fur, rapid pulse, etc.

虛實 [xū shí]
insufficiency (or deficiency) and excessiveness— two of the Eight Principal Syndromes reflecting the condition of the struggle between invading pathogenic factors and body resistance. Insufficiency denotes deficiency of vital energy and lowered body resistance, while excessiveness indicates the presence of excessive pathogenic factors and hyperfunction in the interior.

虛證 [xūzhèng]
insufficiency symptom-complex, including deficiency of Yin (vital essence), Yang (vital function), Qi (vital energy) and blood which is caused by prolonged illness

實證 [shízhèng]

excessiveness symptom-complex, caused by affection due to exogenous pathogenic factors or by accumulation of pathologic products due to dysfunction of internal organs, such as phlegm, stagnant blood, etc., which can bring on further lesions as pathogenic factors

表寒 [biǎohán]

cold in the exterior: the external part of the body being attacked by exogenous wind and cold, marked by chilliness, hypohidrosis, headache, general aching or joint pains, thin and white coat of the tongue, floating and tense pulse, etc.

表热 [biǎorè]

heat in the exterior: the external part of the body being attacked by exogenous wind and heat, marked by fever, intolerance of wind, headache, thirst, floating and rapid pulse, etc.

表虚 [biǎoxū]

insufficiency in the exterior: a type of exterior symptom-complex, marked by lowered superficial resistance, with spontaneous sweating, intolerance of wind, floating, slow and feeble pulse, etc., as its characteristic symptoms

表實 [biǎoshí]

excessiveness in the exterior: a type of exterior symptom-complex, showing the external part of the body being attacked by exogenous factors, yet the patient's vital function is not damaged, with headache, general aching, hypohidrosis, floating and forceful pulse, etc., as its characteristic symptoms

裏寒 [lǐhán]

cold in the interior: a case caused either by endogenous cold, i.e., deficiency of vital energy, or by exogenous cold transmitted to the interior of the body, main symptoms of which are intolerance of cold, pallor, cold limbs, pale tongue with white moistened coat, deep, slow or fine pulse, etc.

裏热 [lǐrè]

heat in the interior: pathologic heat in internal organs, especially in the *stomach, intestines, lung, liver* and *gallbladder*, manifested by fever, intolerance of heat, thirst, irritability, scanty and condensed urine, full, rapid and forceful or taut pulse, reddened tongue with yellow coat, etc.

裏虛 [lǐxū]

deficiency in the interior: a general term for deficiency of vital energy, vital function, essence, or blood of the internal organs

裏實 [lǐshí]; 內實 [nèishí]

excessiveness in the interior: (1) symptom-complex caused by accumulated heat in the *stomach* and intestines after an attack of exogenous pathogenic factors; (2) a general term denoting stagnancy of vital energy and blood (brought about by dysfunction of internal organs), food stagnancy or intestinal parasitosis

表裏同病 [biǎo lǐ tóngbìng]

affection of both the exterior and interior: (1) coexistence of exterior and interior symptom-complex; (2) symptoms and signs of the same nature occurring in the exterior as well as in the interior of the body, e.g., cold or heat in both the exterior and the interior

表寒裏熱 [biǎohán lǐrè]

cold in the exterior and heat in the interior: a complicated condition seen either in cases with pre-existing internal heat and affected by exogenous cold and wind in addition, or in cases with the transformation of exogenous cold into heat after having penetrated into the interior of the body while the pathogenic cold in the exterior of the body being still present, symptoms of which are the coexistance of both exterior coldness (chilliness, headache, hypohidrosis, etc.) and interior heat (fever with irritability, thirst, scanty and condensed urine, constipation, etc.)

表熱裏寒 [biǎorè lǐhán]

heat in the exterior and cold in the interior: a jumbled case with pre-existing deficiency and coldness of the *stomach* and the *spleen* and affected by wind-heat in addition, with symptoms showing the coexistence of exterior heat (fever, headache, intolerance of wind, etc.) and internal cold (cold limbs, loose bowels, etc.)

表虛裏實 [biǎoxū lǐshí]

deficiency in the exterior and excessiveness in the interior, a jumbled case in which symptoms of the former such as intolerance of wind, spontaneous sweating, exist together with symptoms of the

81

latter such as abdominal pain with tenderness, constipation, etc.

表實裏虛 [biǎoshí lǐxū]
excessiveness in the exterior and deficiency in the interior, a jumbled case in which symptoms of the former such as chilliness, headache and general aching exist together with symptoms of the latter such as anorexia, lassitude, palpitation, shortness of breath, etc., seen in cases of chronic disease with new affection due to exogenous factors

由表入裏 [yóu biǎo rù lǐ]
development or transmission of a disease from the exterior to the interior of the body

由裏出表 [yóu lǐ chū biǎo]
recession of a disease from the interior to the body surface, e.g., appearance of skin eruption followed by abatement of fever and irritability in the course of measles, indicating improvement of the case

熱邪傳裏 [rèxié chuán lǐ]; 表熱傳裏 [biǎorè chuán lǐ]
transmission of pathogenic heat from the exterior into the interior of the body, characterized by disappearance of exterior symptoms such as intolerance of cold or wind, and development of interior symptoms: marked by fever, persistent thirst, irritability or even delirium, constipation, scanty and condensed urine, reddened tongue with yellow fur, rapid pulse, etc.

入裏化熱 [rù lǐ huà rè]
transformation of exogenous pathogenic factors into heat after having penetrated into the interior of the body

半表半裏 [bànbiǎo bànlǐ]
affection located between the exterior and interior with symptom-complex marked by alternate fever and chills, fullness and choking feeling in the chest and costal regions, bitter taste in the mouth, dry throat, nausea and loss of appetite, taut pulse, etc. Syndrome of the Yang Minor Channel belongs to this category.

上寒下熱 [shànghán xiàrè]
cold in the upper and heat in the lower part of the body, a jumbled case in which symptoms of cold such as aversion to cold, nausea and

vomiting exist with symptoms of heat such as constipation, scanty
and deep-coloured urine.

上熱下寒 [shàngrè xiàhán]

heat in the upper and cold in the lower part of the body, e.g., acid
regurgitation with annoying sensation of heat in the chest appearing
simultaneously with loose stool and abdominal pain which can be
eased by warmth

上虛下實 [shàngxū xiàshí]

insufficiency in the upper and excessiveness in the lower part of
the body, e.g., frequent passage of bloody mucous stool together with
palpitation of heart and shortness of breath in a patient with insufficient *heart* function contracting dysentery.

上實下虛 [shàngshí xiàxū]

excessiveness in the upper and insufficiency in the lower part
of the body, e.g., insufficient vital essence of the *kidney* (causing
lumbago, weakness of the lower limbs and nocturnal emission) associated with exuberant vital function of the *liver* (causing dizziness, headache, irritability, etc.)

虛中夾實 [xū zhōng jiā shí]

insufficiency symptom-complex complicated by symptoms of
excessiveness

實中夾虛 [shí zhōng jiā xū]

excessiveness symptom-complex complicated by symptoms of
insufficiency

虛寒 [xūhán]

deficiency of vital energy with symptoms of cold, marked by
intolerance of cold, epigastric pain which can be relieved by heat and
pressure, loose bowel, fine, thready pulse, and profuse, whitish and
thin leukorrhea in women

虛熱 [xūrè]

heat symptoms or fever caused by deficiency of vital energy,
essence or blood

虛火 [xūhuǒ]

fire symptoms caused by consumption of vital essence, marked
by afternoon fever, heat sensation in palms and soles, thirst, night

sweat, reddened tongue, fine and rapid pulse

实热 [shírè]

heat symptoms caused by excessive pathogenic factors while the body resistance is still sufficient, such as high fever with restlessness, constipation, gigantic or slippery rapid pulse, etc.

实火 [shíhuǒ]

fire symptoms caused by excessive pathogenic factors, such as blood-shot eyes, bitterness in the mouth, thirst, irritability, constipation, etc.

阴虚 [yīnxū]; 真阴不足 [zhēnyīn bùzú]

deficiency of Yin (vital essence), chiefly referred to that of the *kidney*, usually associated with production of internal heat. Common symptoms are low or hectic fever, feverishness on the palms and soles, emaciation, night sweat, thirst, scanty urine, constipation, reddened and furless tongue, fine and rapid pulse.

阳虚 [yángxū]; 真阳不足 [zhēn yáng bùzú]

deficiency of Yang (vital function), usually accompanied with cold symptoms, marked by pallor, intolerance of cold, cold extremities, loose bowel, feeble pulse, etc.

伤阴 [shāngyīn]

impairment of Yin (vital essence), especially that of the *liver* and *kidney* in advanced cases of febrile disease, symptoms of which are low fever, burning sensation in palms and soles, emaciation, thirst, malar flush, dry and scarlet red tongue, fine, feeble and rapid pulse, etc.

伤津 [shāngjīn]

impairment of body fluid, especially of the *lung* and the *stomach*. The symptoms are thirst, dry cough scanty urine, constipation, etc.

伤阳 [shāngyáng]

impairment of Yang (vital function) leading to its deficiency, resulting from various diseases, overdosage of medicines of cold nature or unchecked psychic reactions, etc.

亡阴 [wángyīn]

perishing of Yin: excessive loss of vital essence due to high fever, profuse sweating, vomiting or diarrhea, etc., manifested by thirst and

84

craving for drink, moist skin covered with sticky sweat, warm limbs, and rapid thready pulse. Perishing of Yin and perishing of Yang are closely related and usually occur in succession.

亡陽 [wángyáng]
perishing of Yang or collapse: critical condition seen in cases of high fever, profuse perspiration, drastic vomiting and diarrhea, etc. The patient lies inert with cold limbs and exceedingly feeble pulse, and dripping cold sweat.

陰證似陽 [yīnzhèng sì yáng]; 陰極似陽 [yīn jí sì yáng]
a case of Yin symptom-complex looking like Yang symptom-complex. For example, an advanced case of deficiency of Yin may show pseudo-heat symptoms such as feeling hot and thirst.

陽證似陰 [yángzhèng sì yīn]; 陽極似陰 [yáng jí sì yīn]
a case of Yang symptom-complex looking like a Yin symptom-complex, a false appearance usually seen in febrile diseases. For example, a severe case of febrile disease may show pseudo-cold symptoms such as intolerance of cold and cold limbs.

假寒 [jiǎhán]
pseudo-cold symptoms, seen in diseases caused by heat. The patient is intolerant of cold but dislikes to be thickly covered; has cold limbs though the chest and abdomen being felt hot.

假熱 [jiǎrè]
pseudo-heat symptoms, seen in diseases caused by cold, such as feeling hot yet wishing to be thickly covered, feeling thirsty yet drinking little, moving restlessly yet being mentally quiescent

真寒假熱 [zhēnhán jiǎrè]
a case of cold showing pseudo-heat symptoms

真熱假寒 [zhēnrè jiǎhán]
a case of heat showing pseudo-cold symptoms

真實假虛 [zhēnshí jiǎxū]
a case of excessiveness in reality showing sham symptoms of insufficiency, e.g., cold limbs found in cases with excessive evil heat. This is also said to be 大實如羸狀 [dàshí rú léi zhuàng] , i.e., great excessiveness looks like debilitation.

真虛假實 [zhēnxū jiǎshí]

a protracted case with insufficiency symptom-complex showing sham symptoms of excessiveness, e.g., severe anemia may bring on high fever and full pulse. This is also said to be 至虛有盛候 [zhì xū yǒu shèng hòu], i.e., extreme insufficiency gives symptoms of exuberance.

六經辨證 [liùjīng biànzhèng]
analysis and differentiation of febrile diseases in accordance with the theory of Six Channels

六經病 [liùjīngbìng]
syndromes of the Six Channels

太陽病 [tàiyángbìng]
syndrome of the Taiyang or Yang Major Channel which lies on the surface of the body, with symptoms such as chills, headache, stiff neck, floating pulse, etc., due to attack of wind and cold on the surface of the body

陽明病 [yángmíngbìng]
syndrome of the Yangming or Splendid Yang Channel running within the interior of the body, which can be subdivided into syndrome of the channel itself and syndrome of the bowel organs to which this pair of channels pertain, i.e., the *stomach* and *large intestine*. Main symptoms of the former are high fever, profuse sweating, persistent thirst, full and gigantic pulse, etc. The latter syndrome is marked by tenderness on the abdomen, constipation, fever, deep and forceful pulse, etc.

少陽病 [shàoyángbìng]
syndrome of the Shaoyang or Yang Minor Channel which runs between the exterior and interior of the body, marked by alternate fever and chills, fullness and choking feeling in the chest and costal regions, bitterness in the mouth, dry throat, taut pulse, etc.

太陰病 [tàiyīnbìng]
syndrome of the Taiyin or Yin Major Channel which pertains to the *spleen*, caused by cold and dampness. Main symptoms are abdominal distension, vomiting, diarrhea with abdominal pain, loss of appetite, pale tongue with white fur, slow pulse, etc.

少陰病 [shàoyīnbìng]

syndrome of the Shaoyin or Yin Minor Channel which pertains to the *heart* and *kidney*, marked by general debility due to lowered vital function of these two organs

厥陰病 [juèyīnbìng]

syndrome of the Jueyin or Shrinking Yin Channel which pertains to the *liver*, marked by a protracted and complicated course and interweaving heat and cold, e.g., fever or burning pain in the epigastrium with cold limbs

經證 [jīngzhèng]

syndrome of channel itself: conditions due to attack of pathogenic factors on one or more of the three Yang Channels while the internal organs linked to them are not affected yet

腑證 [fǔzhèng]

syndrome of the Fu (bowel) organs: conditions showing that pathologic changes of one or more of the Three Yang Channels have already affected the respective internal organs: the *urinary bladder*, the *stomach* and *large intestine*, and the *gallbladder*

并病 [bìngbìng]

overlapping of syndromes of two channels

二陽并病 [èr yáng bìngbìng]

overlapping of syndromes of two Yang Channels, such as Taiyang (headache, chills and fever, joint pains) and Shaoyang (vomiting, fullness in the chest) appearing in succession and then coexisting

合病 [hébìng]

combination of syndromes of two or more channels appearing at the same time

太陽與少陽合病 [tàiyáng yǔ shàoyáng hébìng]

combined syndrome of the Taiyang and Shaoyang Channels: headache and fever occurring together with bitterness in the mouth, dry throat, giddiness, etc.

太陽與陽明合病 [tàiyáng yǔ yángmíng hébìng]

combined syndrome of the Taiyang and Yangming Channels: headache and stiff neck occurring together with general heat sensation, thirst, etc.

陽明與少陽合病 [yángmíng yǔ shàoyáng hébìng]

combined syndrome of the Yangming and Shaoyang Channels: fever and thirst occurring together with bitterness in the mouth, dry throat, fullness in the chest, etc.

三陽合病 [sān yáng hébìng]
combined syndrome of the Three Yang Channels: transmission of evil heat into the Yangming Channel both from the Taiyang and Shaoyang Channels, resulting in a distinctive heat syndrome of the Splendid Yang Channel with fever, thirst, perspiration, abdominal distension, utter loss of appetite, delirium, incontinence of urine, etc.

循經傳 [xúnjīngchuán]
ordinary transmission of a disease from one channel to another, by the order of Taiyang, Yangming, Shaoyang, Taiyin, Shaoyin and Jueyin

越經傳 [yuèjīngchuán]
skip-over transmission of a disease from one channel to another, e.g., to transmit from Taiyang to Shaoyang, instead of by way of the Yangming Channel

表裏傳 [biǎolǐchuán]
transmission of a disease between two exterior-interiorly related channels, e.g., Taiyang and Shaoyin, Yangming and Taiyin, Shaoyang and Jueyin

順傳 [shùnchuán]
normal transmission of a disease, e.g., from Taiyang to Yangming or Shaoyang, or from the superficial defensive system to the Qi (secondary defensive) system

逆傳 [nìchuán]
abnormal transmission of a disease, e.g., from the superficial defensive system directly to the nutrient system and blood system, instead of by way of the Qi (secondary defensive) system

傳經 [chuánjīng]
transmission of a disease from one channel to another, with syndrome of one channel replaced by that of another

傳變 [chuánbiàn]
normal or abnormal development of diseases, particularly referred

to febrile diseases

變證 ［biànzhèng］

complication or deterioration of a case due to improper medication or weakened body resistance

直中 ［zhízhòng］

direct hit or direct attack of exogenous pathogenic factors on the Three Yin Channels (instead of transmission from the Three Yang Channels) or on internal organs

衛氣營血辨證 ［wèi qì yíng xuè biànzhèng］

analysis and differentiation of febrile diseases in accordance with the theory of Wei, Qi, Ying and Xue which indicate the stages of clinical course with corresponding pathological changes

衛分證 ［wèifēnzhèng］

syndrome of the Wei (superficial defensive) system: early stage of a febrile disease when only the superficial part of the defensive energy is being involved, marked by fever and chilliness, headache, general aching, hypohidrosis, whitish fur of the tongue, floating and rapid pulse, etc.

氣分證 ［qìfēnzhèng］

syndrome of the Qi (secondary defensive) system: the second stage of a febrile disease with the Splendid Yang (Yangming) Channel or the *lung, gallbladder, spleen, stomach* or *large intestine* being involved, marked by high fever, sweats, dire thirst, flushed face, scanty urine, constipation, yellow coat of the tongue, and rapid, slippery or gigantic pulse

營分證 ［yíngfēnzhèng］

syndrome of the Ying (nutrient) system: serious development of a febrile disease with the central nervous system being involved, marked by high fever, restlessness, insomnia, delirium, or even loss of consciousness in severe cases

血分證 ［xuèfēnzhèng］

syndrome of the Xue (blood) system: febrile disease at its severest stage, characterized by severe damage of vital essence and blood, with various forms of bleeding such as hemoptysis, epistaxis, hematuria, in addition to high fever, coma, etc.

三焦辨證 [sānjiāo biànzhèng]

analysis and differentiation of febrile diseases in accordance with the theory of Triple Burners

上焦病 [shàngjiāobìng]

syndrome of the Upper Burner, including syndrome of the Lung Channel of Hand Taiyin marked by chills and fever, sweating, headache, cough, etc. and syndrome of the Pericardium Channel of Hand Jueyin marked by delirium, deep red tongue, etc.

中焦病 [zhōngjiāobìng]

syndrome of the Middle Burner, including syndrome of the Stomach Channel of Foot Yangming marked by fever without chilliness, sweating, thirst, gigantic pulse, etc., and syndrome of the Spleen Channel of Foot Taiyin marked by continuous moderate fever, ache and heaviness of the body, stuffiness in the chest with nausea and vomiting, greasy coat of the tongue, etc.

下焦病 [xiàjiāobìng]

syndrome of the Lower Burner, including syndrome of the Kidney Channel of Foot Shaoyin manifested by fever more marked in the palms than on the back of hands, thirst, parched lips, restlessness, etc., and syndrome of the Liver Channel of Foot Jueyin manifested by mental disorders, twitching or convulsion

氣血辨證 [qì xuè biànzhèng]

analysis and differentiation of pathological conditions according to the state of the vital energy and blood

病因辨證 [bìngyīn biànzhèng]

analysing and differentiating pathological conditions attributable to different kinds of etiological factors for making diagnosis, also called 審證求因 [shěn zhèng qiú yīn]

臟腑辨證 [zàngfǔ biànzhèng]

analysis and differentiation of diseases according to pathological changes of the viscera and their interrelations

心虛 [xīnxū]

deficiency in the heart, referred to deficiency of vital energy and blood of the *heart* in general

心氣虛 [xīnqìxū]; 心氣不足 [xīnqì bùzú]

deficiency of Qi (vital energy) of the heart, causing palpitation, shortness of breath (especially on exertion), spontaneous sweating, fine, weak or irregular pulse, usually seen in patients with general debility, neurasthenia, arrhythmia, and heart failure

心陽虛 [xīnyángxū]; 心陽不振 [xīnyángbùzhèn]

deficiency of Yang (vital function) of the heart, marked by aggravated palpitation, cold limbs, profuse sweating, thready and feeble pulse in addition to the symptoms of deficiency of Qi (vital energy) of the *heart*

心血虛 [xīnxuèxū]

deficiency of blood of the heart, marked by giddiness, pallor, palpitation, insomnia, forgetfulness, and fine and feeble pulse, seen usually in patients with neurosis, anemia and general debility

心陰虛 [xīnyīnxū]; 心陰不足 [xīnyīn bùzú]

deficiency of Yin (vital essence) of the heart, manifested by mental irritability, palpitation, insomnia, low fever, night sweating, flushed cheeks, thirst, and fine rapid pulse, seen usually in patients with neurosis, anemia and tuberculosis

心營過耗 [xīnyíng guòhào]

excessive consumption of the nutrients (constructive energy) in the blood, which is kept circulating by the *heart*, as is seen in febrile diseases; marked by debility, night fever, mental irritability, fine and rapid pulse

心火上炎 [xīnhuǒ shàngyán]

flaring up of the fire of the heart, causing ulcers on the tongue, mental irritability, insomnia, red tip of the tongue, etc.

心火内熾 [xīnhuǒ nèichì]; 心火内焚 [xīnhuǒ nèifén]

flaming of the fire of the heart, with symptoms such as mental irritability, insomnia, palpitation, and delirium and mania in severe cases

痰火擾心 [tánhuǒ rǎo xīn]

mental disturbance due to phlegm and fire, with delirium, raving madness, red tongue tip, yellow dense and greasy fur, and slippery rapid pulse, usually seen in schizophrenia and hysteria

痰迷心竅 [tán mí xīnqiào]

The Heart Channel being obstructed by phlegm as a pathogenic factor with symptoms such as phlegmatic sound in the throat, coma, etc., usually seen in cases of apoplexy and epilepsy

水氣凌心 [shuǐqìlíng xīn]

heart trouble caused by retension of water due to dysfunction of the *kidney* and the *spleen*, marked by palpitation and shortness of breath associated with general edema

心脾兩虛 [xīn pí liǎngxū]

deficiency in both the heart and the spleen, giving rise to symptoms such as palpitation, forgetfulness, insomnia, loss of appetite, abdominal distension, loose bowel, lassitude, sallow face and fine pulse, usually seen in patients with neurosis or anemia

心腎不交 [xīn shèn bù jiāo]

breakdown of the normal physiological coordination between the heart and the kidney due to excessive fire of the former and deficiency of essence of the latter, bringing on symptoms such as restlessness, insomnia, palpitation, nocturnal emission, etc.

心移熱於小腸 [xīn yí rè yú xiǎocháng]

transmission of pathologic heat of the heart to the small intestine, resulting in ardor urinae, urodynia, hematuria, etc.

小腸虛寒 [xiǎocháng xūhán]

hypofunction of the small intestine with cold manifestations marked by dull pains in the lower part of the abdomen which may be eased by pressure and heat, borborygmi, diarrhea, frequent urination, slow and weak pulse, etc.

小腸實熱 [xiǎocháng shírè]

excessive heat in the small intestine, manifested by irritability, oral ulceration, red urine and burning pains on urination, abdominal distension, yellow fur of the tongue, slippery and rapid pulse, usually seen in cases of infection of the urinary tract and stomatitis

肝陰虛 [gānyīnxū]; 肝陰不足 [gānyīn bùzú]

deficiency of Yin (vital essence) of the liver, usually due to its being poorly nourished by the blood, marked by dizziness, headache, tinnitus, blurred vision, dry eyes, insomnia, night sweating, feverishness in palms and soles, thirst, dry throat, reddened tongue with scanty fur, taut and fine pulse, etc., seen usually in cases of neurosis, hypertension, and anicteric hepatitis

肝血虚 [gānxuè xū]; 肝血不足 [gānxuè bùzú]

deficiency of blood of the liver, marked by sallow face, failing eye-sight, mental irritability, insomnia, deficient amount or absence of menstruation, pale tongue and lips, seen usually in cases with anemia, neurosis, menopathy and internal eye diseases

肝氣虚 [gānqìxū]

deficiency of Qi (vital energy) of the liver. The symptoms are pallor of the face and lips, lassitude, deteriorated hearing, liability to panic fear, etc.

肝寒 [gānhán]

cold in the liver, caused by (1) deficiency of Yang (vital function) of the *liver*, with symptoms such as depression, timidity, lassitude, cold limbs, deep and fine pulse, etc.;(2) cold being accumulated in the Liver Channel (cf. 寒滯肝脈)

肝热 [gānrè]

heat in the liver caused either by accumulated evil heat or depressed vital energy of the organ, marked by mental irritability, bitter taste in the mouth, thirst, etc. In severe cases, mania may occur.

肝火 [gānhuǒ]

fire (intense heat) in the liver brought about by the gathering and brewing of heat in the Liver Channel or by strong emotional agitations, symptoms of which are headache, dizziness, blood-shot eyes, flushed face, mental irritability, being easily angered, scarlet redness of the tip and sides of the tongue with yellow fur, etc. In severe cases mania, hematemesis, hemoptysis, and rhinorrhagia may occur.

肝陽上亢 [gānyáng shàngkàng]; 肝腸偏旺 [gānyáng piān wàng]

exuberance of Yang (vital function) of the liver due to deficiency of Yin (vital essence) of the *liver* and *kidney*, marked by dizziness, headache, flushed face, blurred vision, tinnitus, bitter taste in the mouth and scarlet redness of the tongue, taut pulse, seen usually in cases of hypertension

肝陽化火 [gānyáng huàhuǒ]
**transformation of Yang (vital function) of the liver into fire;
hyperfunction of the *liver* with manifestations of fire (cf. 肝火)

肝火上炎 [gānhuǒ shàngyán]; 肝經實火 [gānjīng shíhuǒ]
flaming up of excessive fire of the liver, marked by headache,
dizziness, with buzzing in the ears, impairmant of hearing, blood-
shot eyes, mental irritability, bitter taste in the mouth, yellow coat
of the tongue, taut and rapid pulse, and hematuria, hemoptysis or
rhinorrhagia in severe cases

肝風內動 [gānfēng nèidòng]; 肝風 [gānfēng]
endogenous wind stirring in the liver, with symptoms such as
dizziness, convulsion and spasm

肝氣不和 [gānqì bùhé]
disharmonious flow of Qi (vital energy) of the liver, leading to
irritability, being prone to anger, stuffiness feeling in the chest and
costal regions, distension and pain in the lower abdomen, stuffiness
and pain in the breasts and menstruous complaints in women. Functioning of the *spleen* and *stomach* may also be affected.

肝氣鬱結 [gānqì yùjiē]; 肝鬱 [gānyù]; 肝氣不疏 [gānqì
bù shū]
stagnancy of Qi (vital energy) of the liver, often caused by emotional factors, giving rise to symptoms such as fullness feeling in the
chest and costal regions, choking sensations, sighing-like breaths,
dizziness, bitter taste in the mouth, loss of appetite, nausea, and menstruous complaints in women

肝氣犯胃 [gānqì fàn wèi]
**perverted flow of exuberant Qi (vital energy) of the liver leading to
dysfunction of the stomach,** manifested by epigastric pain, belching,
vomiting, acid regurgitation in addition to the symptoms of stagnancy
in the *liver,* which is also called 肝胃不和

肝胃不和 [gān wèi bùhé]
disharmony of the liver and the stomach

肝氣犯脾 [gānqì fàn pí]
**perverted flow of exuberant Qi (vital energy) of the liver leading to
dysfunction of the spleen,** manifested by abdominal pain and distension,

diarrhea, etc., in addition to the symptoms of stagnancy of Qi (vital energy) in the *liver*, which is also called 肝脾不和

肝脾不和 [gān pí bùhé]
disharmony of the liver and the spleen

肝鬱脾虚 [gānyù píxū]
stagnancy in the liver leading to diminished function of the spleen, causing costal pains, abdominal fullness, loose bowel, lassitude, etc.

寒滯肝脈 [hán zhì gānmài]
cold lingering in the Liver Channel, causing spasmodic symptoms in the areas related to this channel, such as stretching pains in the lower abdomen and testicles, etc.

肝腎陰虚 [gān shèn yīnxū]
deficiency of Yin (vital essence) of the liver and kidney. Since the *liver* and the *kidney* have a common source of vital essence, deficiency in one usually leads to deficiency in the other. So symptoms due to deficiency of Yin of these two organs often appear in combination.

肝膽濕熱 [gān dǎn shīrè]
dampness and heat in the liver and gallbladder. Manifestations are fever and chills, jaundice, costal and abdominal pain, bitter taste in the mouth, nausea and slippery, rapid pulse, etc.

膽熱 [dǎnrè]
heat in the gallbladder, often involving the *liver*, marked by mental irritability, bitter taste in the mouth, vomiting of bitter fluid, giddiness, impairment of hearing, alternate chills and fever, and jaundice

脾虚 [píxū]
deficiency in the spleen, referred to deficiency of vital energy and essence of the *spleen* in general

脾氣虚 [píqìxū]; 脾氣不足 [píqì bùzú]
deficiency of Qi (Vital energy) of the spleen manifested by dizziness, fatigue, sallow face, indigestion, abdominal distension, lassitude, anorexia, etc., seen usually in cases with peptic ulcers, gastric neuorsis, chronic dysentery and anemia

脾陽虚 [píyángxū]; 脾陽不足 [píyáng bùzú]
insufficiency of Yang (vital function) of the spleen, marked by cold limbs, cold and pains in the abdomen, anorexia, abdominal fullness,

chronic diarrhea, lassitude, emaciation, edema, etc.

脾胃虛寒 [pí wèi xūhán]

hypofunction of the spleen and stomach with cold manifestation, marked by cold and pains over the stomach, anorexia, abdominal fullness, belching, vomiting thin fluid, chronic diarrhea, lassitude and cold limbs

脾陰虛 [píyīnxū]

deficiency of Yin (vital essence) of the spleen disturbing its normal function of digestion and transportation. As a result, dryness of the lips and mouth, anorexia, and especially constipation may occur.

脾失健運 [pí shī jiànyùn]; 脾不運化 [pí bù yùnhuà]

dysfunction of the spleen in transporting and distributing nutrients and water, resulting in dyspepsia, diarrhea, emaciation, lassitude and even edema of the limbs

脾虛濕困 [píxū shīkùn]

deficiency of Qi (vital energy) of the spleen with stagnancy of dampness induced by it, which further impedes the function of the *spleen*. The symptoms are fullness felt over the epigastric region, poor appetite, borborygmi and diarrhea, nausea, thirst but no desire to drink, lassitude, dense and slippery coat of the tongue, usually seen in chronic gastritis and colitis, chronic hepatitis, etc.

濕困脾陽 [shī kùn píyáng]; 寒濕困脾 [hán shī kùn pí]

disturbance of Yang (vital function) of the spleen owing to external cold dampness, a case which should be cured by removing the external dampness

濕阻中焦 [shī zǔ zhōngjiāo]

dampness lingering in the Middle Burner, obstructing natural flow of the vital energy in the *spleen* (cf. 濕困脾陽，脾虛濕困)

中陽不振 [zhōngyáng bùzhèn]

lowered vital function in the Middle Burner (the spleen and the stomach), resulting in dyspepsia, vomiting, diarrhea, cold limbs, and sallow face, seen in chronic dyspepsia and chronic dysentery

中氣不足 [zhōngqì bùzú]

Deficiency of Qi (vital energy) in the Middle Burner (the spleen and the stomach), leading to hypofunction of the organs , and causing symptoms of indigestion and general debility.

中氣下陷 [zhōngqì xiàxiàn]; 氣虛下陷 [qìxū xiàxiàn]; 脾氣
下陷 [píqì xiàxiàn]

sinking of Qi (vital energy) of the Middle Burner (the spleen), with symptoms such as pallor, dizziness, shortness of breath, lassitude, reduced food intake, loose bowel, bearing down sensation in the abdomen, and frequent urination, usually seen in gastroptosis, hysteroptosis, prolapse of the rectum, chronic diarrhea, etc.

脾氣不升 [píqì bùshēng]

failure of the spleen in sending up food essence, due either to dysfunction of this organ, or impediment of dampness or food stagnancy

脾胃濕熱 [píwèi shīrè]

dampness and heat accumulated in the stomach and spleen: a morbid condition marked by jaundice (bright yellow colour of the skin and the sclera), abdominal distension, loss of appetite, nausea, lassitude, yellow dense and greasy coat of the tongue, etc., seen usually in icteric hepatitis or some other acute diseases of the liver and gallbladder. Skin diseases such as eczema, pustulosis, may also be related to this pathological condition.

脾不統血 [píbùtǒngxuè]

failure of the spleen to keep the blood circulating within the vessels due to its deficiency of Qi (vital energy), resulting in chronic hemorrhage such as menorrhagia and subcutaneous extravasation of blood

脾虛肺弱 [píxū fèiruò]; 脾肺兩虛 [pí fèi liǎng xū]

deficiency in both the spleen and the lung for the condition of the one may influence that of the other. The symptoms are pallor, cold limbs , reduced food intake, loose bowel, dyspnea, cough, profuse phlegm, and emaciation, seen in cases of pulmonary tuberculosis, chronic bronchitis and chronic dyspepsia

脾腎陽虛 [pí shèn yángxū]

insufficiency of Yang (vital function) of the spleen and kidney. The fire of Vital Gate (Yang of the *kidney*) invigorates the vital function of the *spleen*. In case of a decline of this fire, insufficiency of the *spleen* function may occur. The common features are aversion to cold, lumbago, chronic diarrhea before dawn daily.

胃虚 [wèixū]
deficiency in the stomach: a general term for deficiency of Qi (vital energy) or Yin (vital essence) of the *stomach*

胃氣虚 [wèiqìxū]
deficiency of Qi (vital energy) of the stomach, giving rise to symptoms of indigestion

胃陰虚 [wèiyīnxū]; 胃陰不足 [wèiyīn bùzú]
deficiency of Yin (vital essence) of the stomach, with symptoms such as dryness in the mouth, thirst, anorexia, constipation, retching, red and furless tongue, etc., usually seen in cases of chronic gastritis, diabetes mellitus, and in convalescent stage of a febrile disease

胃寒 [wèihán]
cold in the stomach, due to its insufficiency of Yang (vital function) or caused by over-eating of raw or cold food, manifested by stomachalgia relieved by warmth, vomiting of watery fluid, cold feeling over the stomach, preference of hot drinks, etc.

胃熱 [wèirè]; 胃中熱 [wèizhōngrè]
heat in the stomach, usually due to affection by evil heat or over-eating of pungent and hot food, main symptoms of which are thirst, foul breath, hyperorexia, scanty urine and constipation

胃熱壅盛 [wèirè yōngshèng]; 胃火熾盛 [wèihuǒ chìshèng]
intense heat or flaring up of the fire in the stomach, manifested by dire thirst and preference of cold drinks, foul breath, oral ulcer, painful puffy gums, burning sensation in gastric region, scanty brown urine, constipation, red tongue with dense and yellow coat, etc.

胃氣不和 [wèiqì bùhé]; 胃不和 [wèibùhé]
dysfunction of the stomach usually marked by anorexia, nausea, insomnia, etc.

肺虚 [fèi xū]
deficiency in the lung: a general term for deficiency of Qi (vital energy) or Yin (vital essence) of the *lung*

肺氣虚 [fèiqìxū]; 肺氣不足 [fèiqì bùzú]
deficiency of Qi (vital energy) of the lung, marked by pallor, shortness of breath, feeble voice, intolerance of wind, spontaneous sweating, etc.

肺陰虛 [fèiyīnxū]; 肺陰不足 [fèiyīn bùzú]

deficiency of Yin (vital essence) of the lung, manifesting symptoms of dryness and heat, such as unproductive cough, afternoon fever, night sweats, flushed cheeks, dry throat, red and dry tongue, fine and rapid pulse, seen usually in pulmonary tuberculosis, chronic pharyngitis and laryngitis, and diphtheria

肺實 [fèishí]

excessiveness in the lung: the *lung* being attacked by pathogenic factors, e.g., wind and cold, phlegm and heat, phlegm and dampness, manifested by profuse sputum, stuffiness in the chest, heavy coat of the tongue, etc., seen usually in acute bronchitis or pneumonia

風寒束肺 [fēnghán shù fèi]

attack of wind and cold on the lung, such as common cold

風熱乘肺 [fēngrè chèng fèi]

attack of wind and heat on the lung, seen in cases with cough and dyspnea accompanied by fever, chest pain, yellow viscid sputum, etc.

痰濕阻肺 [tánshī zǔ fèi]

block of the lung by phlegm and dampness, bringing on cough, dyspnea, profuse thin white sputum, etc., usually seen in chronic bronchitis or bronchiectasis

痰熱阻肺 [tánrè zǔ fèi]

block of the lung by phlegm and heat, causing cough, dyspnea or asthma, usually accompanied by fever, sputum with blood streaks, costal pains, scarlet red tongue with yellow, smooth fur, slippery and rapid pulse, etc.

肺熱 [fèirè]

heat in the lung, marked by cough with thick or yellow phlegm, chest pains, and shortness of breath and hemoptysis in severe cases

熱傷肺絡 [rè shāng fèiluò]

injury of the pulmonary vascular system by evil fire, bringing on coughing of blood and hemoptysis

肺火 [fèihuǒ]

flaring of pathological fire of the lung, either due to attack of pathogenic factors (seen in acute cases) or due to its deficiency of Yin factor (vital essence) caused by chronic cough

肺燥 [fèizào]

dryness of the lung due either to deficiency of Yin (vital essence) of this organ or to the attack of pathogenic factor of dryness, manifested by dry cough, dryness of the nasal cavity and pharynx, sore throat, thirst, hoarseness, hemoptysis, etc.

陰虛肺燥 [yīnxū fèizào]

dryness of the lung due to deficiency of Yin (vital essence), with symptoms such as dry cough, sore throat, hoarseness, blood-stained phlegmatic discharge, red tongue with scanty fur, fine and rapid pulse, seen in pulmonary tuberculosis, chronic pharyngitis, laryngitis, etc.

水寒射肺 [shuǐhán shè fèi]

the lung being attacked by dampness and cold, usually seen in patients with chronic bronchitis or edema and further affected by exogenous cold. The symptoms are cough, asthma, profuse white thin sputum, white, smooth fur of the tongue, etc.

肺腎兩虛 [fèi shèn liǎngxū]

deficiency of both the lung and the kidney: (1) In cases of deficiency of Qi (vital energy), dyspnea, asthma, shortness of breath, spontaneous sweating, cough with profuse sputum are observed; (2) in cases of deficiency of Yin (vital essence), dry cough, shortness of breath, dryness of the throat, afternoon fever, lumbago, night sweating and nocturnal emission may occur.

大腸虛寒 [dàcháng xūhán]

deficiency of vital energy and presence of cold in the large intestine, manifested by watery stool, anorexia, intolerance of cold, deep and fine pulse, as seen in chronic enteritis, chronic dysentery, etc.

大腸寒結 [dàcháng hánjié]

accumulation of cold in the large intestine, manifested by constipation with dull pains and cold sensations in the abdomen, pale tongue with white moistened fur, etc.

大腸熱結 [dàcháng rèjié]

accumulation of heat in the large intestine, manifested by constipation with abdominal pains and tenderness, yellow and dry fur of the tongue, deep and forceful pulse, etc.

大腸液虧 [dàcháng yèkuī]
fluid deficiency in the large intestine chiefly due to deficiency of vital essence and blood, or attack of febrile disease, marked by constipation or difficulty in defecation, seen usually in cases of senile constipation and habitual constipation

大腸濕熱 [dàcháng shīrè]
dampness and heat accumulated in the large intestine, causing purulent and bloody stool, abdominal pains, tenesmus, scanty and red urine, yellow grimy and smooth fur of the tongue, slippery and rapid pulse, seen usually in dysentery (bacillary and amoebic) and acute enteritis

腎虛 [shènxū]
deficiency in the kidney: a general term for deficiency of Yin (vital essence) and Yang (vital function) of the *kidney*. The common features are asthenia, dizziness, tinnitus, forgetfulness, lumbago, nocturnal emission, impotence, etc.

腎虧 [shènkuī]
waning of the kidney (same as 腎虛)

腎陰虛 [shènyīnxū]; 真陰不足 [zhēnyīn bùzú]; 腎水不足 [shènshuǐ bùzú]; 下元虧損 [xiàyuán kuīsǔn]
deficiency of Yin (vital essence) of the kidney due to chronic disease or immoderate consumption, symptoms of which are lumbago, lassitude, vertigo, tinnitus, nocturnal emission, thirst, flushed cheeks mental irritability, afternoon fever, red and furless tongue, fine and rapid pulse, etc.

腎陽虛 [shènyángxū]; 腎陽不足 [shènyáng bùzú]
deficiency of Yang (vital function) of the kidney, marked by general debility with symptoms such as aversion to cold, lumbago, nocturnal emission, impotence, frequent urination at night, etc. Serious cases are called 腎陽衰微 or 命門火衰 .

真元下虛 [zhēnyuán xiàxū]
deficiency of the genuine vitality of the lower portion of the body (same as 腎陽虛)

命門火旺 [mìngmén huǒ wàng]
intense fire of the Vital Gate, usually due to deficiency of Yin

(vital essence) of the *kidney* marked by hyperaphrodisia, insomnia and dreamfulness, etc.

相火妄動 [xiànghuǒ wàngdòng]

hyperactivity of ministerial fire of the *liver* or *kidney* due to their deficiency of Yin (vital essence), symptoms of the former being dizziness and headache, tinnitus and irritability, while symptoms of the latter are heat sensation felt in the chest, palms and soles, lumbago, hyperaphrodisia, etc.

命門火衰 [mìngménhuǒshuāi]

decline of the fire of the Vital Gate, marked by chronic diarrhea especially before dawn, chilliness in the back, or edema in addition to the symptoms of deficient vital function of the *kidney* (cf. 腎陽虛)

腎陽衰微 [shènyáng shuāiwēi]

failure of Yang (vital function) of the kidney (same as 命門火衰)

腎氣不固 [shènqì bùgù]; 下元不固 [xiàyuán bùgù]

Qi (vital energy) of the kidney being not consolidated, nocturnal and spontaneous emission, frequent urination at night, uroclepsia, and incontinence of urine may occur.

腎虛水泛 [shènxū shuǐfàn]

overflow of water (edema) due to deficiency of Yang (vital function) of the kidney, seen usually in chronic nephritis, cardiac edema, etc.

熱結膀胱 [rè jié pángguāng]

heat accumulated in the urinary bladder, causing fullness and rigidity of the lower abdomen, fever, mental irritability, etc.

腎不納氣 [shèn bù nà qì]

failure of the kidney to maintain normal inspiration, as usually seen in pulmonary emphysema

脬氣不固 [pāoqì bùgù]

diminished function of the urinary bladder, leading to incontinence of urine. This case is usually closely related to deficiency of Yang (vital function) of the *kidney*.

膀胱虛寒 [pángguāng xūhán]

deficiency of vital energy and the presence of cold in the urinary bladder, with frequent urination, incontinence of urine or enuresis as main symptoms

膀胱濕熱 [pángguāng shīrè]

dampness and heat accumulated in the urinary bladder, with symptoms such as frequent, scanty and painful urination, turbid urine or hematuria, scarlet red tongue with yellow greasy fur, and rapid pulse, observed in acute urinary infections

三焦虛寒 [sānjiāo xūhán]

deficiency of vital energy and the presence of cold in the Triple Burners: (1) denoting the deficiency in any of the three portions of the body cavity, viz., in the Upper Burner (上焦虛寒 [shàng jiāo xū hán]) or in the *heart* and *lung* with symptoms such as listlessness, shortness of breath; in the Middle Burner (中焦虛寒 [zhōng jiāo xū hán]) or in the *spleen* and *stomach* with symptoms such as diarrhea, abdominal pain and distension (cf. 脾胃虛寒); in the Lower Burner (下焦虛寒 [xiàjiāo xū hán]) or in the *liver, kidney, intestines* and *urinary bladder* with symptoms such as chronic diarrhea, incontinence of urine, edema, etc.; (2) as one of the causes of edema

三焦實熱 [sānjiāo shírè]

excessive heat in the Triple Burners, denoting: (1) excessive heat in any of the three portions of the body cavity, viz., in the Upper Burner (上焦實熱 [shàngjiāo shírè]) or in the *heart* and *lung* with symptoms such as asthma, stuffiness and fullness in the chest; in the Middle Burner (中焦實熱 [zhōngjiāo, shírè]) or in the *spleen* and *stomach* with symptoms such as abdominal distension with nausea and constipation: in the Lower Burner (下焦實熱 [xiàjiāo shírè]) or in the *urinary bladder, large intestine*, etc. with symptoms such as burning sensation on urination with hematuria, passage of purulent bloody stools; (2) febrile disease with pathogenic factors penetrating into the Qi (secondary defensive) system

VII Principles and Methods of Treatment

辨證施治 [biàn zhèng shī zhì]; 辨證論治 [biàn zhèng lùn zhì]

diagnosis and treatment based on an overall analysis of symptoms and signs, including the cause, nature and location of the illness and the patient's physical condition, according to the basic theories of traditional Chinese medicine

審因施治 [shěn yīn shī zhì]; 審因論治 [shěn yīn lùn zhì]

ascertain the cause (causes) of a disease and give treatment

整體觀念 [zhěngtǐguānniàn]

the conception of the organism as a whole, viewing the various parts of the human body as an organic whole, closely related to the external environment

因時，因地，因人制宜 [yīnshí, yīndì, yīnrén zhì yí]

considerations of medical treatment based on climatic and seasonal conditions, geographical localities, the patient's constitution, etc.

同病異治 [tóngbìng yìzhì]

to apply different methods of treatment to the same kind of disease in the light of different physical reactions and clinical manifestations. For example, in the treatment of gastric pain in peptic ulcer different methods such as warming the *stomach*, tonifying the *spleen*, restoring the normal functioning of the *liver*, etc. should be used, dependent on whether the pain is due to coldness in the *stomach*, deficiency in the *spleen* or stagnancy in the *liver*.

異病同治 [yìbìng tóngzhì]

to treat different diseases by the same method if they are alike in clinical manifestations and pathogeny. For example, chronic dysentery with prolonged diarrhea, prolapse of uterus, chronic infection of urinary tract with urinary incontinence, functional bleeding of the uterus, etc. may all be treated by reinforcing the vital energy and invigorating the function of the *spleen* if they are caused by deficiency of vital energy of the *spleen*.

標本同治 [biāoběn tóngzhì]
to treat a disease by looking into both its root cause and symptoms or complications, which, as a principle of therapy, is applied to cases of severe illness with marked symptoms or complications

標 [biāo]
the incidental, referring to: (1) manifestation (of a disease in relation to its cause); (2) pathogenic factor (in relation to body resistance); (3) complication or relapse (of a disease in relation to its primary onset); (4) disease in the exterior (in relation to that in the interior)

本 [běn]
the fundamental, referring to: (1) root or cause (of a disease in relation to its manifestation); (2) body resistance (in relation to pathogenic factors); (3) primary onset (of a disease in relation to its complication); (4) disease in the interior (in relation to that in the exterior)

治病必求其本 [zhìbìng bì qiú qí běn]
To treat a disease one should find out its root or cause, i.e., to find out the rise and fall of Yin and Yang as the basic pathogenic cause of the disease.

治標不如治本 [zhìbiāo bù rú zhìběn]
to treat the fundamental aspect of the disease rather than provide temporary relief of the symptoms

急則治標, 緩則治本 [jí zé zhì biāo, huǎn zé zhì běn]
In emergency cases treat the acute symptoms first, when these being relieved, treat its fundamental cause.

治未病 [zhì wèibìng]
to treat before disease arises: (1) prevent diseases; (2) give early treatment of a disease for the prevention of its complication; (3) control the advancement of a disease. While treating *liver* disease, for example, reinforce the *spleen* before it is being involved.

上工治未病 [shànggōng zhì wèibìng]
A good doctor prevents the disease or its complication rather than merely cure it.

扶正祛邪 [fúzhèng qūxié]
to strengthen the patient's resistance and dispel the invading patho-

genic factors-to two general principles of treatment which can be applied separately or in combination according to the particular condition of the case

扶正固本 [fúzhèng gùběn]; 扶正培本 [fúzhèng péiběn]

(1) strengthen the patient's resistance and consolidate his constitution; (2) restore the normal functioning of the body to consolidate the constitution

祛邪以扶正 [qū xié yǐ fú zhèng]

to dispel pathogenic factors to restore normal functioning of the human body

正治 [zhèngzhì]

to treat the disease in a routine and regular way, i.e., to use therapy and drugs opposite in nature to the disease, e.g., to treat febrile diseases with medicines cold in nature

反治 [fǎnzhì]

to treat a disease by reverse process, e.g., administering medicines of hot nature to treat pseudofebrile disease

逆從 [nìcóng]; 逆者正治, 從者反治 [nìzhě zhèng zhì, cóngzhě fǎn zhì]

To use drugs opposite in nature to the symptom-complex is the routine or regular treatment, while to use drugs of the same nature as that of the pseudo-symptom-complex is a treatment by reverse process.

反佐 [fǎnzuǒ]

using corrigent, i.e., using drugs with property opposite to that of the principal ingredient being used in order to favorably modify the action of the latter which might otherwise be too powerful or toxicant

實則瀉之 [shí zé xiè zhī]

Excessiveness symptom-complex should be treated with the method of purgation and reduction.

虛則補之 [xū zé bǔ zhī]

Deficiency symptom-complex should be treated with reinforcing or replenishing method.

寒者熱之 [hán zhě rè zhī]

Cold symptom-complex should be treated with drugs warm or hot in property.

热者寒之 [rè zhě hán zhī]

Heat symptom-complex should be treated with drugs cold in property.

客者除之 [kè zhě chú zhī]

External pathogenic factors must be removed.

逸者行之 [yì zhě xíng zhī]

Sluggish flow of vital energy and blood must be treated with activating method, such as activation of the blood circulation, regulation or promotion of the vital energy flow.

留者攻之 [liú zhě gōng zhī]

Lingering pathogenic factors (such as stagnated blood, phlegm and retained water) must be removed with attacking method.

燥者濡之 [zào zhě rú zhī]

Dryness must be cured with moistening method.

急者缓之 [jí zhě huǎn zhī]

Spasms and convulsions must be relieved.

散者收之 [sǎn zhě shōu zhī]

What has come loose (e.g., nocturnal emission) must be consolidated.

劳者温之 [láo zhě wēn zhī]

The debilitated and exhausted must be treated with warm-natured tonics.

坚者削之 [jiān zhě xiāo zhī]

Hard masses must be disintegrated.

结者散之 [jié zhě sàn zhī]

Enlarged nodes (such as scrofula) must be resolved.

下者举之 [xià zhě jǔ zhī]

Prolapse and ptosis must be treated with the lifting method of reinforcing the vital function of the *spleen*.

高者抑之 [gāo zhě yì zhī]

Upward perverted action must be suppressed, e.g., in the treatment of cough, hiccup, etc.

惊者平之 [jīng zhě píng zhī]

Mental stress must be eased with tranquillizers.

微者逆之 [wēi zhě nì zhī]

Mild and simple cases must be treated with drugs opposite in nature to the disease. For example, drugs of warm or hot nature are used for cold symptom-complexes, and those of cold or cool nature for heat symptom-complexes.

甚者從之 [shèn zhě cóng zhī]

Complicated cases with pseudo-symptoms must be treated with drugs similar in nature to the pseudo-symptoms. In treating a febrile case with pseudo-cold symptoms, for example, drugs of cold nature should be used.

木鬱達之 [mù yù dá zhī]

Depression of the liver, which corresponds to wood, should be treated with smoothing method to restore its normal functioning.

火鬱發之 [huǒ yù fā zhī]

Accumulated evil fire should be expelled.

土鬱奪之 [tǔ yù duó zhī]

Dampness accumulated in the spleen, represented by earth, should be removed.

金鬱瀉之 [jīn yù xiè zhī]

Obstruction of the lung, corresponding to metal, must be treated by way of discharging, e.g. with expectorants.

水鬱折之 [shuǐ yù zhé zhī]

Water retention should be treated with draining method, e.g., by administering diuretics to regulate water metabolism.

形不足者溫之以氣 [xíng bù zú zhě wēn zhī yǐ qì]

Patients with flabby outward appearance must be treated with warming nourishing drugs to reinforce their vital energy.

精不足者補之以味 [jīng bù zú zhě bǔ zhī yǐ wèi]

Patients deficient in essence must be treated with nutritious diet or drugs rich in flavour such as *Radix Rehmanniae, Colla Cornus Cervi.*

其高者因而越之 [qí gāo zhě yīn ér yuè zhī]

Troubles lodging in the upper part of the body (e.g., phlegm or stagnant food in the *lung* or *stomach*) may be got rid of by emetic measures.

108

其下者引而竭之 [qí xià zhě yǐn ér jié zhī]
Troubles lodging in the lower part of the body may be got rid of by diuresis or purgation.

壯水之主，以制陽光 [zhuàng shuǐ zhī zhǔ, yǐ zhì yángguāng] replenishing the vital essence to check exuberance of the vital function. When exuberance of the vital function is caused by deficiency of Yin (vital essence), it should be treated by replenishing the vital essence, especially that of the *kidney*, instead of using drugs cold in nature to suppress the vital function.

益火之原，以消陰翳 [yì huǒ zhī yuán, yǐ xiāo yīn yì] reinforceing the fire of the Vital Gate to treat cases of debility with cold symptoms, e.g., by administering warming tonics such as *Radix Aconiti Carmichaeli Praeparata, Cortex Cinnamomi, Cornu Cervi Pantotrichum*, etc., to treat cases of general debility with aversion to cold, lumbago and creeping chill in the back, impotence, frequent urination at night, etc.

陰病治陽 [yīnbìng zhìyáng] to treat the Yang aspect for diseases of Yin nature. (1) Since chronic diseases of cold nature (pertaining to Yin) are apt to damage vital function, the treating method should be invigorating the vital function. (2) Diseases with symptoms on the Yin Channels are treated by needling the points on the Yang Channels, e.g., needling Dashu and Fengmen, belonging to the Urinary Bladder Channel of Foot Taiyang, to treat cough after catching cold, a manifestation of pathological changes in the Lung Channel of Hand Taiyin.

陽病治陰 [yángbìng zhì yīn] to treat the Yin aspect for diseases of Yang nature. (1) A febrile disease (pertaining to Yang) is apt to injure vital essence and should be treated with the method of replenishing Yin (vital essence and blood), in protracted cases. (2) A disease with symptoms of the Yang Channels is treated by needling points of the Yin Channels, e.g., needling Neiguan belonging to the Pericardium Channel of Hand Jueyin, to treat vomiting, a manifestation of pathological changes in the Stomach Channel of Foot Yangming.

虛者補其母，實者瀉其子 [xū zhě bǔ qí mǔ, shí zhě xiè

qí zǐ]

If insufficiency is found in an organ, its generating or "mother" organ should be tonified; if hyperfunction is found in an organ, its "child" organ should be treated with dispelling or inhibiting measures: one of the principles of treatment based upon the theory of the Five Evolutive Phases, e.g., insufficiency of the *liver* is usually treated by tonifying its "mother" organ, the *kidney*, while hyperfunction of the *liver* may be treated by dispelling the fire from its "child" organ, the *heart*.

上病下取, 下病上取 [shàng bìng xià qǔ, xià bìng shàng qǔ]

treat the lower part of the body while symptoms appear in the upper part, and vice versa. (1) In acupuncture, the points on the lower part of the body are needled while symptoms are seen in the upper part, and vice versa, e.g., needle Taichong on the foot to treat dizziness, needle Baihui on the top of the head to treat prolapse of the rectum. (2) In medication, administer proper drugs acting on the lower part of the body while symptoms appear in the upper part, and vice versa, e.g., using Rhubarb to induce catharsis for treating dizziness due to excessive fire, and using drugs to clear up the *lung* for diuresis.

寒因寒用 [hán yīn hán yòng]

to treat pseudo-cold symptoms with drugs cool or cold in property

热因热用 [rè yīn rè yòng]

to treat pseudo-heat symptoms with drugs warm or hot in property

塞因塞用 [sāi yīn sāi yòng]

treat stuffed conditions with filling method, e.g., treat abdominal distension or constipation with tonics if it is caused by insufficient functioning of the *spleen*

通因通用 [tōng yīn tōng yòng]

to treat "open" conditions with "opening" method, one of the unusual ways in treatment. In cases of diarrhea caused by food stagnation, for instance, though the bowels are open, purgatives should be given.

無犯胃氣 [wú fàn wèiqì]

Medication should not impair the functional activities of the stomach.

有胃氣則生, 無胃氣則死 [yǒu wèiqì zé shēng, wú wèiqì zé sǐ]

So long as the functional activities of the stomach remain unimpaired, there is hope of life, otherwise death will occur. This is because all the viscera need fluid and nutrients for their functioning, which can only be acquired from the ingested water and food through the functional activities of the *stomach*.

三法 [sānfǎ]

three therapeutic methods: diaphoresis, emesis and purgation

八法 [bāfǎ]

the eight therapeutic methods: diaphoresis, emesis, purgation, mediation, invigoration, heat reduction, tonification, and resolution

汗法 [hànfǎ]

diaphoretic method, used for anti-pyresis in exterior symptom-complex, for promotion of eruption in measles, for elimination of edema when it is more marked in the upper portion of the body (e.g., in cases of acute nephritis), and for anti-rheumatic treatment

解表 [jiěbiǎo]; 疏表 [shūbiǎo]; 發表 [fābiǎo]

to dispel pathogenic factors from the exterior of the body by diaphoresis, a method commonly used in treating exterior symptom-complex

辛溫解表 [xīnwēn jiě biǎo]

to dispel pathogenic factors from the exterior of the body with sudorifics pungent in flavor and warming in property (such as *Herba Ephedrae, Rhizoma Zingiberis Recens*, etc.)—a method used for treating exterior symptom-complex caused by wind and cold

辛涼解表 [xīnliáng jiě biǎo]

to dispel pathogenic factors from the exterior of the body with drugs pungent in flavor and cooling in property (such as *Flos Lonicerae, Herba Menthae*, etc.)—a method used for treating exterior symptom-complex caused by wind and heat

解肌 [jiějī]

to dispel pathogenic factors from the superficial muscles, a method used in the treatment of exterior symptom-complex with fever and sweating

祛風 [qūfēng]
to dispel pathogenic wind from the exterior of the body, i.e., from the channels, muscles, joints, etc.

祛風止癢 [qūfēng zhǐ yǎng]
to dispelling wind to arrest itching, as in the treatment of urticaria

祛風消腫 [qūfēng xiāo zhǒng]
to dispelling wind to reduce swelling, as in the treatment of migratory edema

疏風 [shūfēng]
to dispel external wind in treating exterior symptom-complex, e.g., administering *Herba Schizonepetae, Radix Ledebouriellae,* etc. to disperse wind and cold, or *Herba Menthae, Fructus Arctii,* etc. to disperse wind and heat

宣肺 [xuānfèi]
to ventilate and smooth a troubled lung, a method to treat disturbances of the functional activities of the *lung* caused by exogenous pathogenic factors, e.g., cough in acute upper respiratory infection, dyspnea in an acute onset of bronchial asthma, or edema in acute nephritis

透表 [tòubiǎo]
to expel pathogenic factors from the exterior of the body

透疹 [tòuzhěn]
to promote eruption, as in the treatment of measles, usually with diaphoretics

透邪 [tòuxié]; 達邪 [dáxié]
expel pathogenic factors (e.g., wind and heat) in treating exterior symptom-complex

調和營衛 [tiáohé yíngwèi]
to rectify derangement of the defensive and constructive energy, a method to relieve exterior symptom-complex associated with spontaneous sweating

開鬼門 [kāi guǐmén]
to open the "devil's gates" (pores), i.e., to induce perspiration

辛開苦洩 [xīnkāi kǔxiè]; 開洩 [kāixiè]

112

to use pungent drugs and bitter drugs in combination: (1) use pungent drugs to disperse external pathogenic factors and bitter drugs to relieve internal heat at the same time; (2) use pungent drugs to remove phlegm-dampness in chest and bitter drugs to remove damp-heat therein

滋陰解表 [zīyīn jiěbiǎo]

to nourish vital essence and resolve exterior symptom-complex, i.e., using both tonifying and sudorific drugs to expel exogenous pathogenic factors attacking the external part of the body from a patient deficient in vital essence

助陽解表 [zhùyáng jiěbiǎo]

to reinforce vital function and resolve exterior symptom-complex, i.e. using stimulating and sudorific drugs to expel exogenous pathogenic factors attacking the external part of the body from patient with insufficient vital function

益氣解表 [yìqì jiěbiǎo]; 補氣解表 [bǔqì jiěbiǎo]

to strengthen vital energy and resolve exterior symptom-complex, i.e., using tonifying and sudorific drugs to expel exogenous pathogenic factors attacking the external part of the body from a patient deficient in vital energy

養血解表 [yǎngxuè jiěbiǎo]

to nourish the blood and resolve exterior symptom-complex, i.e., using blood tonics and sudorific drugs to expel exogenous pathogenic factors attacking the external part of the body from a patient deficient of blood

化飲解表 [huàyǐn jiěbiǎo]

to remove excessive humor and dispel pathogenic factors from the exterior of the body, as in treating acute attacks of chronic bronchitis marked by fever, chills (indicating the presence of exterior symptom-complex), and profuse frothy phlegm (suggesting excess of humor)

表裏雙解 [biǎo·lǐ shuāngjiě]

to dispel pathogenic factors from both the exterior and the interior of the body by administering diaphoretics and purgatives or febrifuges simultaneously

清法 [qīngfǎ]; 清熱法 [qīngrèfǎ]

febrifugal method: administer medicines of cold property to treat acute febrile diseases and other diseases with internal heat

苦寒清热 [kǔhán qīng rè]; 苦寒泄热 [kǔhán xiè rè]

to relieve internal heat by using drugs bitter in flavor and cold in property

清热生津 [qīngrè shēngjīn]

to clear up evil heat and improve secretion by administering febrifugal and secretion-promoting drugs such as *Rhizoma Phragmitis*

除烦止渴 [chúfán zhǐkě]

to ease restlessness and quench thirst

清热解毒 [qīngrè jiědú]

to remove toxic heat with febrifugal and detoxicant drugs such as *Flos Lonicerae* and *Fructus Forsythiae* in treating febrile diseases and pyogenic inflammation

清热解暑 [qīngrè jiěshǔ]

to relieve summer heat with febrifugal drugs such as *Herba Artemisiae Chinghao* and *Folium Nelumbinis*

清热祛湿 [qīngrè qū shī]

to remove evil heat and dispel dampness for treating illnesses caused by evil heat and dampness in combination

清热化湿 [qīngrè huàshī]

to remove evil heat and resolve dampness, which in combination cause tightness of the chest, abdominal distension, poor appetite, bitterness in the mouth or sore throat, scanty red urine, yellow dense fur, soft and rapid pulse

清营 [qīngyíng]; 清营泄热 [qīngyíng xièrè]

to dispel pathogenic heat from the Ying (nutrient) system for treating febrile disease marked by high fever, using febrifugal drugs such as rhinoceros horn

清营透疹 [qīngyíng tòuzhěn]

to remove pathogenic heat from the Ying (nutrient) system and promote skin eruption

清热凉血 [qīngrè liángxuè]; 凉血 [liángxuè]

to dispel pathogenic heat from blood with drugs cold in property, such as Decoction *Corni Rhinoceri* et *Radicii Rehmanniae* (犀角地黄汤),

114

for treating febrile diseases with bleeding symptoms or petechial eruptions

凉血解毒〔liángxuè jiědú〕
to dispel noxious heat from blood to control inflammation and fever in treating pyogenic infections

清热開竅〔qīngrè kāi qiào〕; 清心開竅〔qīngxīn kāi qiào〕
to remove evil heat to cause resuscitation from coma in acute febrile diseases, usually by administering aromatic and febrifugal drugs, e.g., Bezoar Resurrection Pills (安宮牛黃丸)

清臟腑熱〔qīngzàngfǔrè〕
to remove evil heat from the viscera and bowels

瀉肝〔xiègān〕; 清肝火〔qīnggānhuǒ〕; 清肝瀉火〔qīng gān xièhuǒ〕
to quench fire in the liver, a method to cure hyperactivity of the vital function of the organ by administering drugs bitter in taste and cold in property such as *Herba Gentianae, Radix Scutellarie,* etc.

清心〔qīngxīn〕
to dispel pathogenic heat from the heart or pericardium, a method of treating acute febrile diseases when the high fever is accompanied by impairment of consciousness, deep red tongue and rapid pulse

清心瀉火〔qīngxīn xièhuǒ〕
to remove intense heat (fire) from the heart, a method to cure illnesses such as oral ulceration and hematemesis caused by intense heat in the *heart* or the *stomach*

瀉心〔xièxīn〕
to remove excessive fire from the stomach, by using purgative drugs such as Rhubarb

清胃熱〔qīngwèirè〕
to remove evil heat from the stomach

清肺熱〔qīngfèirè〕
to remove evil heat from the lung, a method to cure illnesses such as cough and asthma caused by excessive heat in the *lung*

瀉肺〔xièfèi〕
to quench fire in the lung by administering drugs such as *Cortex Mori Radicis, Cortex Lycii Radicis,* etc., a method to cure accumulated

heat or fire with phlegm in the *lung* marked by persistent fever, cough and dyspnea or hemoptysis

清腸潤燥 [qīngcháng rùn zào]

removing evil heat from the intestines to relieve dryness, a method to cure constipation due to excessive heat manifested by herpes on lips, foul breath, etc.

清瀉相火 [qīngxiè xiānghuǒ]

to remove "ministerial fire", a method to cure nocturnal emission or hyperaphrodisia due to hyperactivity of the Vital Gate

下法 [xiàfǎ]; 瀉下 [xièxià]; 攻下 [gōngxià]; 通下 [tōngxià]; 通裏 [tōnglǐ]

purgation method: to relieve constipation, clear stagnation of food or blood and expel internal heat and excessive fluid through purgation

寒下 [hánxià]

to purge with purgatives cold in nature to treat constipation caused by excessive internal heat, dysentery caused by dampness and heat, stagnation of undigested food, and water retention in some cases

溫下 [wēnxià]

to purge with drugs of warm nature: administering purgatives warm in property or administering warm drugs together with other laxatives cold in nature to treat illness with stagnation of food or accumulation of other pathogenic factors marked by cold symptom-complex, e.g., to remove constipation and abdominal pain with cold extremities, white-coated tongue, deep and taut pulse, etc.

緩下 [huǎnxià]; 潤下 [rùnxià]

to administer mild laxatives to relieve constipation, usually using drugs of lubricating property such as *Fructus Cannabis, Semen Pruni,* Honey, etc., for old people and drugs that can promote secretion of fluid in the intestine for patients with febrile diseases

峻下 [jùnxià]

to purge with drastic purgatives such as *Radix et Rhizoma Rhei, Fructus Crotonis,* etc.

急下存陰 [jí xià cún yīn]; 急下存津 [jí xià cún jīn]

to administer drastic purgatives to prevent further loss of fluid.
In febrile diseases with persistent high fever and impairment of body
fluid as manifested by thirst, constipation, yellow and dry fur of the
tongue, etc., use drastic cathartics to purge off the excessive heat,
thus preventing further loss of fluid. This is not indicated to typhoid
fever.

增液瀉下 [zēngyè xièxià]
to administer secretion-promoting drugs together with purgatives
to remove persistent constipation due to impairment of body fluid
in febrile diseases

通洩[tōngxiè]; 通腑洩熱[tōngfǔ xièrè]
to purge off the internal heat by administering purgatives

逐水 [zhúshuǐ]
to expel the retained water with purgatives, i.e., to relieve water
retention (e.g., edema, especially ascites) by means of purgation

去菀陳莝 [qù wǎn chén cuò]
to eliminate the stale and the stagnant, e.g., the abnormally retained water in anasarca, the stagnant blood, etc.

攻瘀 [gōngyū]; 逐瘀 [zhúyū]
to attack blood stasis, usually for treating amenorrhea with fullness, rigidity and tenderness in the lower abdomen

攻痰 [gōngtán]
to attack phlegm, usually for treating mania or cough with sticky
sputum and stuffiness in the chest

先攻後補 [xiān gōng hòu bǔ]
administering medicines to drive out the pathogenic agents first
and then give tonics for recuperation

先補後攻 [xiān bǔ hòu gōng]
administering tonics first to improve the patient's general condition and then give drastic drugs to drive out the pathogens

攻補兼施 [gōng bǔ jiān shī]
administering medicines to drive out invading pathogenic agents
and tonics to reinforce the body resistance at the same time

誤下 [wùxià]
erroneous administration of purgatives in cases where purgation

is contraindicated, as a result of which complications may ensue

和法 [héfǎ]; 和解法 [héjiěfǎ]

mediation method: using drugs of regulating or intermediating action to restore normal correlation between the internal organs or eliminate the pathogenic factors from the part between the exterior and interior of the body

和解表裏 [héjiě biǎolǐ]

to mediate the exterior and interior, a method to treat febrile diseases while the pathogenic factors are located between the exterior and interior of the body

和解少陽 [héjiě shàoyáng]

to mediate the Yang Minor Channel; using medicines to combat pathogenic factors lingering at the Yang Minor Channel and at the same time to strengthen the body resistance in treating febrile diseases while the harmful factors are neither superficial nor deeply entrenched

開達膜原 [kāidá móyuán]; 開達募原 [kāidá mùyuán]

dredge the Mo Yuan (or Mu Yuan) : administering drugs to rout out pathogenic factors which are said to have lodged between the pleural membrane and the diaphragm, with irregular spells of alternative fever and chills occurring once to thrice a day, accompanied by chest tightness, nausea, headache, irritability, taut and rapid pulse, etc.

和胃 [héwèi]; 和中 [hézhōng]

to regulate the vital function of the stomach, a method to cure dysfunction of the *stomach* with symptoms such as nausea and vomiting

理中 [lǐzhōng]

to regulate the functions of the spleen and stomach, usually referring to invigorating the functions of these organs with warming drugs

調和肝胃 [tiáohé gān wèi]

to coordinate the functioning of the liver and the stomach, i.e., treat dysfunction of the *stomach* caused by perverted flow of exuberant vital energy of the *liver*

調和肝脾 [tiáohé gān pí]

to coordinate the functioning of the liver and the spleen, i.e.,

118

treat dysfunction of the *spleen* caused by perverted flow of exuberant vital energy of the *liver*

交通心肾 [jiāotōng xīn shèn]

to restore balanced physiological relationship between the heart and the kidney to cure palpitation, insomnia, nocturnal emission, etc., caused by the breakdown of the normal coordination of the two organs

温法 [wēnfǎ]; 祛寒法 [qūhánfǎ]

warming method; method to dispel internal cold, including restoration of vital function from collapse, warming the *spleen* and *stomach*, warming the channels, and dispelling cold from them

温心阳 [wēnxīnyáng]

to warm up vital function of the heart, e.g., by administering warming drugs such as *Radix Aconiti Praeparata, Rhizoma Zingiberis*, etc., in the treatment of functional insufficiency of the *heart*

回阳救逆 [huíyáng jiùnì]

to restore Yang (vital function) from collapse, a method of treating collapse or shock by administering warming drugs, such as *Radix Aconiti Praeparata* and *Radix Ginseng*

救脱 [jiùtuō]

emergency treatment of prostration

通阳 [tōngyáng]

remove obstruction in the flow of vital energy and reinforce vital function

宣痹通阳 [xuānbì tōngyáng]

to remove obstruction of vital energy and blood flow in the chest to reinforce vital function, as in the treatment of angina pectoris

通脉 [tōngmài]

(1) to invigorate the pulse-beat by warming up and restoring natural flow of the vital energy; (2) to promote lactation after childbirth by administering tonics

温中祛寒 [wēnzhōng qūhán]; 温中散寒 [wēnzhōng sànhán]

to warm the spleen and stomach and dispel cold from them, a method by administering drugs of warm nature to treat insufficient functional activities of these organs, such as indigestion with watery stools, or epigastric pain aggravated by exposure to cold or after a cooling drink

温胃建中 [wēnwèi jiànzhōng]

to warm up the stomach and invigorate its vital function, a method to treat hypofunction of the *stomach* with cold symptoms as marked by dull pain and cold feeling in the epigastrium which can be lessened by food, pressing and warmth

温肾 [wēnshèn]; 温肾阳 [wēnshènyáng]

to warm the kidney, i.e., invigorate vital function of the *kidney* by administering warming drugs such as *Radix Aconiti Praeparata, Cortex Cinnamomi, Cornu Cervi Pantotrichum, Herba Epimedii,* etc.

温肾缩尿 [wēnshèn suō niào]

warming the kidney (invigorate vital function of the *kidney***) to reduce excessive urination,** e.g., by administering *Fructus Rubi, Radix Linderae,* etc.

温肾止泻 [wēnshèn zhǐ xiè]

warming the kidney to cure diarrhea due to hypofunction of the *kidney,* which usually occurs before dawn daily, accompanied with abdominal pain, borborygmi and intolerance of cold

温肾健脾 [wēnshèn jiànpí]

warming the kidney (invigorate vital function of the *kidney***) to activate the functioning of the spleen** (cf. 补火生土)

温经祛寒 [wēnjīng qūhán]

to warm the channels and dispel cold from them, a method to cure joint pains and menstruous complaints due to cold

甘温除热 [gānwēn chú rè]

to relieve fever by administering sweet and warming-up drugs if the fever is caused by deficiency of vital energy

补法 [bǔfǎ]

(1) **tonifying method,** a general term for the methods of treating various deficiency symptom-complexes by using tonics; (2) **method of reinforcing in acupuncture**

补气[bǔqì]; 益气 [yìqì]

to reinforce the vital energy with tonics, a method to cure deficiency of vital energy, usually with drugs such as *Radix Ginseng, Radix*

120

Astragali, Rhizoma Atractylodis Alba, etc.

補氣固表 [bǔ qì gù biǎo]

replenishing vital energy to strengthen superficial resistance, in treating spontaneous sweating and aversion to wind

補益心氣 [bǔyì xīnqì]

to reinforce functional activities of the heart, e.g., by administering *Radix Ginseng* in the treatment of diminished activities of the *heart* marked by palpitation, shortness of breath and spontaneous sweating

健脾 [jiànpí]; 培土 [péitǔ]; 補脾 [bǔpí]

to reinforce or invigorate the function of the spleen (corresponding to Earth) with tonifying drugs

運脾 [yùnpí]

to promote functioning of the spleen, a method of treatment chiefly by administering drugs to dispel dampness for activating functioning of the *spleen* when it is depressed by dampness, marked by indigestion with nausea, abdominal distension, diarrhea, white greasy fur of the tongue, soft pulse, etc.

醒脾 [xǐngpí]

to enliven the spleen, a method to treat dyspepsia due to diminished function of the *spleen* marked by anorexia, dull abdominal pain, loose bowel, pale tongue, feeble pulse, etc.

健脾止瀉 [jiànpí zhǐ xiè]

invigorating functioning of the spleen to cure diarrhea when it is caused by hypofunction of the *spleen,* which usually takes a chronic course with emaciation, anorexia, abdominal distention and presence of undigested food in the stool

健脾和胃 [jiànpí héwèi]

to invigorate functioning of the spleen and normalize the functioning of the stomach, i.e., treat diminished function of the *spleen* and *stomach* with tonics and stomachics

溫補脾胃 [wēnbǔ píwèi]

to warm and tonify the spleen and stomach, i.e., using tonics warm in nature (e.g., *Fructus Amomi, Rhizoma Zingerberis*) to treat diminished functioning of the *spleen* and *stomach* with manifestations of coldness such as cold and pains over the stomach, chronic diarrhea,

121

etc.

開胃 [kāiwèi]
to improve appetite

升提中氣 [shēngtí zhōngqì]
to invigorate the function of the spleen in sending vital energy and nutrients upward for treating chronic diarrhea, prolapse of the anus and uterus, etc.

升陽舉陷 [shēngyáng jǔxiàn]
invigorating vital function (of the *spleen*) to cure drooping and ptosis, e.g., prolapse of uterus, menorrhagia, bleeding per rectum, prolapse of rectum, etc.

補脾益肺 [bǔpí yì fèi]; 培土生金 [péitǔ shēng jīn]
to strengthen the lung (corresponding to Metal) by way of reinforcing the function of the spleen (corresponding to Earth), a method to cure chronic consumptive diseases of the *lung*

補肺 [bǔfèi]
to tonify the lung; replenish vital essence and energy of the *lung*

補益肺氣 [bǔyì fèiqì]
to replenish vital energy of the lung, e.g., by administering drugs such as *Radix Codonopsis Pilosulae, Radix Astragali*

補血 [bǔxuè]
tonify the blood

補養心血 [bǔyǎng xīnxuè]
to nourish the blood of the heart, a method to treat palpitation, insomnia or dreamfulness due to deficiency of blood in the *heart*

養血柔肝 [yǎngxuè róngān];養肝 [yǎnggān]; 柔肝 [róugān]
to nourish and soothe the liver by administering blood tonics, a method to treat diseases due to deficiency of essence and blood in the *liver*. Since the *liver* is believed to be "a viscus of temperament" and deficiency of essence and blood in this organ brings on irritability, so it should be "soothed".

補益心脾 [bǔyì xīnpí]
to tonify the heart and the spleen in treating illnesses due to insufficient functioning of the two organs marked by palpitation or insomnia associated with lassitude, anorexia, loose bowel or menorr-

122

hagia in women patients

氣血雙補 [qì xuè shuāngbǔ]
tonify both the vital energy and the blood

補陰 [bǔyīn]
to replenish vital essence, a general method to cure deficiency of Yin by administering tonics

酸甘化陰 [suāngān huà yīn]
to replenish Yin with drugs sour and sweet in taste, a method to cure deficiency of Yin especially of the *heart* marked by insomnia, forgetfulness, oral ulceration, etc., by administering sour-tasting drugs such as *Semen Zizyphi Jujubae* and *Fructus Schizandrae* together with sweet-tasting drugs such as *Radix Ophiopogonis* and *Bulbus Lilii*

滋養肝腎 [zīyǎng gān shèn]
to nourish Yin of the liver and kidney: (1) to reinforce vital essence of the *liver* by replenishing the vital essence of the *kidney*; (2) using tonics to cure diseases due to deficiency of vital essence of both the *liver* and the *kidney*

補養心陰 [bǔyǎng xīnyīn]
to replenish vital essence of the heart, a method to treat palpitation, insomnia or dreamfulness caused by deficiency of vital essence in the *heart*

滋養胃陰 [zīyǎng wèiyīn]; 養胃 [yǎngwèi]
to nourish vital essence of the stomach, a method to cure deficiency of vital essence in the *stomach* marked by discomfort and burning pain in the gastric region, constipation, dryness in the mouth, red and furless tongue, etc., by administering drugs such as *Radix Glehniae, Radix Ophiopogonis, Herba Dendrobii*

補養肺陰 [bǔyǎng fèiyīn]
to replenish vital essence of the lung, e.g., by administering drugs such as *Radix Asparagi, Radix Ophiopogonis, Bulbus Lilii, Radix Adenophorae*

養陰清肺 [yǎngyīn qīngfèi]
to replenish Yin (vital essence) of the lung, and remove pathogenic heat from this organ, a method to treat deficiency of vital essence of

the *lung* with heat symptoms such as dry cough with hectic fever, or scanty sputum with blood streaks, hoarseness of voice, etc., usually by administering *Radix Rehmanniae, Radix Ophiopogonis,* etc.

滋補肺腎 [zībǔ fèi shèn]

to tonify the lung and the kidney by administering drugs to replenish vital essence of these two organs

補陽 [bǔyáng]; 助陽 [zhùyáng]

to reinforce vital function, a general method to cure insufficient vital function of the *heart, spleen* and *kidney* with tonics

壯陽 [zhuàngyáng]

invigorate Yang by administering warm-natured drugs to promote vital function, especially virility in the treatment of sexual impotence

補腎 [bǔshèn]

to replenish vital energy or essence of the kidney

溫補命門 [wēnbǔ mìngmén]

to reinforce the fire of the Vital Gate, a method to invigorate vital function of the *kidney* with warming and tonifying drugs, used in the treatment of declining fire of the Vital Gate with aversion to cold, chronic diarrhea before dawn, sexual impotence, etc., as symptoms

補腎納氣 [bǔshèn nàqì]

tonifying the kidney to invigorate inspiration process, e.g., by administering *kidney* tonics to treat chronic bronchitis or pulmonary emphysema

補火生土 [bǔ huǒ shēng tǔ]

to restore normal functioning of the spleen (corresponding to Earth) by reinforcing the fire of the Vital Gate, a method commonly used to cure chronic diarrhea occurring before dawn daily

溫腎健脾 [wēnshèn jiànpí]

warming and tonifying the kidney to invigorate the functioning of the spleen (cf. 補火生土)

強筋健骨 [qiángjīn jiàngǔ]

to strengthen the tendons and the bones, e.g., by administering *Cortex Eucommiae, Radix Dipsaci, Rhizoma Cibotii,* etc.

消法 [xiāofǎ]

elimination method, including removing stagnation of food, disintegrating masses formed by stagnated vital energy and blood, etc.

消导 [xiāodǎo]; 消食导滞 [xiāoshí dǎozhì]

to promote digestion and remove food stagnancy, a method to cure dyspepsia caused by improper diet or overeating in its early stage with stomachics and laxatives

消痞 [xiāopǐ]

(1) to disintegrate masses in hypochondria; (2) to remove stuffiness in the chest and epigastrium caused by stagnancy of phlegm and food

理气 [lǐqì]

to regulate the flow of vital energy, a general term for treating disorders in the flow of vital energy

行气 [xíngqì]

to promote the normal flow of the vital energy in treating conditions such as fullness in the chest and abdominal distension

顺气 [shùnqì]

to smooth the flow of vital energy, a method for treating symptoms due to upward perverted flow of the vital energy in the *lung* and *stomach*, such as cough, asthma, hiccup, etc.

降气 [jiàngqì]; 下气 [xiàqì]

to keep air or gas going downward, a method to cure perversive upward flow of air or gas such as coughing, gasping and belching

调气 [tiáoqì]

to adjust the flow of vital energy in order to guarantee a smooth normal circulation, a term for promoting natural flow of vital energy in general, and keeping it going downward in particular

破气 [pòqì]

to disintegrate aggregated and stagnated vital energy with drastic carminatives such as *Pericarpium Citri Reticulatae Viride*

疏肝 [shūgān]; 舒肝 [shūgān]; 疏肝理气 [shūgān lǐqì]

to soothe the liver; restore the normal functioning of a depressed liver (cf. 疏肝解郁)

疏肝解郁 [shūgān jiěyù]

to relieve stagnancy of vital energy of the liver, i.e., to restore
the normal function of a depressed *liver* due to emotional depression
by administering carminative drugs such as *Radix Bupleuri*

疏肝和胃 [shūgān héwèi]
(1) to soothe the liver and regulate the functioning of the stomach;
(2) soothing the liver (i.e., remove stagnancy of vital energy of the
liver) to normalize the functioning of the stomach (cf. 調和肝胃)

疏肝健脾 [shūgān jiànpí]
(1) to soothe the liver and invigorate the functioning of the spleen;
(2) soothing the liver (i.e., remove stagnancy of vital energy of the
liver) to invigorate the functioning of the spleen (cf. 調和肝脾)

降逆止吐 [jiàng nì zhǐ tù]
putting down upward perverted flow of vital energy to stop vomiting

理氣消脹 [lǐqì xiāo zhàng]
normalizing the flow of vital energy to relieve distension, e.g.,
distension in the abdomen, stuffiness in the chest, etc.

理血 [lǐxuè]
to treat blood disorders. The treatment consists mainly in tonification of the blood, activation of the blood and hemostasis.

活血 [huóxuè]
to invigorate blood circulation; activate the blood

活血化瘀 [huóxuè huà yū]
activating the blood circulation to eliminate blood stasis

祛瘀活血 [qūyū huó xuè]
to promote or activate blood circulation by removing blood
stasis

祛瘀消腫 [qūyū xiāo zhǒng]
removing blood stasis to cure traumatic swelling

祛瘀生新 [qūyū shēng xīn]
removing blood stasis to promote regeneration (of blood, tissues,
etc.)

破瘀消癥 [pòyū xiāo zhēng]
to disintegrate mass caused by blood stasis, chiefly in the abdomen or uterus

126

破血 [pòxuè]

to eradicate blood stasis with drastic drugs such as *Radix et Rhizoma Rhei, Semen Persicae, Flos Carthami*, etc.

止血 [zhǐ xuè]

to stop bleeding, hemostasis

清热止血 [qīngrè zhǐ xuè]

removing evil heat to stop bleeding, e.g., to treat hematemesis due to excessive heat in the *stomach* with febrifugal drugs such as *Radix Scutellariae, Radix Rubiae, Hebra Cephalanoplosis*, etc.

凉血止血 [liángxuè zhǐ xuè]

to stop bleeding by dispelling pathogenic heat from blood with cooling drugs such as *Radix Sanguisorbae*

補氣攝血 [bǔqì shè xuè]

replenishing vital energy to stop chronic hemorrhage such as uterine hemorrhage due to deficiency of vital energy by administering tonics

祛瘀止血 [qūyū zhǐ xuè]

to stop bleeding by removing blood stasis, e.g., in case of functional uterine hemorrhage or bleeding after childbirth with blood clots, abdominal pain and tenderness

祛痰 [qūtán]

to dispel phlegm, a general term for measures of treating diseases caused by phlegm

化痰 [huàtán]

to resolve phlegm, one of the measures to dispel phlegm, usually by administering expectorants

清热化痰 [qīngrè huàtán]

to clear up heat and resolve phlegm, a method to treat diseases caused by heat-phlegm, e.g., bronchitis or pulmonary infection marked by fever, expectoration of yellow sticky phlegm, thirst, reddened tongue with yellow fur, and rapid pulse

宣肺化痰 [xuānfèi huàtán]

to ventilate and smooth the lung and resolve phlegm, a method to cure affection by wind and cold with productive cough, e.g., cough in common cold

潤肺化痰 [rùnfèi huàtán]

to moisten the lung and resolve phlegm, a method to treat diseases caused by dryness-phlegm with symptoms such as dry throat, unproductive cough or expectoration of thick sticky phlegm which is difficult to cough up

燥濕化痰 [zàoshī huàtán]

to eliminate dampness and resolve phlegm, a method to treat diseases caused by dampness-phlegm, e.g., chronic bronchitis with expectoration of profuse foamy phlegm and slippery white-coated tongue

祛寒化痰 [qūhán huàtán]; 溫化寒痰 [wēnhuà hántán]

to dispel cold and resolve phlegm, a method to treat diseases caused by cold phlegm, e.g., chronic bronchitis with expectoration of watery thin phlegm, intolerance of cold, pale tongue and slippery white fur

治風化痰 [zhìfēng huàtán]

to relieve wind and resolve phlegm, a method to treat diseases caused by wind-phlegm, marked by headache and vertigo as seen in certain cases of hypertension and Meniere's syndrome

滌痰 [dítán]

to expel stubborn phlegm by administering drastic expectorants, a method of treating illnesses caused by "stubborn phlegm" such as pleurisy with effusion and depressive-maniac insanity

豁痰 [huòtán]

to break through the phlegm, a method to treat complicated conditions caused by the phlegm, e.g., loss of consciousness in apoplexy

祛濕 [qūshī]

to dispel dampness, a method to cure diseases caused by dampness, such as typhoid fever, dysentery, diarrhea, edema, leukorrhea, etc., by using various kinds of drugs including diuretics to remove the dampness, pungent drugs to resolve it, and bitter drugs to eliminate it

化濕 [huàshī]

to resolve dampness, one of the measures to dispel dampness, especially that lodging in the upper part or exterior of the body, by using pungent drugs such as *Herba Agastachis Rugosa*, *Herba Eupa-*

torii, etc.

清热化湿 [qīngrè huàshī]

to clear up heat and resolve dampness, a method to treat diseases with dampness and heat in the upper or middle part of the body usually seen in acute gastritis

燥湿 [zàoshī]

to eliminate dampness by drying, one of the measures to dispel dampness, especially that lodging in the middle part of the body, by using bitter drugs either warm in nature such as *Rhizoma Atractyloidis* and *Cortex Magnolia Officinalis*, or cold in nature such as *Radix Scutellariae* and *Rhizoma Coptidis*

苦温燥湿 [kǔwēn zào shī]

to eliminate dampness by drying method with bitter drugs warm in nature (cf. 燥湿)

苦寒燥湿 [kǔhán zào shī]

to eliminate dampness by drying method with bitter drugs cold in nature (cf.燥湿)

利湿 [lìshī]; 利尿 [lìniào]; 利水 [lìshuǐ]

to remove dampness through diuresis; diuresis: one of the measures to dispel dampness by using diuretics

清热利湿 [qīngrè lìshī]; 清利湿热 [qīnglì shīrè]

to remove or clear up heat and eliminate dampness with febrifugal and diuretic drugs, a method to cure diseases with dampness and heat accumulated in the lower portion of the body, such as urinary infection

清暑利湿 [qīngshǔ lìshī]

to remove or clear up summer damp-heat by refrigerant and diuretic drugs

淡渗利湿 [dànshèn lì shī]; 渗湿 [shèn shī]

dispel dampness through diuresis by using mild-flavored drugs, one of the common measures to treat diarrhea with watery stools, and edema with oliguria

温阳利水 [wēnyáng lì shuǐ]

to invigorate or promote Yang (vital function) for diuresis, one of the measures to remove dampness through diuresis, usually used in cases of water retention due to insufficient function of the *spleen* and *kidney*

温肾利水 [wēnshèn lì shuǐ]
warming the kidney to relieve water retention, a method to cure edema due to deficiency of Yang (vital function) of the *kidney*

利小便，实大便 [lì xiǎobiàn, shí dàbiàn]
to treat watery diarrhea with diuretic drugs

潔净府 [jié jìngfǔ]
to cause diuresis. 净府 is referred to the urinary bladder

芳香化浊 [fāngxiāng huàzhuó]
to resolve damp turbidity with aromatic drugs, a method to cure diseases caused by internal dampness with symptoms such as epigastric fullness, nausea, regurgitation, greasy coat of the tongue, etc.

固涩 [gùsè]; 收涩 [shōusè]
to cause contraction and arrest discharges; administer styptic or astringent agents for the treatment of spontaneous sweating, seminal emission, chronic diarrhea, menorrhagia, etc.

敛汗 [liǎnhàn]; 止汗 [zhǐhàn]
to check profuse sweating, e.g., by administering *Fructus Tritici Levis* and *Concha Ostreae* in treating spontaneous sweating and night sweating

敛汗固表 [liǎnhàn gùbiǎo]
to arrest abnormal sweating and strengthen superficial resistance; check spontaneous sweating due to deficiency of vital function, or night sweating due to deficiency of vital essence by administering astringent drugs

敛气 [liǎnqì]
to consolidate vital energy, as in treating impaired vital energy due to profuse sweating, with drugs such as *Fructus Schizandrae*

敛阴 [liǎn yīn]
to consolidate Yin (vital essence and body fluid) so as to replenish and preserve it, chiefly with *Radix Paeoniae Alba*

敛肺止咳 [liǎnfèi zhǐ ké]
to relieve cough with astringent drugs, a method to treat persistent unproductive cough

敛肺止喘 [liǎnfèi zhǐ chuǎn]

130

consolidating vital energy of the lung to relieve asthma, a method
to treat asthma by using astringent drugs

固精［gùjīng］；澀精［sèjīng］
to arrest seminal emissions with styptic or astringent drugs

固肾澀精［gùshèn sè jīng］
consolidating vital energy of the kidney to arrest seminal emissions

固肾缩尿［gùshèn suō niào］
strengthening functional activities of the kidney to reduce urination to normal

固崩止帶［gùbēng zhǐdài］
to check profuse uterine bleeding and leukorrhea

澀腸止瀉［sècháng zhǐ xiè］；澀腸固脱［sècháng gù tuō］
administering styptic or astringent drugs to treat incontinence
of stool due to chronic diarrhea

潤燥［rùnzào］
moistening, a measure to treat illnesses caused by dryness

潤肺［rùnfèi］
to moisten the lung, remove dryness of the *lung*, usually by administering drugs to replenish vital essence of this organ

甘寒潤燥［gānhán rùn zào］
to relieve symptoms of dryness by administering drugs sweet
in taste and cold in nature such as *Radix Ophiopogonis* and *Radix
Glehniae*, a method of treating deficiency of fluid of the *lung* and
kidney, marked by sore throat, dry cough or bloody sputum, etc.

養陰潤燥［yǎngyīn rùn zào］
nourishing Yin (vital essence) to relieve symptoms of dryness,
a method of treating injured body fluid in the *stomach* and *lung* caused
by pathogenic factors of heat and dryness

養血潤燥［yǎngxuè rùn zào］
nourishing the blood to relieve symptoms of dryness, a method
of treating constipation due to blood deficiency, i.e., constipation
accompanied by pallor, dizziness, palpitation, pale tongue, rapid and
fine pulse

甘寒生津［gānhán shēng jīng］
to replenish the body fluid by administering drugs sweet in flavor

131

and cold in property, such as *Rhizoma Phragmitis, Herba Dendrobii,* or pear juice, lotus root juice, sugarcane juice, etc.

益氣生津［yìqì shēngjīn］

to replenish vital energy and body fluid with tonifying drugs, a method to cure the prostrated state after profuse sweating

安神［ānshén］

to soothe the nerves by tonifying the blood and Yin or subduing exuberance of Yang (with weighty drugs) in the *heart* and the *liver*

養心安神［yǎngxīn ānshén］

to nourish the heart and soothe the nerves, a method of treating nervous excitement due to deficiency of vital essence with tonifying and tranquillizing medicines

潛陽［qiányáng］

to check exuberance of Yang (vital function) due to deficiency of Yin (vital essence) usually with symptoms such as headache, dizziness, tinnitus, numbness or tremor of limbs, by using weighty drugs such as *Os Draconis Concha Ostreae,* etc.

滋陰潛陽［zīyīn qián yáng］; 育陰潛陽［yùyīn qián yáng］

nourishing vital essence to subdue exuberant Yang, a method to check hyperactivity of the *liver* due to deficiency of its Yin (vital essence)

平肝［pínggān］

to subdue hyperactivity of the liver, a general term for methods of treating hyperactivity of the *liver* including checking its functioning with weighty and calmative drugs and reducing its functioning with cooling drugs

鎮肝［zhèngān］

to check hyperactivity of the liver with weighty and calmative drugs such as *Os Draconis* and *Concha Haliotidis*

鎮肝潛陽［zhèngān qiányáng］; 鎮潛［zhènqián］; 潛鎮 ［qiánzhèn］

to subdue exuberance of Yang of the liver marked by nervous tension, palpitation, insomnia, dizziness, headache, etc., by administering sedatives and tranquillizers such as cinnabar, magnetite, together with other drugs to check exuberance of Yang

132

熄風 [xīfēng]
to subdue endogenous wind, i.e., to relieve vertigo, tremor, infantile convulsion, epilepsy, etc., by administering sedatives

滋陰熄風 [zīyīn xī fēng]
nourishing the Yin (vital essence) to subdue endogenous wind due to serious impairment of vital essence and fluid at a later stage of febrile disease

平肝熄風 [pínggān xīfēng]
to subdue hyperfunction of the liver and the endogenous wind, a method of treating endogenous wind caused by hyperfunction of the *liver*

清熱熄風 [qīngrè xī fēng]
clearing up heat to relieve convulsion, a method of treating convulsion due to high fever

養血熄風 [yǎngxuè xī fēng]
nourishing blood to subdue endogenous wind, a method of treating endogenous wind caused by blood deficiency marked by dizziness, involuntary movement of the limbs, etc., as seen in chronic case of blood deficiency

開竅 [kāiqiào]; 醒神 [xǐngshén]
to resuscitate; i.e., to bring one back to consciousness from coma

芳香開竅 [fāngxiāng kāi qiào]
to cause resuscitation by administering aromatic drugs such as *Borneolum, Moschus, Rhizoma Acori Graminei*, etc., in the emergency treatment of loss of consciousness due to apoplexy, epilepsy or high fever

滌痰開竅 [dítán kāi qiào]
clearing off phlegm to cause resuscitation, a method to treat impairment of consciousness caused by apoplexy or psychosis

清熱化痰開竅 [qīngrè huàtán kāi qiào]
to restore the patient to consciousness by clearing up heat and resolving phlegm, a method to relieve convulsion and coma due to high fever in children by administering febrifugal and phlegm-resolving drugs

豁痰醒腦 [huōtán xǐng nǎo]

removing the phlegm to bring resuscitation. It is believed that loss of consciousness is often associated with presence of phlegm, so removal of the phlegm should be stressed in the treatment

吐法 [tùfǎ]
emetic method, a method to expel noxious substances with emetics or mechanical stimulation to induce vomiting

探吐 [tàntù]
to cause vomiting artificially with mechanical means, such as brushing the soft palate with feather

安胎 [āntāi]
to prevent miscarriage

催生 [cuīshēng]
to expedite child delivery

通經 [tōngjīng]
stimulate menstrual discharge in cases of pathological amenia

調經 [tiáojīng]
to regulate menstruation

催乳 [cuīrǔ]
to stimulate lactation

內消 [nèixiāo]
to administer antiphlogistics per os to cure a sore before it undergoes suppuration

內托 [nèituō]; 托法 [tuōfǎ]
to administer tonifying drugs in favour of discharging pus as a method of treating sores

排膿 [páinóng]
to drain pus

生肌 [shēngjī]
promote granulation, promote the growth of new tissue

攻潰 [gōngkuì]
to administer suppurantia such as pangolin scale and Chinese honey locust in treating ulcer and boils

以毒攻毒 [yǐ dú gōng dú]
to combat poison with poison; treat malignant or poisoning diseases with poisonous drugs, e.g., chaulmoogra for leprosy, gamboge for

carbuncle

解毒 [jiědú]

(1) **to relieve pyogenic inflammation;** (2) **to detoxicate;** neutralize the toxic property of poisons, e.g., venom

利咽 [lìyān]

to ease the stiffiness or pain of a sore throat, cure sore throat, e.g., by administering *Radix Platycodi, Rhizoma Belamcandae*, etc.

明目 [míngmù]

to improve or restore eyesight

驱虫 [qūchóng]

to expel parasites, especially of the intestines

杀虫 [shāchóng]

to destroy intestinal parasites, e.g., by administering *Fructus Quisqualis* or *Cortex Meliae* for ascaris, and *Semen Arecae* for taenia

化石 [huàshí]

to resolve stone (biliary or urinary)

排石 [páishí]

to expel stone from the biliary duct or urinary tract

外治 [wàizhì]

external treatment

敷 [fū]; 外敷 [wàifū]

external application

罨 [yǎn]

compression: hot compression, e.g., in treating rheumatic arthritis and cold compression, e.g., over the forehead to stop epistaxis

熨法 [yùnfǎ]

hot compression with rubbing, press and rub the diseased area with hot medical substance or salt wrapped in cloth

熏蒸 [xūnzhēng]

fuming or steaming: treat a disease with fumes from a burning roll of medicated paper or with the steam from boiling medicinal ingredients

吸入 [xīrù]

to inhale fume or steam

热烘 [rèhōng]

to warm over fire the diseased part after administering medical ointment

烙 [lào]
cauterization, a surgical procedure used in ancient times, e.g., application of a hot iron to a maturated abscess to make it burst for draining pus

渭浴 [tāyù]
medicated immersion

發泡 [fāpào]
to stimulate blister formation with drugs for curing purpose

膏摩 [gāomó]
to rub the affected area with ointment for curing rheumatic or skin disease

點眼 [diǎnyǎn]
to apply medicine to the eye

嚏鼻 [xùbí]
inhale or blow into the nose powdered medicine

漱滌 [shùdí]; 含漱 [hánshù]
to gargle

吹藥 [chuīyào]
to blow powdered medicine into the throat or inner part of the mouth with a sprayer, a tube or a paper roll

撲粉 [pūfěn]
to powder the skin with finely powdered medicine

導法 [dǎofǎ]; 導便 [dǎobiàn]
enema, made of condensed honey or pig bile in ancient times

塞法 [sāifǎ]
application of suppository

枯痔法 [kūzhìfǎ]
necrosis therapy of hemorrhoids, causing necrosis of the hemorrhoids by applying a special drug

掛綫法 [guàxiànfǎ]
ligating method for treating anal fistula

拔罐療法 [báguàn liáofǎ]
cupping therapy, medical treatment with vacuumized cup or

small jar sucked on the skin to cause local congestion

刮痧 [guāshā]

scraping therapy, a popular treatment for sunstroke or other febrile diseases by scraping the patient's neck, chest or back with a coin or something hard and smooth moistened with water or vegetable oil until local congestion is achieved

捏脊 [niējí]; 捏积 [niējī]

chiropractic along the spine, a method of treating children's digestive disorders by kneading and lifting the skin along the spine

导引 [dǎoyǐn]

breathing and physical exercise to build up health and also to treat illness in ancient times

气功疗法 [qìgōngliáofǎ]

breathing exercise therapy

正骨法 [zhènggǔfǎ]

bone-setting

推拿 [tuīná]

(1) massage; (2) pushing and holding, two instances of manipulation in traumatology

食治 [shízhì]; 食疗 [shíliáo]

food therapy; diet therapy

VIII Chinese Materia Medica

中藥 [zhōngyào]
Chinese drugs or Chinese traditional drugs, usually referring to those recorded in Chinese Materia Medica

草藥 [cǎoyào]
herbal drugs or medicinal herbs, usually referring to those not recorded in Chinese Materia Medica or only used in folk medicine. A clear-cut differentiation between medicinal-herbs in folk medicine and regular traditional drugs is difficult to make and so they are usually called 中草藥 [zhōng cǎo yào]or Chinese herbal drugs in combination.

藥材 [yàocái]
medicinal substance; crude drug

藥味 [yàowèi]
(1) medicinal ingredients in a prescription; (2) taste or flavour of a drug

氣味 [qìwèi]; 性味 [xìngwèi]
properties and flavours of drugs. Drugs of different flavour have different effects though they may be of the same property, and vice versa.

四氣 [sìqì]; 四性 [sìxìng]
the four properties of drugs, i.e., cold, hot, warm and cool, classified according to their therapeutic effects. Drugs effective for the treatment of heat symptom-complexes are endowed with cold or cool properties, while those effective for cold symptom-complexes, with warm or hot properties.

五味 [wǔwèi]
the five tastes (flavours) of durgs: pungent, sweet, sour, bitter and salty. The tastes of drugs are different as are their properties, e.g., most of the carminatives are pungent, tonifying drugs are usually sweet in taste and sour drugs have the property of astringency.

五味所入 [wǔwèisuǒ rù]

viscera on which drugs of different tastes act selectively—an ancient hypothesis in Chinese pharmacology based upon the theory of Five Evolutive Phases

苦入心 [kǔ rù xīn]
Drugs bitter in taste act on the heart.

酸入肝 [suān rù gān]
Drugs sour in taste act on the liver.

甘入脾 [gān rù pí]
Drugs sweet in taste act on the spleen.

辛入肺 [xīn rù fèi]
Drugs pungent in taste act on the lung.

鹹入腎 [xián rù shèn]
Drugs salty in taste act on the kidney.

歸經 [guījīng]
classification of drugs according to the channel(s) on which their therapeutic action is manifested. For instance, *Radix Platycodi, Flos Farfarae, Radix et Rhizoma Asteris,* etc., are grouped under the drugs of the Lung Channel owing to their antitussive effect in *lung* diseases.

升降浮沉 [shēng jiàng fú chén]
ascending and descending, floating and sinking—direction of the action of drugs. The ascending and floating drugs have an upward and outward effect and are used for activating vitality, inducing sweat and dispelling cold, while the descending and sinking drugs, having a downward and inward effect, are used for tranquillizing, causing contraction, relieving cough, arresting emesis, and promoting diuresis or purgation.

大毒、常毒、小毒、無毒 [dàdú、chángdú、xiǎodú、wúdú]
extremely poisonous, moderately poisonous, slightly poisonous and non-poisonous drugs—a classification of drugs according to their toxicity

三品 [sānpǐn]
three grades of drugs—an ancient classification of drugs chiefly based upon their toxicity

上品 [shàngpǐn]
high grade drugs, which are supposed to be non-toxic, possessing

139

rejuvenating properties and can be taken frequently and for long periods of time without harm

中品 [zhōngpǐn]
medium grade drugs, which are said to have no or slight toxic effects and are used for symptom-complexes of deficiency

下品 [xiàpǐn]
low grade drugs, which are toxic and should not be taken for long periods of time

解表藥 [jiěbiǎoyào]
diaphoretics or drugs for treating exterior symptom-complex, which have the effect to dispel pathogenic factors from the exterior of the body by diaphoresis. They are divided into two categories according to their properties: warm or cold.

辛溫解表藥 [xīnwēn jiěbiǎoyào]
diaphoretics with pungent and warm properties, such as *Herba Ephedrae, Ramulus Cinnamomi*, etc., which are usually used for treating exterior symptom-complex caused by wind and cold

辛涼解表藥 [xīnliáng jiěbiǎoyào]
diaphoretics with pungent and cold properties, such as *Herba Menthae, Fructus Arctii*, etc., which are usually used for treating exterior symptom-complex caused by wind and heat

溫化寒痰藥 [wēnhuàhántányào]
phlegm-resolving drugs with warm properties, such as *Rhizoma Pinelliae, Flos Inulae*, etc., which are usually used for treating symptom-complex caused by cold phlegm or phlegm-dampness, marked by expectoration of watery thin phlegm or profuse foamy phlegm when the *lung* is involved, nausea and vomiting when the stomach is involved, and so forth

清化熱痰藥 [qīnghuàrètányào]
phlegm-resolving drugs with cold properties, such as *Fructus Trichosanthis, Caulis Bambusae in Taenis*, etc., which are usually used for treating symptom-complex caused by heat-phlegm, marked by expectoration of yellow thick phlegm with other symptoms showing heat in the *lung*. Some of these drugs are also used for the treatment of goiter, scrofula, impairment of consciousness, convulsion or even

140

mania if these conditions are caused by phlegm.

止咳藥 [zhǐkéyào]

antitussives: drugs for relieving cough

平喘藥 [píngchuǎnyào]

anti-asthmatics; antasthmatics, drugs for relieving asthmatic symptoms. Since most of the antitussives may have some effect on asthma while anti-asthmatics also relieve cough, they are usually called in combination 止咳平喘藥。

清熱藥 [qīngrèyào]

antipyretics; febrifuges, drugs which, being cool or cold in property, have the action to clear up internal heat, and are usually used in febrile or inflammatory conditions and other heat symptom-complexes

清熱瀉火藥 [qīngrè xièhuǒyào]

drugs for reducing intense internal heat, such as *Gypsum* and *Rhizoma Anemarrhenae*, which are usually used to clear up the heat in the Qi system, especially in the *lung* and the *stomach*, marked by high fever, dire thirst, delirium, dry yellow fur of the tongue, rapid gigantic pulse, and also used to treat other symptom-complexes of excessive heat and fire

清熱涼血藥 [qīngrè liángxuèyào]

drugs for eliminating pathological heat from blood, such as *Cornu Rhinoceri* and *Cortex Moutan Radicis*, which are usually used in the treatment of febrile diseases with bleeding symptoms or petechial eruptions, and also of hemorrhagic disorders due to excessive heat in the blood

清熱燥濕藥 [qīngrè zàoshīyào]

febrifugal and antipyic drugs; drugs for eliminating heat and dampness, such as *Rhizoma Coptidis* and *Radix Sophorae Flavescentis*, which are bitter in taste and cold in property, usually used in the treatment of diseases caused by dampness and heat, e.g., acute jaundice, acute dysentery, urinary infection, eczema, boils and carbuncles

清熱解毒藥 [qīngrè jiědúyào]

febrifugal and detoxicant drugs; drugs for eliminating toxic heat. Toxic heat as a pathogenic factor causes inflammation, mostly pyogenic. Some of the febrifugal and detoxicant drugs such as *Herba Andrograph-*

itis, Radix Isatidis and *Rhizoma Paridis* have been shown to have anti-pyretic, antibacterial or antiviral actions, while others have the effect to enhance immune function.

祛風濕藥 [qūfēngshīyào]

antirheumatics, drugs for relieving rheumatic conditions. Most of the antirheumatics are pungent in flavor and warm in property, such as *Rhizoma seu Radix Notopterygii* and *Radix Clematidis*, and have the actions to dispel wind, remove dampness, eliminate cold, activate blood circulation in collaterals and relieve pain.

溫寒藥 [wēnhányào]

drugs for dispelling internal cold, which are warm or hot in property and are used for treating symptom-complexes of internal cold either due to direct attack of the interior of the body by exogenous cold or due to hypofunction of the *kidney* and *spleen*. The representative drugs are *Radix Aconiti* and *Cortex Cinnamomi*.

芳香化濕藥 [fāngxiāng huàshīyào]

dampness-resolving drugs with fragrant odour. Most of them have a pungent flavor and warm property, and are used in the treatment of symptom-complexes of dampness marked by anorexia, lassitude, nausea and vomiting, distension in the chest and abdomen, white greasy fur of the tongue, and slippery pulse either in febrile diseases or in other miscellaneous diseases.

利尿逐水藥 [lìniào zhúshuǐyào]

diuretics and hydragogues. Diuretics are drugs that promote the secretion of urine, such as *Polyporus Umbellatus* and *Rhizoma Alismatis*. They are used in the treatment of various diseases caused by accumulation of water or dampness, e.g., edema, rheumatism, urinary disturbances, jaundice. Hydragogues are drugs that remove water from the body not only by increasing the secretion of urine but mainly by causing diarrhea. Thus, hydragogues are also drastic purgatives.

理氣藥 [lǐqìyào]

carminatives, drugs for regulating the flow of vital energy. Most of them are aromatic in odour, pungent in flavor and warm in property and have the action to promote the normal flow of the vital energy, remove obstruction or stagnation of the vital energy, alleviate pain, activate the function of stomach, and relieve nausea, vomiting and hiccough.

理血藥 [lǐxuèyào]
drugs for regulating blood conditions, drugs to arrest bleeding, to invigorate blood circulation and to eliminate blood stasis

止血藥 [zhǐxuèyào]
hemostatics; drugs for arresting bleeding

活血化瘀藥 [huóxuè huàyūyào]
drugs for invigorating blood circulation and eliminating blood stasis. Some of these drugs such as *Rhizoma Ligustici Chuanxiong* and *Rhizoma Corydalis* have milder actions and are usually used for activating blood circulation in collaterals, e.g., in the treatment of dysmenorrhea or pains due to blood stasis, while others such as *Flos Carthami* and *Rhizoma Sparganii* have stronger actions and are usually used for eliminating blood stasis, e.g., in the treatment of tumors or masses in the abdomen.

芳香開竅藥 [fāngxiāng kāiqiàoyào]
aromatic stimulants, drugs which have resuscitating actions and are usually used for treating loss of consciousness, delirium, and convulsions in acute febrile diseases and apoplexy. Most of the drugs are only for emergency use.

安神藥 [ānshényào]
sedatives and tranquilizers

平肝熄風藥 [pínggān xīfēngyào]
anticonvulsives, drugs for subduing the hyperactivity of the *liver* and endogenous wind. The main symptoms of hyperactivity of the *liver* with endogenous wind are dizziness, vertigo, convulsion and spasm. These drugs are chiefly used for symptomatic treatment.

補養藥 [bǔyǎngyào]
tonics, drugs which have tonifying actions for the treatment of deficiencies of Yin, Yang, Qi and blood and therefore can be classified into four groups: Yin tonics, Yang tonics, Qi tonics and blood tonics

補氣藥 [bǔqìyào]
Qi tonics, drugs for replenishing the vital energy, usually used in the treatment of deficiency of Qi (functional activities) of the *spleen*

and the *lung*; also used in the treatment of blood deficiency together with blood tonics. The representative drugs are *Radix Ginseng* and *Radix Astragali*.

補血藥 [bǔxuèyào]
blood tonics; drugs for nourishing the blood, mainly used in the treatment of deficiency of blood. Most of these drugs are also Yin tonics used for replenishing the vital essence.

補陰藥 [bǔyīnyào]
Yin tonics, drugs for replenishing the vital essence and fluid, used in the treatment of deficiency of vital essence and fluid marked by thirst, tidal fever, malar flush, heat sensation in palms and soles, fidget and insomnia, red and furless tongue, fine and rapid pulse, etc.

補陽藥 [bǔyángyào]
Yang tonics, drugs for reinforcing the vital function (chiefly of the *kidney*), used in the treatment of insufficient vital function of the *kidney* marked by chilliness in the back and loins, impotence, urorrhea, chronic diarrhea occurring daily before dawn, chronic asthmatic conditions, etc.

固澀藥 [gùsèyào]
astringents and hemostatics, drugs which have the actions to arrest or reduce perspiration, diarrhea, seminal emission, urorrhea, bleeding, leukorrhea, coughing, etc. These drugs are chiefly used for symptomatic treatment.

消導藥 [xiāodǎoyào]
stomachics and evacuants, drugs for improving appetite and digestion and removing stagnated food, usually used in the treatment of dyspepsia or indigestion.

瀉下藥 [xièxiàyào]
purgatives; cathartics, drugs which promote defecation or even cause diarrhea. These drugs are used not only in the treatment of constipation, but also for removing the evil heat or fire from the body.

驅蟲藥 [qūchóngyào]
anthelmintics

劑型 [jìxíng]
forms of prepared medicines; preparation forms; dosage forms

丸 [wán]

(1) **pill**: a small globular mass made of powdered medicine with water and flour paste or rice paste as excipient, also called 水丸 [shuǐ wán] or "watered pill"; (2) **bolus**: a rounded medicated mass larger than a pill, usually with honey as excipient and thus called 蜜丸 [mì wán] or "honeyed bolus"

散 [sǎn]

medicinal powder, for internal administration or topical application

膏 [gāo]

soft extract; ointment or adhesive plaster (1) 煎膏 [jiāngāo]; 膏滋 [gāozī] soft extracts for oral administration, usually made by concentrating a decoction to a syrupy consitency with the addition of sugar or honey; (2) 膏藥 [gāoyào] ointment or adhesive plasters for external application

丹 [dān]

pellet or powder (1) for topical application, usually made from minerals by sublimation; (2) for internal administration

露 [lù]

distillate or essence of herbal medicine, usually aromatic

烘 [hōng]

to bake with mild heat, to dry drugs in a drying cabinet or room with mild heat

焙 [bèi]

to bake, to dry medical substances on a clean tile or in a pan over a slow fire

煨 [wēi]

to roast in hot ashes, to bake drugs wrapped in wet paper or coated with dough in hot ashes till the paper or coat turns black

炒 [chǎo]

to stir-bake, to bake drugs in a pan with constant stirring

微炒 [wēichǎo]

to stir-bake to just dry, to bake drugs in a pan over a slow fire with constant stirring to make them dry

炒爆 [chǎobào]

to stir-bake to cracking, to bake a drug (usually seeds) in a pan with constant stirring till it cracks

炒黄 [chǎohuáng]

to stir-bake to yellowish, to bake a drug in a pan till it turns yellowish and gives off a scent

炒焦 [chǎojiāo]

to stir-bake to brown, to bake a drug in a pan with constant stirring till it turns brown

片 [piàn]

tablet, small, flattened pellet of compressed powdered medicines or extract of medicines with starch as formative agent

冲服劑 [chōngfùjì]

medicinal granules, made of extract of the drug with sugar as corrigent, to be dissolved in boiling water before taking

炮 [páo]

to stir-bake at high temperature, to prepare a drug by baking with stirring (usually together with hot sand) at a high temperature for a short while so as to reduce its violent action

炮製 [páozhì]

process of preparing Chinese medicine, e.g., soaking, drying, calcining, baking, steaming, simmering, carbonizing, roasting, etc.

泡 [pào]; 浸 [jìn]; 漬 [zì]

to macerate, to immerse drugs in water to soften them before peeling or cutting

水飛 [shuǐfēi]

to elutriate, to remove impurities from a powdered drug and at the same time to obtain finer grade of powder (such as talc powder) by mixing it with water and allowing the turbid fluid to settle in tanks and then collecting the deposit

煅 [duàn]

to calcine: to burn a drug on fire to make it crispy

錠 [dìng]

pastil; lozenge; troche; ingot-shaped tablet of medicine used internally or externally

藥酒 [yàojiǔ]

medicated liquor, wine or spirits in which medicinal ingredients
have been steeped

湯藥 [tāngyào]; 湯劑 [tāngjì]

decoction of medicinal ingredients, a medicine prepared by boiling,
to be taken after the dregs are removed

飲 [yǐn]

cold decoction, decoction of Chinese drugs to be taken cold

飲片 [yǐnpiàn]

medicinal herbs in small pieces or slices

藥面 [yàomiàn]

medicinal powder; powdered drugs

茶 [chá]

medicinal tea, drugs in crude powder or made into small cakes,
taken as tea after being infused with boiling water or boiled in water

曲 [qǔ]

leaven, powdered drugs mixed with wheat flour and beaten into
cakes for fermentation, usually used as stomachics

製炭 [zhìtàn]

to carbonize, to heat a vegetable drug in an air-tight container
or by stir-baking with a strong fire till its outer part is charred while
its inner part becomes yellowish-brown so that its original property
is retained

炙 [zhì]

to stir-bake with adjuvant, to bake a drug mixed with a fluid
adjuvant such as wine, vinegar salt water, honey, ginger juice, suet,
etc., until the latter is infiltrated into the drug

蒸 [zhēng]

to steam, to prepare a drug by steaming

燉 [dùn]

to simmer in bath, to put a drug and fluid adjuvant in an airtight
container and heat it in a water bath or with steam until the fluid
adjuvant has been absorbed

熬 [āo]

to stew, to stew a drug with adjuvants for concentration

煮 [zhǔ]

147

to boil, to boil a drug with water or fluid adjuvant

烊化 ［yánghuà］

to melt, to melt or dissolve a drug (such as honey, ass-hide glue) with hot water or decoction before taking

燒存性 ［shāo cún xìng］

to burn with the original property retained, to burn a vegetable drug till its outer part is charred while its inner part becomes yellowish-brown so that its original property is retained

去油 ［qùyóu］

to defat, to remove fat or oil from drugs (such as Croton Seed) to reduce their toxicity

去火毒 ［pù huǒdú］

to remove the irritating quality of newly prepared plaster base by placing it in shady cool place or in water for a period of time before using it to make plasters

煎藥法 ［jiānyàofǎ］

method of making a decoction. The usual process is to mix the ingredients with adequate amount of water, boil them for a certain period of time and remove the drugs from the liquid before taking.

文火 ［wénhuǒ］

a small or slow fire used for making decoctions which need longer period of boiling, such as tonics

武火 ［wǔhuǒ］

a large or strong fire used for making decoctions such as diaphoretics and carminatives for which only short period of boiling is allowed

先煎 ［xiānjiān］

to decoct first. While making a decoction certain drugs (chiefly minerals and shells with active constituents difficult to be extracted) should be boiled first before other ingredients are thrown in.

後下 ［hòuxià］

to decoct later. Drugs with active constituents ready to diffuse or evaporate should be thrown in when the decoction is nearly done.

包煎 ［bāojiān］

to decoct a drug wrapped. Downy or powdered drugs or drugs containing much mucilage are usually wrapped with a piece of cloth

148

or gauze when the decoction is made.

冲服 [chōngfù]

to take (medicine) after pouring liquid on it, to take medicine (usually aromatics or powders) by pouring hot water or hot decoction of other drugs over it with stirring

調服 [tiáofù]

to take (medicinal powder) after mixing it with liquid such as a portion of hot decoction of other drugs, water, wine, etc.

吞服 [tūnfù]

(pills) to be swallowed

送服 [sòngfù]

(pills) to be swallowed with liquids such as warm boiled water in most cases, dilute decoction of fresh ginger for warming drugs, tea or mint solution for febrifuges, dilute salt water for tonics, weak tea for antidinic pills, etc.

嚼化 [qínhuà]

(pills or pastil) to be melted in mouth and then swallowed or spat out

食遠服 [shíyuǎnfù]

to be taken away from the mealtime

臨睡前服 [línshuìqiánfù]

to be taken before bed time

空腹服 [kōngfùfù]

to be taken with an empty stomach, e.g., before breakfast

頓服 [dùnfù]

(decoction) to be taken at one draught

頻服 [pínfù]

(decoction) to be taken in small portions at frequent intervals

溫服 [wēnfù]

to be taken warm

熱服 [rèfù]

to be taken hot. Decoctions with ingredients hot in nature and to be taken hot are good for symptom-complex of extreme cold.

冷服 [lěngfù]

to be taken cold. Decoctions with ingredients cold in nature and to

149

be taken cold are good for symptom-complex of extreme heat.

忌口 [jìkǒu]

food taboo on patient's diet

解表藥
Diaphoretics or Drugs for the Treatment of Exterior Symptom-Complex

辛溫解表藥 Diaphoretics with Pungent and Warm Properties

麻黄 [máhuáng]

Ephedra; *Herba Ephedrae.* The drug consists of the dried herbaceous twigs of *Ephedra sinica* Stapf, *Ephedra equisetina* Bunge or *Ephedra intermedia* Schrenk et Meyer (family Ephedraceae). It is used as (1) diaphoretic for affection due to wind and cold without sweat, (2) antiasthmatic, and (3) diuretic for edema caused by wind, e.g., acute nephritic edema.

桂枝 [guìzhī]

Cinammon Twigs, Cassia Twigs; *Ramulus Cinnamomi.* The drug consists of the twigs of *Cinnamomum cassia* Blume (family Lauraceae). It is used (1) as diaphoretic for affection due to wind and cold, (2) to warm and clear out the channels for treating rheumatic arthritis, and (3) to promote blood circulation for amenorrhoea and angina pectoris.

生薑 [shēngjiāng]

Fresh Ginger; *Rhizoma Zingiber is Recens.* The drug consists of the fresh rhizome of *Zingiber officinale* (Willd.) Rosc. (family Zingiberaceae). It is used (1) as diaphoretic for affection due to wind and cold, and (2) as antemetic.

防風 [fángfēng]

Ledebouriella Root; *Radix Ledebouriellae,* The drug consists of the dried root of *Ledebouriella divaricata* (Turcz.) Hiroe (family Umbelliferae). It is used (1) as diaphoretic for affection due to wind and cold and rheumatic pain; (2) as spasmolytic for tetanus.

白芷 [báizhǐ]

Dahurian Angelica Root; *Radix Angelicae Dahuricae.* The drug con-

150

sists of the dried root of *Angelica dahurica* (Fisch. ex Hoffm.) Benth. et Hook. f. or *Angelica dahurica* var. *formosana* Boiss. (family Umbelliferae). It is used (1) in the treatment of affection due to wind, cold or dampness, as anodyne for frontal headache, supra-orbital neuralgia, etc. and (2) to discharge pus and to reduce swellings for the treatment of boils, carbuncles, rhinitis and nasosinusitis.

荆芥 [jīngjiè]

Schizonepeta; *Herba Schizonepetae.* The drug consists of dried aerial parts of *Schizonepeta tenuefolia* Briq. (family Labiatae). It is used (1) as diaphoretic for affection due to wind and cold, (2) to promote eruption in treating measles, urticaria, etc. The spike (called 荆芥穗 [jing jiè suì]) is used similarly with stronger actions. The carbonized drug is used as hemostatic for the functional bleeding of uterus and hematochezia.

紫蘇葉 [zǐsūyè]

Perilla Leaf; *Folium Perillae.* The drug consists of the dried leaves of *Perilla frutescens* var. *acuta* (Thunb) Kudo. (family Labiatae). It is used as (1) diaphoretic to disperse the external wind and cold for the treatment of common cold without sweat; (2) antidote for fish and crab poisoning.

細辛 [xìxīn]

Asarum Herb, Wild Ginger; *Herba Asari.* The drug consists of the dried entire plant of *Asarum heterotropoides* var. *manschuricum* (Maxim.) Kitagawa and *Asarum sieboldii* Miq. (family Aristolochiaceae). It is used (1) to relieve pain by dispersing the external cold for the treatment of headache in common cold, severe toothache, or rheumatic pain; (2) to reduce copious, thin phlegm in chronic bronchitis.

藁本 [gǎoběn]

Ligusticum Root; *Rhizoma et Radix Ligustici.* It is the dried rhizome and root of *Ligustrum sinense* Oliver or *Ligustrum jeholense* Nakai et Kitagawa (family Umbelliferae). It is used to relieve headache due to affection by wind and cold.

辛夷 [xīnyí]

Magnolia Flower; *Flos Magnoliae.* The drug consists of the dried flowerbuds of *Magnolia liliflora* Desr., *Magnolia biondii* Pamp. or

Magnolia denudata Desr. (family Magnoliaceae). It is used for stuffy nose due to rhinitis and nasosinusitis.

苍耳子 [cāngěrzǐ]

Xanthium Fruit; Cochlebur Fruit; *Fructus Xanthii.* The drug consists of the dried fruit of *Xanthium sibiricum* Patrin. (family Compositae). It is used as antiallergic, antipruritic and antirheumatic for the treatment of allergic rhinitis,nasosinusitis, pruritus of the skin, and rheumatism.

鹅不食草 [ébùshícǎo]

Centipeda Herb; *Herba Centipedae.* The drug consists of the dried entire plants of *Centipeda minima* (L.) A. Braum et Aschers (family Compositae). It is used (1) for the treatment of acute or chronic rhinitis; (2) to stop cough for whooping cough.

辛凉解表藥 **Diaphoretics with Pungent and Cold Properties**

柴胡 [cháihú]

Bupleurum Root, Thorowax Root; *Radix Bupleuri.* The drug consists of the dried root of *Bupleurum chinense* DC. or *Bupleurum scorzonerifolium* Willd. (family Umbelliferae). It is used (1) as antipyretic for intermittent fever, such as malaria; (2) to relieve stagnancy of vital energy of the *liver* for pains in the sides and chest; and (3) to elevate the vital energy of the *spleen* for visceroptosis.

薄荷 [bòhé]

Peppermint; *Herba Menthae.* The drug consists of the dried aerial parts of the Field Mint, *Mentha arvensis* L. (family Labiatae). It is used for affection due to wind and heat with fever, headache, stuffy nose and sore throat.

桑葉 [sāngyè]

Mulberry Leaf, *Folium Mori.* The drug consists of the dried leaves of White Mulberry, *Morus alba* L. (family Moraceae). It is used for affection due to wind and heat with headache and acute conjunctivitis.

菊花 [júhuā]

Chrysanthemum Flower; *Flos Chrysanthemi.* The drug consists of the dried flower-head of Florists Chrysanthemum. *Chrysanthemum morifolium Ramat.* (family Compositae). It is used for affection due to wind and heat with fever, bloodshot eyes and headache, and as anti-

152

hypertensive for hypertension.

葛根 [gěgēn]

Pueraria Root, Kudzuvine Root; *Radix Puerariae.* The drug consists of the dried root of *Pueraria lobata* (Willd.) Ohwi or *Pueraria thomsanii* Benth. (family Leguminosae). It is used (1) as diaphoretic for fever with discomfort and pain in the neck and back; (2) to relieve thirst for febrile conditions, (3) for hypertensive headache and coronary heart disease, (4) to promote eruption for measles.

牛蒡子 [niúbàngzǐ]

Arctium Fruit, Burdock Fruit; *Fructus Arctii.* The drug consists of the fruit of Great Burdock, *Arctium lappa* L. (family Compositae). It is used for inflammation of the throat, such as acute pharyngitis and acute tonsillitis.

蔓荆子 [mànjīngzǐ]

Chaste-tree Fruit; *Fructus Viticis.* The drug consists of the dried ripe fruit of Simple-leaved Chaste Tree, *Vitex trifolia* L. var. *simplicifolia* Cham. or Three-leaved Chaste Tree, *Vitex trifolia* L. (family Verbenaceae). It is used for affection due to wind and heat with fever, headache, dizziness, acute conjunctivitis or neuro-muscular pains.

野菊花 [yějúhuā]

Mother Chrysanthemum Flower, Indian Chrysanthemum Flower; *Flos Chrysanthemi Indici.* The drug consists of the dried flower-heads of *Chrysanthemum indicum* L. (family Compositae). It is used for relieving pyogenic inflammations, such as carbuncles and furnncles, acute conjunctivitis, headache and dizziness. It may also be used for influenza, tuberculosis, hepatitis, dysentery and hypertension.

蝉蜕 [chán tuì]; 蝉衣 [chán yī]

Ciccada Slough, Ciccada Skin; *Periostracum Cicadae.* The drug consists of the slough shed by the ciccada nymph, *Cryptotypana pustulata* Fabr. (family Cicadidae). It is used for hoarseness in phonation due to infections of upper respiratory tract, measles, pruritus of the skin, spasm and convulsion due to high fever or tetanus.

升麻 [shēngmá]

Cimicifuga Rhizome, Bugbane Rhizome; *Rhizoma Cimicifugae.* The drug consists of the dried rhizome of Large-trileaf Bugbane, *Cimi-*

153

cifuga heracleifolia Kom., Dahurian Bugbane, *Cimicifuga dahurica* (Turcz.) Maxim. or Fetid Bugbane, *Cimicifuga foetida* L. (family Ranunculaceae). It is used (1) to promote eruption in the treatment of measles; (2) as detoxicant for sore-throat and stomatitis; (3) to restore normal position of the viscera for splanchnoptosis.

淡豆豉 〔dàndòuchǐ〕

Prepared Soybean; *Semen Sojae Praeparatum.* The drug consist of the prepared seed of *Glycine max* (L.) Merr. (family Leguminosae). It is used in early stage of febrile diseases to cause diaphoresis and in late stage for the treatment of fidget and insomnia.

西河柳 〔xīhéliǔ〕

Tamarisk Tops; *Cacumen Tamaricis.* The drug consists of the dried young green twigs of *Tamarix chinensis* Lour. (family Tamaricaceae). It is used in the treatment of measles to promote eruption.

浮萍 〔fúpíng〕

Spirodela; Ducksmeat; *Herba Spirodelae.* The drug consists of the dried entire plant of *Spirodela polyrrhiza* (L.) Schneid. (family Lemnaceae). It is used as diaphoretic and diuretic for fever without sweat, measles and edema.

常山 〔chángshān〕

Dichroa Root; *Radix Dichroae.* The drug consists of the dried root of *Dichroa febrifuga* Lour. (family Saxifragaceae). It is used for the treatment of malaria.

<h1 style="text-align:center">止咳化痰平喘藥</h1>

Antitussives, Expectorants and Anti-asthmatics

溫化寒痰藥 Drugs for Resolving Cold - Phlegm

半夏 〔bànxià〕

Pinellia Tuber; *Rhizoma Pinelliae.* The drug consists of the dried tuber of *Pinellia ternata* (Thunb.) Breit. (family Araceae). It is used as antibechic and expectorant for cough with profuse thin phlegm; as antiemetic for nausea, vomiting and morning sickness.

天南星 〔tiānnánxīng〕

Arisaema Tuber, Jack-in-the-Pulpit Tuber; *Rhizoma Arisaematis.*

The drug consists of the dried tuber of *Arisaema consanguineum* Schott, *Arisaema heterophyllum* Bl. or *Arisaema amurense* Maxim. (family Araceae). It is used as expectorant and anticonvulsive for cough with profuse phlegm and for convulsion at high fever or epilepsy.

白芥子 [báijièzǐ]

White Mustard Seed; *Semen Sinapis Albae.* The drug consists of the seed of *Brassica alba* (L.) Boiss. (family Cruciferae). It is used for cough with profuse phlegm and stuffy feeling in the chest, for cold (tuberculous) abscess and liquid accumulation in the thoracic cavity.

白附子 [báifùzǐ]

Typhonium Tuber; *Rhizoma Typhonii.* The drug consists of the dried tuber of *Typhonium giganteum* Engl. (family Araceae). It is used as expectorant and anticonvulsive for cough with profuse phlegm and for epilepsy or tetanus.

旋覆花 [xuánfùhuā]

Inula Flower; *Flos Inulae.* The drug consists of the dried flower head of Japanese Inula, *Inula japonica* Thunb. (family Compositae). It is used for asthmatic bronchitis with excessive phlegm; also for belch and vomiting.

紫菀 [zǐwǎn]

Aster Root; *Radix Asteris.* The drug consists of the dried root and rhizome of Tatarian Aster, *Aster tataricus* L.f. (family Compositae). It is used as expectorant and antitussive for cough with thick phlegm in chronic bronchitis and for prolonged cough.

桔梗 [jiégěng]

Platycodon Root, Balloonflower Root; *Radix Platycodi.* The drug consists of the dried roots of Balloonflower, *Platycodon grandiflorum* (Jacq.) A.DC. (family Campanulaceae). It is used as expectorant and to eliminate pus for cough due to infection in the respiratory tract or pulmonary abscess; also for inflammation of the throat.

清化熱痰藥 **Drugs for Resolving Heat - Phlegm**

瓜蔞 [guālóu]; 栝樓 [guālóu]

Trichosanthes Fruit, Snakegourd Fruit; *Fructus Trichosanthis.* The drug consists of the dried fruit of *Trichosanthes kirilowii* Maxim.

or *Trichosanthes uniflora* Hao (family Cucurbitaceae). It is used for pulmonary infections with yellow and thick (mucopurulent) phlegm, stuffy feeling in the chest, chest pain and dry stools.

天花粉 [tiānhuāfěn]
Trichosanthes Root, Snake-gourd Root; *Radix Trichosanthis.* The drug consists of the dried root of Mongolian Snakegourd, *Trichosanthes kirilowii* Maxim. or Japanese Snakegourd, *Trichosanthes japonica* Regel (family Cucurbitaceae). It is used for relieving thirst (such as in diabetes mellitus) and inflammatory swellings. An injection prepared from it is used for artificial abortion.

竹茹 [zhúrú]
Bamboo Shavings; *Caulis Bambusae in Taenis.* The drug consists of the culm shavings of *Bambusa breviflora* Munro, *Sinocalamus beecheyanus* (Munro) McClure var. *pubescens* P.F. Li or *Phyllostachys nigra* var. *henonis* Stapf (family Gramineae). It is used as antipyretic, expectorant and antiemetic agent for pulmonary infections with cough and yellow phlegm, and for vomiting due to heat in stomach (e.g. chronic gastritis).

南沙参 [nánshāshēn]
Adenophora Root, Ladybell Root; *Radix Adenophorae.* The drug consists of the dried root of *Adenophora tetraphylla* (Thunb.) Fisch. or *Adenophora stricta* Miq. or related species (family Campanulaceae). It is used for pulmonary infections with cough and yellow thick phlegm, chronic bronchitis with dry cough.

海藻 [hǎizǎo]
Sargassum, Seaweed; *Sargassum.* The drug consists of the dried seaweed of *Sargassum pallidum* (Turn.) G. Ag. or *Sargassum fusiforme* (Harv.) Setch. (family Sargassaceae). It is used as expectorant for chronic bronchitis, but more frequently used for goitre, tuberculosis of lymph-nodes and hypertension.

昆布 [kūnbù]
Laminaria or Ecklonia; *Thallus Laminariae seu Eckloniae.* The drug consists of the dried thallus of Japanese Sea Tangle, *Laminaria japonica* Aresch. or *Ecklonia kurome* Okam, (family Laminariaceae). It is used as expectorant for chronic bronchitis but more frequently

used for goitre and chronic inflammation of the lymph-node.

前胡 [qiánhú]

Peucedanum Root, Hogfennel Root; *Radix Peucedani.* The drug consists of the dried root of *Peucedanum praeruptorum* Dunn or *Peucedanum decursivum* Maxim. (family Umbelliferae). It is used for cough with thick phlegm and asthmatic symptom due to infections in the upper respiratory tract.

止咳藥 Antitussives

苦杏仁 [kŭxìngrén]

Bitter Apricot Kernel, Bitter Apricot Seed; *Semen Armeniacae Amarum.* The drug consists of the bitter seed of Ansu Apricot, *Prunus armeniaca* L. var. *ansu* Maxim., Siberian Apricot, *Prunus sibirica* L., Manchurian Apricot, *Prunus mandshurica* (Maxim.) Koehne or Apricot, *Prunus armeniaca* L. (family Rosaceae). It is used to relieve cough and asthma for acute or chronic bronchitis.

枇杷葉 [pípāyè]

Loquat Leaf; *Folium Eriobotryae.* The drug consists of the dried leaves of *Eriobotrya japonica* (Thunb.) Lindl. (family Rosaceae). It is used as antitussive, expectorant and antiemetic for acute or chonic bronchitis and vomiting due to heat in stomach, such as gastritis.

白果 [báiguŏ]

Ginkgo Seed; *Semen Ginkgo.* The drug consists of the seed of Maidenhair Tree, *Ginkgo biloba* L. (family Ginkgoaceae). It is used for prolonged cough or asthma, also used as antisecretory agent for leukorrhea, and to reduce urination in cases of frequent micturition.

款冬花 [kuǎndōnghuā]

Coltsfoot Flower, *Flos Farfarae.* The drug consists of the dried flower buds of *Tussilago farfara* L. (family Compositae). It is used for chronic cough with profuse phlegm, and hemoptysis.

百部 [bǎibù]

Stemona Root; *Radix Stemonae.* The drug consists of the dried root of *Stemona sessilifolia* (Miq.) Miq., *Stemona japonica* (Bl.) Miq. or *Stemona tuberosa* Lour. (family Stemonaceae). It is used to relieve cough for acute and chronic bronchitis, and to treat tuberculosis. It is also used externally as anthelmintic and insecticide for enterobiasis and lice.

浙貝母 [zhèbèimǔ]

Thunberg Fritillary Bulb, *Bulbus Fritillariae Thunbergii.* The drug consists of the dried bulb of Thunberg Fritillary, *Fritillaria thunbergii* Miq. (family Liliaceae). It is used for cough with thick phlegm due to heat in the *lung* (such as acute bronchitis and pneumonia), and subcutaneus swellings (such as scrofula).

川貝母 [chuānbèimǔ]

Tendrilled Fritillary Bulb; *Bulbus Fritillariae Cirrhosae.* The drug consists of the dried bulb of Tendril-leaf Fritillary, *Fritillaria cirrhosa* D. Don, *Fritillaria unibracteata* Hsiao et K. C. Hsia, *Fritillaria przewalskii* Maxim. or *Fritillaria delavayi* Franch. (family Liliaceae). It is used for dry cough and cough with little phlegm due to deficiency of vital essence in the *lung* (such as pulmonary tuberculosis).

罌粟殼 [yīngsùqiào]; 米殼 [mǐ qiào]

Poppy Capsules, Poppy Heads; *Pericarpium Papaveris.* The drug consists of the dried capsules of *Papaver somniferum* L. (family Papaveraceae) with seeds removed. It is used as antitussive, antidiarrhetic and analgesic for chronic cough, chronic diarrhea and all kinds of pain.

滿山紅 [mǎnshānhóng]

Dahurian Rhododendron Leaf; *Folium Rhododendri Daurici.* The drug consists of the dried leaves of *Rhododendron dauricum* L. (family Ericaceae). It is used as antitussive and expectorant for chronic bronchitis.

百合 [bǎihé]

Lily Bulb; *Bulbus Lilii.* The drug consists of the dried bulb of *Lilium lancifolium* Thunb., *Lilium brownii* F.E. Brown var. *viridulum* Baker or *Lilium pumilum* DC. (family Liliaceae). It is used as antitussive and sedative for cough and hemoptysis due to deficiency of vital essence of the lung, insomnia and fidget in the late stage of febrile disease with residual heat or due to neurosis.

桑白皮 [sāngbáipí]

Mulberry Bark; *Cortex Mori Radicis.* The drug consists of the dried rootbark of *Morus alba* L. (family Moraceae). It is used (1) as antitussive for cough due to heat in the *lung*; (2) as diuretic for edema.

158

It is also used for hypertension.

暴馬子皮 [bàomǎzǐ pí]
Manchurian Lilac Bark; *Cortex Syringae.* The drug consists of the dried stembark of *Syringa reticulata* (Bl.) Hara var. *mandshurica* (Maxim.) Hara (family Oleaceae). It is used as antipyretic, antitussive and diuretic agent for acute or chronic bronchitis, asthma and cardiac edema.

胖大海 [pàngdàhǎi]
Boat Sterculia Seed; *Semen Sterculiae Scaphigerae.* The drug consists of the dried seeds of *Sterculia scaphigera* Wall. (family Sterculiaceae). It is used for inflammation of throat and hoarseness in phonation; also used for constipation.

平喘藥 **Anti-asthmatics**

洋金花 [yángjīnhuā]
Datura Flower; *Flos Daturae.* The drug consists of the dried flowers of *Datura metel* L. (family Solanaceae). It is used to relieve cough and asthma for bronchial asthma; also used as analgesic to relieve gastralgia and rheumatalgia.

葶藶子 [tínglìzǐ]
Lepidium Seed or **Descurainia Seed;** *Semen Lepidii seu Descurainiae.* The drug consists of the seeds of *Lepidium apetalum* Willd. or *Descurainia sophia* (L.) Webb et Prantl (family Cruciferae). It is used for cough and asthma with excessive phlegm and as diuretic for edema or liquid accumulation in thoraco-abdominal cavity.

馬兜鈴 [mǎdōulíng]
Aristolochia Fruit, Birthwort Fruit; *Fructus Aristolochiae.* The drug consists of the dried capsules of *Aristolochia contorta* Bge. or *Aristolochia debilis* Sieb. et Zucc. (family Aristolochiaceae). It is used for cough and asthmatic conditions due to heat in the *lung.*

紫蘇子 [zǐsūzǐ]
Perilla Seed; *Fructus Perillae.* The drug consists of the fruits of Purple Common Perilla, *Perilla frutescens* (L.) Britt. var. *acuta* (Thunb.) It is used as antiasthmatic and expectorant for chronic bronchitis with thin white phlegm and stuffy feeling in the chest.

莨菪子 [làngdàngzǐ]; 天仙子 [tiānxiānzǐ]

159

Henbane Seed; *Semen Hyoscyami.* The drug consists of the dried seeds of Black Henbane, *Hyoscyamus niger* L. (family Solanaceae). It is used to relieve cough and asthma for bronchial asthma and to relieve gastralgia and rheumatalgia.

華山參 [huáshānshēn]; 热參 [rèshēn]

Funnel Physochlaina Root; *Radix Physochlainae.* The drug consists of the dried root of Funnel Physochlaina, *Physochlaina infundibularis* Kuang (family Solanaceae). It is used to relieve cough and asthma for asthmatic bronchitis and to relieve gastric or abdominal pain.

芸香草 [yúnxiāngcǎo]

Lemongrass; *Herba Cymbopogonis.* The drug consists of the dried aerial parts of *Cymbopogon distans* (Nees) A. Camus (family Gramineae). It is used to relieve cough and asthma for chronic bronchitis and also as carminative for stuffy feeling in chest and abdomen.

清熱藥

Antipyretics or Febrifuges Drugs for Clearing up Internal Heat

清熱瀉火藥 Drugs for Reducing Intense Internal Heat

石膏 [shígāo]

Gypsum; *Gypsum Fibrosum.* The drug consists of a soft mineral composed of hydrated calcium sulphate. It is used as antipyretic for heat in the *lung* and *stomach* with high fever, fidget and thirst.

知母 [zhīmǔ]

Anemarrhena Rhizome; *Rhizoma Anemarrhenae.* The drug consists of the dried rhizomes of *Anemarrhena asphodeloides* Bge. (family Liliaceae). It is used for high fever with dire thirst in acute infectious diseases and for low febrile condition in chronic diseases.

决明子 [juémíngzǐ]

Cassia Seed; *Semen Cassiae.* The drug consists of the dried seed of *Cassia obtusifolia* L. or *Cassia tora* L. (family Leguminosae). It is used frequently in ophthalmology for acute inflammations and is also used for reducing blood pressure and blood cholesterol.

木賊 [mùzéi]

Shave Grass; *Herba Equiseti Hiemalis*. The drug consists of the aerial parts of Common Scouring Rush (Shave Grass), *Equisetum hiemale* L. (family Equisetaceae). It is used in ophthalmology for acute infections such as conjunctivitis, also for acute hepatitis and jaundice.

淡竹葉 [dàzhúyè]

Lophatherum; *Herba Lophatheri*. The drug consists of the dried aerial parts of *Lophatherum gracile* Brongn. (family Gramineae). It is used as antipyretic and diuretic for febrile condition with oliguria and acute infections of the urinary tract.

蘆根 [lúgēn]

Reed Rhizome; *Rhizoma Phragmitis*. The drug consists of the dried rhizomes of Common Reed, *Phragmites communis* (L.) Trin. (family Gramineae). It is used to reduce fever and to promote secretions in cases of high fever with thirst and for pulmonary abscess.

羅布麻葉 [luóbùmá yè]

Dogbane Leaf; *Folium Apocyni Veneti*. The drug consists of the dried leaves of Red Dogbane, *Apocynum venetum* L. (family Apocynaceae). It is used to clear up heat from the *liver* and as antihypertensive for headache and dizziness due to hypertension.

夏枯草 [xiàkūcǎo]

Prunella Spike, Selfheal Spike; *Spica Prunellae*. The drug consists of the spike of Common Selfheal, *Prunella vulgaris* L. (family Labiatae). It is used to clear up heat from the *liver* for the treatment of acute conjunctivitis, hypertension with headache; also used to eliminate nodulation for the treatment of acute mastitis, mumps, scrofula and goitre.

清熱涼血藥 **Drugs for Eliminating Pathological Heat from Blood**

犀角 [xījiǎo]

Rhinoceros Horn; *Cornu Rhinoceri*. The drug consists of the horn of Asiatic Rhinoceros, *Rhinoceros unicornis* L., *Rhinoceros sondaicus* Desmarest or *Rhinoceros sumatrensis* Cuvier (family Rhinocerotidae). It is used for the treatment of impaired consciousness and maculation with high fever in acute infectious diseases, also used for bleeding

161

due to existence of pathological heat.

水牛角 [shuǐniújiǎo]

Buffalo Horn; *Cornu Bubali.* The drug consists of the horn of *Bubalus bubalis* L. (family Bovidae). It is used similarly as 犀角 [xījiǎo] and also for thrombocytopenic purpura and acute hepatitis.

地黄 [dìhuáng]; 生地 [shēngdì]

Rehmannia Root; *Radix Rehmanniae.* The drug consists of the dried tuberous root of *Rehmannia glutinosa* Libosch (family Scrophulariaceae). The fresh root is used for the treatment of thirst, exanthesis and bleeding due to existence of pathological heat. The dried root has similar effect, and is also used to nourish the vital essence for the treatment of its deficiency.

牡丹皮 [mǔdānpí]

Moutan Bark; Tree Peony Bark; *Cortex Moutan Radicis.* The drug consists of the dried root-bark of Tree Peony, *Paeonia suffruticosa* Andr. (family Ranunculaceae). It is used (1) to eliminate heat from the blood for the treatment of bleeding in high febrile conditions; (2) to promote blood circulation and remove blood stasis for appendicitis, boils, carbuncles and amenorrhea.

紫草 [zǐcǎo]

Arnebia or Lithosperm Root, Purple Gromwell Root; *Radix Arnebiae seu Lithospermi.* The drug consists of the dried roots of *Arnebia euchroma* (Royle) Johnst. or *Lithospermum erythrorhizon* Sieb. et Zucc. (family Boraginaceae). It is used to promote exanthesis in measles, used externally for burns, frostbite, dermatitis and eczema.

地骨皮 [dìgǔpí]

Wolfberry Bark; *Cortex Lycii Radicis.* The drug consists of the dried root-bark of Chinese Wolfberry, *Lycium chinense* Mill. or *Lycium barbarum* L. (family Solanaceae). It is used for chronic febrile diseases, hematemesis and epistaxis.

銀柴胡 [yíncháihú]

Stellaria Root; *Radix Stellariae.* The drug consists of the dried roots of *Stellaria dichotoma* L. var. *lanceolata* Bge. (family Caryophyllaceae). It is used for hectic fever or residual heat in the late stage of febrile diseases.

162

青蒿 [qīnghāo]
Chinghao, Sweet Wormwood, *Herba Artemisiae Chinghao*. The drug consists of the dried aerial parts of Sweet Wormwood, *Artemisia annua* L. or *Artemisia apiacea* Hance (family Compositae). It is used for febrile diseases when Yin (vital essence) is invaded and fever due to deficiency of vital essence. It is also used for malaria.

白薇 [báiwēi]
Swallowwort Root; *Radix Cynanchi Atrati*. The drug consists of the dried root and rhizome of *Cynanchum atratum* Bge. or *Cynanchum versicolor* Bge. (family Asclepiadaceae). It is used for hectic fever or fever due to deficiency of Yin (vital essence).

白茅根 [báimáogēn]
Imperata Rhizome, Cogongrass Rhizome; *Rhizoma Imperatae*. The drug consists of the dried rhizomes of *Imperata cylindrica* Beauv. var. *major* (Nees) C.E. Hubb. (family Graminae).It is used as a febrifugal, diuretic and hemostatic agent for the treatment of epitaxis, hematuria, edema, jaundice, urodynia, etc. associated with heat symptom-complexes.

清熱燥濕藥 Febrifugal and Antipyic Drugs or Drugs for Eliminating Heat and Dampness

黃芩 [huángqín]
Scutellaria Root, Baikal Skullcap Root; *Radix Scutellariae*. The drug consists of the dried roots of Baikal Skullcap, *Scutellaria baicalensis* Georgi (family Labiatae). It is used (1) to eliminate heat in the *lung* for cough with yellow thick phlegm; (2) to eliminate heat and dampness in the large intestine for acute enteritis and dysentery; (3) for the treatment of pyogenic infections of skin and (4) for the treatment of hypertension and threatened abortion.

黃連 [huánglián]
Coptis Root; *Rhizoma Coptidis*. The drug consists of the dried rhizomes of Chinese Goldthread, *Coptis chinensis* Franch., *Coptis deltoidea* C.Y. Cheng et Hsiao or *Coptis teetoides* C.Y. Cheng (family Ranunculaceae). It is used to (1) eliminate heat in the *heart* for insomnia, fidget, delirium due to high fever, inflammation of the mouth and tongue; (2) stop diarrhea for acute enteritis and dysentery.

163

黄柏 [huángbǎi]
Phellodendron Bark; *Cortex Phellodendri.* The drug consists of the dried barks of Chinese Corktree, *Phellodendron chinense* Schneid. or Amur Corktree, *Phellodendron amurense* Rupr. (family Rutaceae). It is used (1) to eliminate heat and dampness for acute dysentery, jaundice, leukorrhea, infection of the urinary system, etc, and (2) as detoxicating or antibacterial agent for boils and furuncles.

三颗針 [sānkēzhēn]
Berberis Root, Barberry Root; *Radix Berberidis.* The drug consists of the roots of *Berberis soulieana* Schneid, *Berberis wilsonae* Hemsl., *Berberis poiretii* Schneid. or *Berberis vernae* Schneid. (family Berberidaceae). It is used similarly as 黄連 [huáng lián]

龍膽 [lóngdǎn]; 龍膽草 [lóngdǎncǎo]
Chinese Gentian; *Radix Gentianae.* The drug consists of the dried root and rhizome of *Gentiana manshurica* Kitag., *Gentiana scabra* Bge., *Gentiana triflora* Pall. or *Gentiana regescens* Franch. (family Gentianaceae). It is used to eliminate intense heat or fire in the *liver* and *gallbladder* for the treatment of hypertension with dizziness and tinnitus, conjunctivitis, sore-throat, bitterness in mouth and pain in ear, and to clear up damp heat in the lower part of the body cavity for acute infections of the urinary system, and eczema of scrotum.

苦參 [kǔshēn]
Flavescent Sophora Root; *Radix Sophorae Flavescentis.* The drug consists of the dried roots of *Sophora flavescens* Ait. (family Leguminosae). It is used as cholagogue and antidysenteric for jaundice and acute dysentery; also used externally as parasiticide and antipruritic for eczema, ringworm with pruritus.

秦皮 [qínpí]
Ash Bark; *Cortex Fraxini.* The drug consists of the dried bark of Korean Ash, *Fraxinus rhynchophylla* Hance, Chinese Ash, *Fraxinus chinensis* Roxb. or *Fraxinus stylosa* Lingelsh. (family Oleaceae). It is used as antidysenteric for acute dysentery.

白蘚皮 [báixiǎnpí]
Dittany Bark; *Cortex Dictamni Radicis.* The drug consists of the dried rootbark of *Dictamnus dasycarpus* Turcz. (family Rutaceae).

It is used for skin diseases with excessive secretion and itching.

鴉膽子 [yādǎnzǐ]

Brucea Fruit; *Fructus Bruceae.* The drug consists of the dried fruit of *Brucea javanica* (L.) Merr. (family Simarubaceae). It is used for amebic dysentery and malaria. It is also used externally for warts, clavus and trichomonas vaginitis.

白頭翁 [báitóuwēng]

Pulsatilla Root; *Radix Pulsatillae.* The drug consists of the dried root of *Pulsatilla chinensis* (Bge.) Regel (family Ranunculaceae). It is used for bacterial and amebic dysentery, and externally for trichomonas vaginitis

椿皮 [chūnpí]; 椿根白皮 [chūngēnbáipí]; 樗白皮 [chūbái pí]

Ailanthus Bark, Tree of Heaven Bark; *Cortex Ailanthi.* The drug consists of the dried root-or stem-bark of Tree of Heaven, *Ailanthus altissima* (Mill.) Swingle (family Simarubaceae). It is used for diarrhea, chronic dysentery, emission and leukorrhea.

茵陳 [yīnchén]

Oriental Wormwood; *Herba Artemisiae Scopariae.* The drug consists of the dried young shoots of *Artemisia scoparia* Waldst. et Kit. or *Artemisia capillaris* Thunb. (family Compositae). It is used to eliminate damp heat in the *liver* and *gallbladder* for the treatment of jaundice, such as icteric hepatitis and cholecystitis.

土茯苓 [tǔfúlíng]

Smilax Glabra Rhizome, Glabrous Greenbrier Rhizome; *Rhizoma Smilacis Glabrae.* The drug consists of the dried rhizomes of *Smilax glabra* Roxb. (family Liliaceae). It is used for the infection of the urinary system, leptospirosis, rheumatoid arthritis, furuncles and carbuncles. It was used for the treatment of syphilis in ancient times.

馬齒莧 [mǎchǐxiàn]

Portulaca, Purslane; *Herba Portulacae.* The drug consists of the dried aerial parts of Purslane, *Portulaca oleracea* L. (family Pottulacaceae). It is used for dysentery, enteritis, leukorrhea and hookworm disease (ancylostomiasis).

黃櫨 [huánglú]

Cotinus Twigs, Smoketree Twigs. *Folium et Ramulus Cotini.*
The drug consists of the dried leaves and branches of *Cotinus coggygria* Scop. var. *cinerea* Engl. (family Anacardiaceae). It is used for hepatitis, jaundice, dysentery, pruritus, skin eczema, etc.

拳参 [quánshēn]
Bistort Rhizome; Snakeweed Rhizome; *Rhizoma Bistortae.* The drug consists of the dried rhizomes of *Polygonum bistorta* L. (family Polygonaceae). It is used for dysentery, enteritis; also used as hemostatic for gastro-intestinal and vaginal bleeding; used externally for bleeding and burns.

虎杖 [hǔzhàng]
Giant Knotweed Rhizome; *Rhizoma Polygoni Cuspidati.* The drug consists of the dried rhizomes of Giant or Japanese Knotweed, *Polygonum cuspidatum* Sieb. et Zucc. (family Polygonaceae). It is used for hepatitis, jaundice, enteritis, dysentery, also used for bronchitis, pneumonia, various kinds of pyogenic infection and externally for burns to prevent infection.

翻白草 [fānbáicǎo]
Potentilla Discolor, Diversecolour Cinquefoil, *Herba Potentillae Discoloris.* The drug consists of the dried entire plant of *Potentilla discolor* Bge. (family Rosaceae). It is used for enteritis; dysentery, pharyngitis, bleeding of the gastro-intestinal tract.

栀子 [zhīzǐ]
Capejasmine Fruit; *Fructus Gardeniae.* The drug consists of the dried fruits of Capejasmine, *Gardenia jasminoides* Ellis var. *radicans* (Thunb.) Makino (family Rubiaceae). It is used as (1) antipyretic and sedative for fever with fidget and insomnia; (2) cholagogue for acute icteric hepatitis; (3) antifebrile and hemostatic for bleeding in febrile diseases.

清熱解毒藥 Febrifugal and Detoxicant Drugs or Drugs for Eliminating Heat-Toxics
金銀花 [jīnyínhūa]
Honeysuckle Flower; *Flos Lonicerae.* The drug consists of the dried flower-buds of *Lonicera japonica* Thunb., *Lonicera hypoglauca* Miq., *Lonicera confusa* DC. or *Lonicera dasystyla* Rehd. (family Capri-

166

foliaceae). It has a strong antibacterial action and is used as antipyretic and anti-inflammatory agent for pyogenic infections such as inflammation of the upper respiratory tract, boils and furuncles, enteritis, dysentery, etc.

金銀藤 [jīnyínténg]; 忍冬藤 [rěndōngténg]

Honeysuckle Stem; *Caulis Lonicerae.* The drug consists of the dried stem and branch of Japanese Honeysuckle, *Lonicera japonica* Thunb. (family Caprifoliaceae). Its actions are similar to those of 金銀花 but it is more frequently used for clearing up evil heat in channels and collaterals for the treatment of acute rheumatic arthritis.

連翹 [liánqiào]

Forsythia Fruit, *Fructus Forsythiae.* The drug consists of the dried fruits of Weeping Forsythia, *Forsythia suspensa* (Thunb.) Vahl (family Oleaceae). Its actions are similar to those of 金銀花 , with which it is usually prescribed in combination to achieve a stronger action.

板藍根 [bǎnlángēn]

Isatis Root, Dyer's Woad Root; *Radix Isatidis.* The drug consists of the dried root of Dyer's Woad, *Isatis tinctoria* L. (family Cruciferae). It has a strong action of relieving fever and pyogenic inflammations, frequently used for influenza and other virus infections. It is also used for the treatment of maculation in acute infectious diseases.

大青葉 [dàqīngyè]

Isatis Leaf, Dyer's Woad Leaf; *Folium Isatidis.* The drug consists of the dried leaf of *Isatis tinctoria* L. (family Cruciferae). Its actions are similar to those of *Radix Isatidis* but it is more frequently used for reducing maculation in febrile cases.

青黛 [qīngdài]

Natural Indigo; *Indigo Naturalis.* The drug consists of a blue powder prepared from the leaves of *Baphicacanthus cusia* (Ness) Bremek. (family Acanthaceae), *Indigofera suffruticosa* Mill.(family Leguminosae), *Polygonum tinctorium* Ait. (family Polygonaceae) or *Isatis tinctoria* L. (family Cruciferae). It is used for eliminating internal heat, chiefly for the treatment of high febrile conditions of children. It is used externally for thrush, mumps (epidemic parotitis), and infections of the skin.

蒲公英 [púgōngyīng]

Dandelion Herb; *Herba Taraxaci.* The drug consists of the dried aerial parts of *Taraxacum mongolicum* Hand. -Mazz., *Taraxacum sinicum* Kitag. or *Taraxacum heterolepis* Nakai et H. Koidz. (family Compositae). It is used for boils, furuncles and other pyogenic infections.

紫花地丁 [zǐhuādìdīng]

Viola Herb, Yedoens Violet; *Herba Violae.* The drug consists of the dried entire plant of *Viola yedoensis* Makino (family Violaceae). It is used for the treatment of acute pyogenic infections such as boils and carbuncles.

魚腥草 [yúxīngcǎo]

Houttuynia; *Herba Houttuyniae.* The drug consists of the dried aerial parts of *Houttuynia cordata* Thunb. (family Saururaceae). It is frequently used for the treatment of pulmonary infections such as pneumonia and pulmonary abscess.

重樓 [chónglóu]; 蚤休 [zǎoxiū]

Paris Rhizome; *Rhizoma Paridis.* The drug consists of the dried rhizomes of *Paris chinensis* Franch. or *Paris yunnanensis* Franch. (family Liliaceae). It is used for acute pyogenic inflammations and septicopyemia; also used as anticonvulsive for the treatment of convulsions in high febrile conditions of children.

败醬草 [bàijiàngcǎo]

Patrinia Herb; *Herba Patriniae.* The drug consists of the dried entire plant of *Patrinia scabiosaefolia* Fisch. or *Patrinia villosa* Juss. (family Valerianaceae). It is used to reduce inflammations and eliminate pus for the treatment of carbuncles and acute appendicitis.

穿心蓮 [chuānxīnlián]

Green Chiretta; Kariyat; *Herba Andrographitis.* The drug consists of the dried aerial parts of *Andrographis paniculata* (Burm. f.) Nees (family Acanthaceae). It is used as febrifugal detoxicant, antiphlogistic and analgesic agent for the treatment of acute infections of the gastro-intestinal tract, respiratory organs and urinary system.

白花蛇舌草 [báihuāshéshécǎo]

Oldenlandia; *Herba Oldenlandiae.* The drug consists of the dried entire plants of *Oldenlandia diffusa* (Willd.) Roxb., *Oldenlandia corym-*

168

bosa L. and possibly other related species (family Rubiaceae). It is used as detoxicant, antiphlogistic and anticancer agent for the treatment of acute appendicitis, infections of the urinary system and cancer of the gastro-intestinal tract. It is also used for the treatment of snakebite.

龍葵 [lóngkuí]

Black Nightshade; *Herba Solani Nigri.* The drug consists of the dried aerial parts of Black Nightshade, *Solanum nigrum* L. (family Solanaceae). It is used as diuretic, antihypertensive and anticancer agent for the treatment of acute infections of the urinary system, hypertension and cancer of the digestive system.

半枝蓮 [bànzhīlián]

Barbat Skullcap; *Herba Scutellariae Barbatae.* The drug consists of the dried entire plant of *Scutellaria barbata.* D. Don (family Labiatae). It is used as febrifugal, detoxicant, anti-inflammatory and diuretic agent for the treatment of hepatitis, cirrhosis of the liver with ascites, snake and insect-bites.

半邊蓮 [bànbiānlián]

Radical Lobelia; *Herba Lobeliae Radicantis.* The drug consists of the dried entire plant of *Lobelia radicans* Thunb. (family Campanulaceae). It is used as anti-inflammatory and diuretic agent for enteritis, cirrhosis of the liver with ascites and nephrotic edema.

土牛膝 [tǔniúxī]

Native Achyranthes Root; *Radix Achyranthis Asperae.* The drug consists of the dried roots of *Achyranthes aspera* L. and possibly other related species (family Amaranthaceae). It is used for sore-throat and diphtheria.

山豆根 [shāndòugēn]; 廣豆根 [guǎngdòugēn]

Subprostrate Sophora Root; *Radix Sophorae Subprostratae.* The drug consists of the dried root and rhizome of *Sophora subprostrata* Chum et T. Chen (family Leguminosae). It is used as detoxicating, anti-inflammatory and anticancer agent for the treatment of sore-throat, gingivitis and cancer of the respiratory tract.

射干 [shègàn]

Belamcanda Rhizome, Blackberrylily Rhizome, *Rhizoma Belam-*

candae. The drug consists of the dried rhizomes of *Belamcanda chinensis* (L.) DC. (family Iridaceae). It is used as febrifugal, detoxicating and anti-inflammatory agent for acute tonsillitis, acute laryngitis and edema of the glottis.

馬勃 [mǎbó]

Puff-ball; *Lasiosphaera seu Calvatia.* The drug consists of the fructification of *Lasiosphaera fenzlii* Reich., *Calvatia gigantea* (Batsch ex Pers.) Lloyd or *Calvatia lilacina* (Mont. et Berk.) Lloyd (family Lycoperdaceae). It is used as febrifugal, anti-inflammatory and hemostatic agent for acute inflammation of the throat and hoarseness in phonation, and for hematemesis and nose-bleeding.

青果 [qīngguǒ]

Chinese Olive; *Fructus Canarii.* The drug consists of the dried fruit of *Canarium album* Raeusch. (family Burseraceae). It is used for dryness in pharynx, hoarseness in phonation and sore-throat.

錦燈籠 [jǐndēnglóng]; 酸漿 [suānjiāng]

Winter-cherry Fruit or Calyx; *Calyx seu Fructus Physalis.* The drug consists of the dried persistent calyx with fruit or the dried calyx only of Winter Cherry, *Physalis alkekengi* L. var. *franchetii* (Mast.) Makino (family Solanaceae). It is used for sore-throat.

葎草 [lǜcǎo]

Scandent Hops; *Herba Humuli Scandentis.* The drug consists of the dried aërial parts of *Humulus scandens* (Lour.) Merr. (family Moraceae). It is used as febrifugal, detoxicating, diuretic and sedative agent for the treatment of enteritis, dysentery, acute infection of urinary system and insomnia.

祛風濕藥

Antirheumatics or Drugs for Relieving Rheumatic Conditions

羌活 [qiānghuó]

Notopterygium Root; *Rhizoma seu Radix Notopterygii.* The drug consists of the dried rhizomes or roots of *Notopterygium incisum* Ting ex H.T. Chang or *Notopterygium forbesii* Boiss. (family Umbelliferae). It is used as antirheumatic and analgesic agent for the treatment of rheumatic pain especially that of the upper part of body.

独活 [dúhuó]

Pubescent Angelica Root; *Radix Angelicae Pubescentis.* The drug consists of the dried root of *Angelica pubescens* Maxim. f. *biserrata* Shan et Yuan (family Umbelliferae). It is used as antirheumatic and analgesic agent for the treatment of rheumatic pain especially that of the lower part of body.

威灵仙 [wēilíngxiān]

Clematis Root; *Radix Clematidis.* The drug consists of the dried root and rhizome of *Clematis chinensis* Osbeck, *Clematis hexapetala* Pall. or *Clematis manshurica* Rupr. (family Ranunculaceae). It is used as antirheumatic and analgesic agent for the treatment of rheumatic pain especially that of the whole body; and also for the treatment of fish bone stuck in the throat.

秦艽 [qínjiāo]

Large-leaf Gentian Root; *Radix Gentianae Macrophyllae.* The drug consists of the dried root of *Gentiana macrophylla* Pall., *Gentiana straminea* Maxim., *Gentiana crassicaulis* Duthie ex Burk. or *Gentiana dahurica* Fisch. (family Gentianaceae). It is used as antirheumatic agent for the treatment of rheumatic pain of the whole body; also used for fever in chronic diseases, for allergic inflammation, for hepatitis and jaundice.

木瓜 [mùguā]

Chaenomeles Fruit, Flowering-quince Fruit; *Fructus Chaenomelis.* The drug consists of the dried fruits of *Chaenomeles speciosa* (Sweet) Nakai or *Chaenomeles sinensis* (Thouin) Koehne (family Rosaceae). It is used as antirheumatic and anti-spasmodic agent for the treatment of rheumatic pain and convulsion of the calf muscles; also used for the treatment of vomiting, diarrhea and dyspepsia.

豨莶草 [xīxiāncǎo]

Siegesbeckia Herb, St. Paulswort; *Herba Siegesbeckiae.* The drug consists of the dried aerial parts of Common St. Paulswort, *Siegesbeckia orientalis* L., *Siegesbeckia pubescens* Makino or *Siegesbeckia glabrescens* Makino (family Compositae). It is used (1) as antirheu-

171

matic agent for the treatment of rheumatism and (2) as antihypertensive for the treatment of hypertension.

海風藤 [hǎifēngténg]
Futokadsura Stem; *Caulis Piperis Futokadsurae.* The drug consists of the dried stem of *Piper futokadsura* Sieb. et Zucc. (family Piperaceae). It is used as antirheumatic and anti-arthritic agent for the treatment of rheumatalgia of joints and muscles.

絡石藤 [luòshíténg]
Chinese Starjasmine; *Caulis Trachelospermi.* The drug consists of the dried foliferous stem of Chinese Starjasmine, *Trachelospermum jasminoides* (Lindl.) Lem. (family Apocynaceae). It is used as antirheumatic and antiarthritic agent for the treatment of rheumatalgia of joints and muscles, difficulty in bending and stretching of limbs.

白花蛇 [báihuāshé]
When this is prescribed, 蘄蛇 or 金錢白花蛇 may be supplied.

蘄蛇 [qíshé]
Long-noded Pit Viper; *Agkistrodon.* The drug consists of the dried body of *Agkistrodon acutus* (Guenther) (family Crotalidae). It is used as (1) antirheumatic for chronic and stubborn rheumatalgia and (2) anticonvulsive for hemiplegia, convulsion and epilepsy.

金錢白花蛇 [jīnqiánbáihuāshé]
Multibanded Krait; *Bungarus Parvus.* The drug consists of the dried body of the young snake, *Bungarus multicinctus* Blyth (family Elapidae). It is used similarly as 蘄蛇 [qíshé]

烏梢蛇 [wūshāoshé]
Black-tailed Snake; *Zaocys.* The drug consists of the dried body of *Zaocys dhumnades* (Cantor) (family Colubridae). It is used as antirheumatic for severe cases of rheumatalgia and urticaria.

五加皮 [wǔjiāpí]
Acanthopanax Bark; *Cortex Acanthopanacis Radicis.* The drug consists of the dried root bark of *Acanthopanax gracilistylus* W. W. Smith (family Araliaceae). It is used as (1) antirheumatic for the treatment of rheumatic arthritis and (2) diuretic for the treatment of edema and oliguria.

海桐皮 [hǎitóngpí]

Erythrina Bark, Coral-bean Bark; *Cortex Erythrinae*. The drug consists of the dried bark of *Erythrina variegata*. L. var. *orientalis* (L.) Merr. or *Erythrina arborescens* Roxb. (family Leguminosae). It is used as antirheumatic agent for the treatment of rheumatalgia, and also externally for neurodermatitis and chronic eczema.

絲瓜絡 [sīguāluò]

Vegetable Sponge; *Retinervus Luffae Fructus*. The drug consists of the dried skeleton (vascular bundles) of the mature towel gourd, *Luffa cylindrica* (L.) Roem. (family Cucurbitaceae). It is used as antiinflammatory and antirheumatic agent for the treatment of rheumatism and arthritis. It is also used as diuretic.

伸筋草 [shēnjīncǎo]

Club-moss, *Herba Lycopodii*. The drug consists of the dried Common Clubmoss, *Lycopodium clavatum* L. (family Lycopodiaceae). It is used as antirheumatic agent and to clear out channels and collaterals for the treatment of rheumatic arthritis and difficulty in bending and stretching of the body and limbs after hemiplegia.

老鸛草 [lǎoguàncǎo]

Erodium (Heronbill) or Geranium, *Herba Erodii seu Geranii*. The drug consists of the dried aerial parts of *Erodium stephanianum* Willd. or *Geranium wilfordii* Maxim. (family Geraniaceae). It is used as antirheumatic and circulation-promoting agent for the treatment of acute and chronic rheumatalgia; also used as detoxicant for enteritis and dysentery.

接骨木 [jiēgǔmù]

Elder Stem and Leaf; *Caulis et Folium Sambuci*. The drug consists of the dried stem and leaves of *Sambucus williamsii* Hance and related species (family Caprifoliaceae). It is used as antirheumatic and circulation-promoting agent for the treatment of rheumatalgia and pain due to injuries.

蠶砂 [cánshā]

Silkworm Excrement; *Excrementum Bombycis*. The drug consists of the dried excrement of healthy silkworm, *Bombyx mori* L. (family Bombycidae). It is used to dispel wind and dampness for the treatment of rheumatic pain and swelling and urticaria.

173

臭梧桐葉 [chòuwútóngyè]

Glorybower Leaf; *Folium Clerodendri Trichotomi.* The drug consists of the dried leaf of Harlequin Glorybower, *Clerodendrum trichotomum* Thunb. (family Verbenaceae). It is used as antirheumatic and antihypertensive agent for the treatment of rheumatism and hypertension.

穿山龍 [chuānshānlóng]; 穿地龍 [chuāndìlóng]

Japanese Dioscorea Rhizome; *Rhizoma Dioscoreae Nipponicae.* The drug consists of the dried rhizome of *Dioscorea nipponica* Makino (family Dioscoreaceae). It is used as antirheumatic and analgesic agent for the treatment of rheumatalgia, numbness of limbs and sprain of body and limbs.

徐長卿 [xúchángqīng]

Paniculate Swallowwort Root; *Radix Cynanchi Paniculati.* The drug consists of the dried root and rhizome of *Cynanchum paniculatum* (Bge.) Kitag. (family Asclepiadaceae). It is used (1) as antirheumatic and analgesic agent for the treatment of rheumatalgia, toothache and abdominal pain; (2) as detoxicant and antiphlogistic for snake bites and insect stings.

青風藤 [qīngfēngténg]

Orientvine; *Caulis Sinomenii.* The drug consists of the dried stem of Orientvine, *Sinomenium acutum* (Thunb.) Rehd. et Wils. or *Sinomenium acutum* var. *cinereum* Rehd. et Wils. (family Menispermaceae). It is used as antirheumatic and analgesic agent for the treatment of rheumatic arthritis, articular swelling and pain.

香加皮 [xiāngjiāpí]

Silkvine Bark; *Cortex Periplocae Radicis.* The drug consists of the dried root bark of Chinese Silkvine, *Periploca sepium* Bge. (family Asclepiadaceae). It is used as (1) antirheumatic for rheumatic arthritis; (2) cardiotonic and diuretic for cardiac edema.

防己 [fángjǐ]; 粉防己 [fěnfángjǐ]

Tetrandra Root; *Radix Stephaniae Tetrandrae.* The drug consists of the dried tuberous root of *Stephania tetrandra* S. Moore (family Menispermaceae). It is used as antirheumatic, analgesic and diuretic for the treatment of rheumatic arthritis, edema and oliguria.

溫寒藥
Drugs for Dispelling Internal Cold

附子 ［fùzǐ］

Prepared Aconite Root; *Radix Aconiti Praeparata.* The drug consists of the prepared root of *Aconitum carmichaeli* Debx. (family Ranunculaceae). It is used (1) as cardiotonic to restore the vital function of the *heart* and the *kidney* for the treatment of collapse and shock; (2) to relieve pain by dispelling coldness for the treatment of cold sensation of patients with chronic diseases, gastralgia, rheumatalgia with aversion to cold; and (3) for the treatment of edema, diarrhea, etc., due to hypofunction of the *kidney* and *spleen.*

肉桂 ［róuguì］

Cinnamon Bark, Cassia Bark; *Cortex Cinnamomi.* The drug consists of the dried barks of *Cinnamomum cassia* Presl. (family Lauraceae). It is used (1) to warm up Yang (vital function) of the *kidney* for the treatment of chronic diarrhea with coldness of the limbs, oliguria and edema due to hypofunction of the *kidney;* (2) to relieve pain by dispelling cold for the treatment of gastro-in-testinal pain due to cold.

乾薑 ［gānjiāng］

Dried Ginger; *Rhizoma Zingiberis.* The drug consists of the dried rhizome of Common ginger, *Zingiber officinale* (Willd.) Rosc. (family Zingiberaceae). It is used (1) to warm up the *stomach* and the *spleen* for the treatment of nausea, vomiting, abdominal pain and diarrhea; (2) to warm up the *lung* for chronic bronchitis with thin, white and foamy phlegm.

高良薑 ［gāoliángjiāng］

Galangal Rhizome; Lesser galangal; *Rhizoma Alpiniae officinarum; Rhizoma Galangae.* The drug consists of the dried rhizome of *Alpinia officinarum* Hance (family Zingiberaceae). It is used to warm up the *stomach* for the treatment of gastralgia due to cold in the *stomach.*

花椒 ［huājiāo］; 川椒 ［chuānjiāo］

Prickly-ash Peel; *Pericarpium Zanthoxyli.* The drug consists of the dried pericarp of Chinese Prickly-ash. *Zanthoxylum schinifolium* Sieb.

et Zucc. or Bunge's Prickly-ash, *Zanthoxylum bungeanum* Maxim. (family Rutaceae). It is used (1) to invigorate the vital function of the *stomach* by dispelling cold for the treatment of gastralgia and dyspepsia due to cold, and (2) as ascaricide.

吴茱萸〔wúzhūyú〕

Evodia Fruit; *Fructus Evodiae.* The drug consists of the dried fruit of *Evodia rutaecarpa* (Juss.) Benth. var. *officinalis* (Dode) Huang or *Evodia rutaecarpa* (Juss.) Henth. var. *bodinieri* (Dode) Huang (family Rutaceae). It is used to warm up the stomach and relieve pain for the treatment of gastralgia, abdominal pain, acid regurgitation and vomiting.

丁香〔dīngxiāng〕

Cloves; *Flos Caryophylli.* The drug consists of the dried flower-bud of *Eugenia caryophyllata* Thunb. (family Myrtaceae). It is used to warm up the *stomach* and relieve hiccup due to cold in the *stomach.*

小茴香〔xiǎohuíxiāng〕

Fennel Fruit; *Fructus Foeniculi.* The drug consists of the dried fruits of Common Fennel, *Foeniculum vulgare* Mill. (family Umbelliferae). It is used to dispel cold, regulate the flow of vital energy and relieve pain for the treatment of cold and pain in the lower abdomen, distension and pain of the testis.

艾叶〔àiyè〕

Argyi Leaf; Chinese Mugwort Leaf; *Folium Artemisiae Argyi.* The drug consists of the dried leaves of *Artemisia argyi* Levl. et Vant. (family Compositae). It is used to warm up the uterus and stop bleeding for the treatment of functional bleeding of the uterus, sterility and dysmenorrhea.

川乌〔chuānwū〕

Sichuan Aconite Root; *Radix Aconiti.* The drug consists of the dried parent root of *Aconitum carmichaeli* Debx. (family Ranunculaceae). It is used to dispel cold and wind and to relieve pain for the treatment of serious rheumatalgia, cold and pain in the abdomen. For internal use, the prepared root is usually employed.

草乌〔cǎowū〕

Wild Aconite Root; *Radix Aconiti Kusnezoffii.* The drug consists of the dried tuberous root of *Aconitum kusnezoffii* Reichb. (family

Ranunculaceae). It is used similarly as 川烏 , but the dose is usually much smaller.

蓽撥 [bìbō]

Long Pepper; *Fructus Piperis Longi.* The drug consists of the dried fruit-spike of Long Pepper, *Piper longum* L. (family Piperaceae). It is used to warm up the *stomach* for the treatment of cold and pain in the stomach.

芳香化濕藥
Drugs with Fragrant Odour
for Resolving Dampness

廣藿香 [guǎnghuòxiāng]

Cablin Pachouli; *Herba Pogostemonis.* The drug consists of the dried aerial parts of *Pogostemon cablin* (Blanco) Benth. (family Labiatae). It is used as 藿香 [huòxiāng].

藿香 [huòxiāng]; 土藿香 [tǔhuòxiāng]

Agastache, Wrinkled Giant-hyssop; *Herba Agastachis.* The drug consists of the dried aerial parts of *Agastache rugosus* (Fisch. et Mey.) O. Ktze. (family Labiatae). It is used to (1) dispel summer heat and dampness for the treatment of acute gastro-enteritis in summer; (2) as stomachic and antiemetic for nausea, vomiting poor appetite and diarrhea due to accumulation of dampness.

佩蘭 [pèilán]

Eupatorium; *Herba Eupatorii.* The drug consists of the aerial parts of *Eupatorium fortunei* Turcz. (family Compositae). It is used as stomachic and antiemetic agent for the treatment of poor appetite and gastro-intestinal fullness due to accumulation of dampness.

蒼朮 [cāngzhù]

Atractylodes Rhizome; *Rhizoma Atractylodis.* The drug consists of the dried rhizome of *Atractylodes lancea* (Thunb.) DC. or *Atractylodes chinensis* (DC.) Koidz. (family Compositae). It is used as stomachic and antirheumatic by drying dampness for the treatment of dyspepsia due to heavy dampness, rheumatic arthritis, and also for night blindness.

白豆蔻仁 [bái dòukòurén]; 白蔻仁 [báikòurén]

Round Cardamom Seed; *Semen Cardamomi Rotundi.* The drug consists of the dried seeds of *Amomum cardamomum* L. (family Zingiberaceae). It is used as stomach-warming and carminative agent for the treatment of gastro-intestinal fullness, nausea, vomiting, with white and slippery coat of tongue due to cold and dampness in the *spleen* and *stomach.*

砂仁 [shārén]

Amomum Fruit; *Fructus Amomi.* The drug consists of the dried fruit of *Amomum villosum* Lour. or *Amomum longiligulare* T. L. Wu (family Zingiberaceae). It is used as antidiarrhetic by warming up the *spleen* for the treatment of chronic diarrhea, and to prevent miscarriage in threatened abortion.

草豆蔻 [cǎo dòukòu]

Katsumadai Seed; *Semen Alpiniae katsumadai.* The drug consists of the dried seeds of *Alpinia katsumadai* Hayata (family Zingiberaceae). It is used (1) as stomachic by promoting the function of *spleen* and drying dampness for the treatment of poor appetite; (2) as antiemetic agent by warming up the *stomach* for the treatment of gastralgia and vomiting.

草果 [cǎoguǒ]

Tsaoko; *Fructus Tsaoko.* The drug consists of the dried fruits of *Amomum tsao-ko* Crevost et Lemaire (family Zigiberaceae). It is used to dry dampness and warm up *stomach* for gastro-intestinal fullness and pain, or vomiting. It is also used for the treatment of malaria.

利尿逐水藥
Diuretics and Hydragogues

利尿滲濕藥 Diuretics

茯苓 [fúlíng]

Fu-ling, Poria, Tuckahoe; *Poria.* The drug consists of the dried sclerotium of the fungus, *Poria cocos* (Schw.) Wolf (family Polyporaceae). It is used as (1) diuretic for dropsy and oliguria, and (2) stomachic and sedative for poor appetite, palpitation and insomnia.

豬苓 [zhūlíng]

Zhu-ling, Umbellate Pore-fungus; *Polyporus Umbellatus.* The drug consists the dried sclerotium of the fungus, *Polyporus umbellatus* (Pers.) Fries (family Polyporaceae). It is used as diuretic for visceral dropsy, edema and oliguria.

澤瀉 [zéxiè]

Alismatis Rhizome, Water-plantain Tuber; *Rhizoma Alismatis.* The drug consists of the dried tuber of Oriental Water-plantain, *Alisma orientalis* (Sam.) Juzep. (family Alismaceae). It is used (1) as diuretic for oliguria and edema, also (2) for acute diarrhea, (3) for reducing blood cholesterol level, and (4) for the treatment of fatty liver.

車前子 [chēqiánzǐ]

Plantain Seed; *Semen Plantaginis.* The drug consists of the seeds of Asiatic Plantain, *Plantago asiatica* L. or *Plantago depressa* Willd. (family Plantaginaceae). It is used as (1) diuretic and antidiarrhetic for watery diarrhea, edema and oliguria, (2) anti-inflammatory for infection of the urinary system, and (3) antitussive and expectorant for coughs with profuse phlegm.

車前草 [chēqiáncǎo]

Plantain Herb; *Herba Plantaginis.* The drug consists of the dried entire plant of Asiatic Plantain, *Plantago asiatica* L. or *Plantago depressa* Willd. (family Plantaginaceae). It is used as (1) diuretic for edema and oliguria, and (2) antimicrobial for furuncles, carbuncles, acute dysentery and acute infections of the lung and urinary system.

滑石 [huáshí]

Talc; *Talcum.* It is a very soft mineral composed mainly of hydrous magnesium silicate. It is used as diuretic and to clear up summer damp-heat for the treatment of acute diseases due to summer heat, acute enteritis, watery diarrhea, oliguria and infections of the urinary system.

薏苡仁 [yìyǐrén]

Coix Seed, Job's-tears Seed; *Semen Coicis.* The drug consists of the dried seeds obtained by removing the hard husk of the fruit of *Coix lacryma-jobi* L. var. *ma-yuen* (Roman.) Stapf (family Graminae). It is used (1) to improve the function of the *spleen* and dispel damp-ness for the treatment of diarrhea due to weakness of the *spleen*, (2) to eliminate inflammation and discharge pus for the treatment of abscess of the lung and acute appendicitis, and (3) as anti-cancer agent.

冬瓜皮 [dōngguāpí]

Benincasa Peel, Chinese Wax-gourd Peel; *Exocarpium Benincasae.*
The drug consists of the dried exocarp of *Benincasa hispida* (Thunb.)
Cogn. (family Cucurbitaceae). It is used as febrifuge and diuretic for
the treatment of oliguria and edema.

大腹皮 [dàfǔpí]

Areca Peel; *Pericarpium Arecae.* The drug consists of the dried pericarp of Betel Palm, *Areca catechu* L. (family Palmae). It is used as diuretic and carminative for the treatment of abdominal distension and
edema.

木通 [mùtōng]

When this is prescribed, either 川木通 or 關木通 may be supplied.

川木通 [chuānmùtōng]

Sichuan Clematis Stem; *Caulis Clematidis Armandii.* The drug consists of the dried lianoid stem of *Clematis armandii* Franch. or *Clematis
montana* Buch.-Ham. (family Ranunculaceae). It is used (1) as anti-
inflammatory and diuretic for acute infections of the urinary system,
and (2) as emmenagogue and galactagogue for amenorrhea and scanty
lactation.

關木通 [guānmùtōng]

Manshurian Aristolochia Stem; *Caulis Aristolochiae Manshuriensis.*
The drug consists of the dried stem of *Aristolochia manshuriensis* Kom.
(family Aristolochiaceae). Its uses are the same as that of 川木通 .

通草 [tōngcǎo]

Ricepaper Pith; *Medulla Tetrapanacis.* The drug consists of the pith
of Ricepaper plant, *Tetrapanax papyriferus* (Hook.) K. Koch (family
Araliaceae). It is used as febrifuge and diuretic for oliguria with signs of
heat, and as galactagogue for scanty lactation.

萹蓄 [biǎnxū]

Common Knot-grass; *Herba Polygoni Avicularis.* The drug consists
of the dried aerial parts of *Polygonum aviculare* L. (family Polygonaceae). It is used as diuretic and to eliminate damp-heat for acute urinary
infection, burning pain of the urethera (urethritis), also for the treatment of jaundice and skin infections.

瞿麥 [qūmài]

Pink; *Herba Dianthi*. The drug consists of the dried aerial parts of Fringed Pink, *Dianthus superbus* L. or Chinese Pink, *Dianthus chinensis* L. (family Caryophyllaceae). It is used as diuretic and to eliminate damp-heat for the treatment of acute urinary infections and hematuria.

冬葵子 [dōngkuízǐ]
Abutilon Seeds; *Semen Abutili*. The drug consists of the dried seeds of *Abutilon theophrasti* Medic. (family Malvaceae). It is used to eliminate damp-heat, as detoxicant and lactogenic for the treatment of urinary infections, oliguria, edema of pregnancy and mastitis, also for constipation and calculi of urinary tract.

萆薢 [bìxiè]
When this is prescribed, either 綿萆薢 or 粉萆薢 may be supplied.

綿萆薢 [mián bìxiè]
Seven-lobed Yam; *Rhizoma Dioscoreae Septemlobae*. The drug consists of the dried rhizome of *Dioscorea septemloba* Thunb. or *Dioscorea futschauensis* Uline (family Dioscoreaceae). It is used (1) to eliminate damp-turbidity for chyluria and infections of the urinary system with turbid urine and (2) as antirheumatic for rheumatic arthritis.

粉萆薢 [fěn bìxiè]
Hypoglauca Yam; *Rhizoma Dioscoreae Hypoglaucae*. The drug consists of the dried rhizome of *Dioscorea hypoglauca* Palib. (family Dioscoreaceae). Its uses are the same as that of 綿萆薢 .

地膚子 [dìfūzǐ]
Broom Cypress Fruit; *Fructus Kochiae*. The drug consists of the dried fruit of *Kochia scoparia* (L.) Schrad. (family Chenopodiaceae). It is used to eliminate damp-heat, as diuretic and antipruritic for pruritus, urticaria, eczema, and acute infections of the urinary system and acute nephritis.

金錢草 [jīnqiáncǎo]
Lysimachia; *Herba Lysimachiae*. The drug consists of the dried entire plant of *Lysimachia christinae* Hance (family Primulaceae). It is used as febrifuge, cholagogue, lithagogue and diuretic for the treatment of acute icteric hepatitis, calculi of the biliary and urinary tracts.

海金沙 [hǎijīnshā]
Lygodium Spores, Japanese Fern Spores; *Spora Lygodii*. The drug

consists of the spores of Japanese fern, *Lygodium japonicum* (Thunb.) Sw. (family Schizaeaceae). It is used to eliminate damp-heat and as lithagogue for the treatment of acute infections of urinary system and calculi of the urinary tract.

赤小豆 [chìxiǎodòu]

Phaseolus Seeds, Adsuki Bean; *Semen Phaseoli.* The drug consists of the dried seeds of *Phaseolus angularis* Wight or *Phaseolus calcalatus* Roxb. (family Leguminosae). It is used as (1) diuretic for edema and oliguria; (2) to detoxicate and dispel pus for suppurative infections of the skin.

石韦 [shí wěi]

Pyrrosia Leaf; *Folium Pyrrosiae.* The drug consists of the dried leaf of *Pyrrosia sheareri* (Bak.) Ching, *Pyrrosia lingua (Thunb.)* Farwell or *Pyrrosia petiolosa* (Christ) Ching (family Polypodiaceae). It is used (1) as febrifuge, diuretic and lithagogue for acute infections of the urinary system, calculi of the urinary tract and also for nephritic albuminuria; (2) as antitussive and expectorant for chronic bronchitis with cough and profuse phlegm.

葫蘆 [húlú]; 抽葫蘆 [chōuhúlú]

Calabash Gourd; *Pericarpium Lagenariae.* The drug consists of the dried pericarps of *Lagenaria siceraria* (Molina) Standl. var. *depressa* (Ser.) Hara (family Cucurbitaceae). It is used as diuretic for severe edema and ascites.

螻蛄 [lóugū]

Mole Cricket; *Gryllotalpa .* The drug consists of the dried body of *Gryllotalpa africana* Palisot et Beaurois (family Gryllotalpidae). It is used as diuretic for severe edema, ascites and retention of urine.

路路通 [lùlùtōng]

Sweetgum Fruit; *Fructus Liquidambaris.* The drug consists of the dried strobile (cone) of *Liquidambar formosana* Hance (family Hamamelidaceae). It is used (1) as diuretic for edema and oliguria; (2) to clear out the channels and collaterals for the treatment of rheumatalgia and abnormal menstruation.

玉米鬚 [yùmǐxū]

Corn Stigma; *Stigma Maydis.* The drug consists of the dried styles

182

and stigmata of Indian Corn, *Zea mays* L. (family Gramineae). It is used as (1) diuretic for acute and chronic nephritic edema; (2) cholagogue for icteric hepatitis, cholecystitis, etc.; (3) antihypertensive for hypertension.

燈芯草 [dēngxīncǎo]

Rush Pith; *Medulla Junci.* The drug consists of the dried pith of Common Rush, *Juncus effusus* L. (family Juncaceae). It is used as diuretic and febrifuge for the treatment of infections of urinary system.

逐水藥 **Hydragogues or Drastic Purgatives**

牽牛子 [qiānniúzǐ]

Pharbitis Seed; *Semen Pharbitidis.* The drug consists of the dried seeds of *Pharbitis nil* (L.) Choisy or *Pharbitis purpurea* (L.) Voigt (family Convolvulaceae). It is used as hydragogue for edema, oliguria and as anthelmintic for ascariasis.

商陸 [shānglù]

Phytolacca Root, Poke Root, *Radix Phytolaccae.* The drug consists of the dried root of Indian Pokeberry, *Phytolacca acinosa* Roxb. or American Pokeberry, *Phytolacca americana* L. (family Phytolaccaceae). It is used as diuretic and hydragogue for edema and oliguria.

巴豆 [bādòu]

Croton Seed; *Semen Crotonis.* The drug consists of the dried seed of Purging Croton, *Croton tiglium* L. (family Euphorbiaceae). It is used as a drastic purgative for the treatment of constipation with gastro-intestinal distension and pain due to accumulation of cold and stagnation of food; also used externally for furuncles, dermatitis and warts.

甘遂 [gānsuì]

Kansui Root; *Radix Euphorbiae Kansui.* The drug consists of the dried tuberous root of *Euphorbia kansui* T.N. Liou ex T.P. Wang (family Euphorbiaceae). It is used as hydragogue and purgative for hydrothorax and ascites.

芫花 [yuánhuā]

Genkwa Flower; *Flos Genkwa.* The drug consists of the dried flower-bud of Lilac Daphne, *Daphne genkwa* Sieb. et Zucc. (family Thymelaeaceae). It is used as hydragogue and purgative for severe edema of hydrothorax, ascites.

黄芫花 [huángyuánhuā]

Chamaedaphne Leaf and Flower, Yellow Genkwa Leaf and Flower; *Folium et Flos Wikstroemiae Chamaedaphnis.* The drug consists of the leaves and flower-buds of *Wikstroemia chamaedaphne* Meisn. (family Thymelaeaceae). It is used similarly as 芫花. The leaf is effective for certain mental disorders.

京大戟 [jīngdàjǐ]; 龍虎草 [lónghǔcǎo]

Reking Spurge Root; *Radix Euphorbiae Pekinensis.* The drug consists of the dried roots of *Euphorbia pekinensis* Rupr. (family Euphorbiaceae). It is used as a hydragogue and purgative for severe edema, hydro-thorax and ascites; used externally for scrofula.

狼毒 [lángdú]

Ebracteolate Euphorbia Root; *Radix Euphorbiae Ebracteolatae.* The drug consists of the dried roots of *Euphorbia ebracteolata* Hayata or *Euphorbia fischeriana* Steud. (family Euphorbiaceae). It is used as drastic purgative to remove stagnated food, and as anthelmintic for the treatment of intestinal parasites; also used for scrofula.

理氣藥

Carminatives or Drugs for Regulating the Flow of Vital Energy

陳皮 [chénpí]

Tangerine Peel; *Pericarpium Citri Reticulatae.* The drug consists of the dried pericarp of Tangerine (Mandarin Orange), *Citrus reticulata* Blanco (family Rutaceae). It is used as carminative, stomachic and expectorant for the treatment of gastro-intestinal distension, vomiting, hiccup and cough with profuse phlegm.

青皮 [qīngpí]

Green Tangerine Peel, *Pericarpium Citri Reticulatae Viride.* The drug consists of the dried green exocarp of Mandarin Orange, *Citrus reticulata* Blanco (family Rutaceae). It is used as carminative to restore the normal flow of vital energy in the *liver* for the treatment of pain in the chest and hypochondrium, gastro-intestinal distension, swelling of the liver and spleen, etc.

桔核 [júhé]

Tangerine Seed; *Semen Citri Reticulatae.* The drug consists of the dried seeds of *Citrus reticulata* Blanco (family Rutaceae). It is used as carminative to promote the flow of vital energy in the *liver* for the treatment of mastitis and swelling and pain of the testis.

桔紅 [júhóng]

Pummelo Peel; *Exocarpium Citri Grandis.* The drug consists of the dried exocarps of Pummelo (Shaddock), *Citrus grandis* Osbeck var. *tomentosa* Hort. or *Citrus grandis* Osbeck (family Rutaceae). It is used as 陳皮 with stronger action.

枳實 [zhǐshí]

Immature Bitter Orange; *Fructus Aurantii Immaturus.* The drug consists of the dried immature fruits of *Citrus aurantium* L. (family Rutaceae). It is used as carminative to disperse the stagnated vital energy and remove the stagnated food in the gastro-intestinal tract for the treatment of dyspepsia, constipation and abdominal distension due to food stagnation; large dose for visceroptosis.

枳殼 [zhǐqiào]

Bitter Orange; *Fructus Aurantii.* The drug consists of the dried fruits of *Citrus aurantium* L. (family Rutaceae). The endocarp and seeds should be removed before use. It is used as 枳實 with milder effect.

厚朴 [hòupò]; 川朴 [chuān pò]

Magnolia Bark; *Cortex Magnoliae Officinalis.* The drug consists of the dried barks of *Magnolia officinalis* Rehd. et Wils. or *Magnolia officinalis* var. *biloba* Rehd. et Wils. (family Magnoliaceae). It is used (1) to promote the flow of vital energy for the treatment of gastro-intestinal distension with pain due to food stagnation; (2) to invigorate the function of the *spleen* by drying up the dampness for the treatment of vomiting, diarrhea due to dyspepsia, and (3) to relieve cough and asthmatic conditions with profuse phlegm.

木香 [mùxiāng]

Aucklandia Root, Costus Root; *Radix Aucklandiae.* The drug consists of the dried root of *Aucklandia lappa* Decne. (*Saussurea* *lappa* Clarke) (family Compositae). It is used as carminative, antispasmodic and anodyne for the treatment of abdominal distension with pain and tenesmus due to stagnation of vital energy in the gastrointestinal tract, cholecystalgia.

香附 [xiāngfù]
Cyperus Tuber, Flatsedge Tuber; *Rhizoma Cyperi.* The drug consists of the dried tubers of Nutgrass Flatsedge, *Cyperus rotundus* L. (family Cyperaceae). It is used as carminative, antispasmodic and anodyne for the treatment of chest and abdominal distension with pain, menorrhalgia and abnormal menstruation.

烏藥 [wūyào]
Lindera Root, Spicebush Root; *Radix Linderae.* The drug consists of the dried tuberous roots of *Lindera strychnifolia* (Sieb. et Zucc.) Vill. (family Lauraceae). It is used (1) as carminative and anodyne by dispelling cold for the treatment of distension with pain of the lower abdomen due to cold; (2) to warm up the *kidney* to stop urorrhagia for the treatment of frequent micturition.

香櫞 [xiāngyuán]
Citron; *Fructus Citri.* The drug consists of the dried fruit of *Citrus medica* L. or *Citrus wilsonii* Tanaka (family Rutaceae). It is used as carminative for the treatment of gastric distension with pain and fullness sensation in the chest.

佛手 [fúshǒu]
Finger Citron; *Fructus Citri Sarcodactylis.* The drug consists of the dried fruit of *Citrus medica* L. var. *sarcodactylis* Swingle (family Rutaceae). It is used as carminative and stomachic for the treatment of fullness sensation in the chest and stomach, gastralgia, eructation and poor appetite.

薤白 [xièbái]
Macrostem Onion; *Bulbus Allii Macrostemi.* The drug consists of the dried bulb of *Allium macrostemon* Bge. (family Liliaceae). It is used as carminative (1) to warm up (invigorate) and regulate the vital energy in the chest for the treatment of stuffiness sensation and pain in the chest, and angina pectoris. It is also used for the treatment of diarrhea and tenesmus in cases of dysentery.

186

甘松 [gānsōng]

Nardostachys Rhizome, Spikenard Rhizome; *Rhizoma Nardostachyos*. The drug consists of the dried rhizome and root of *Nardostachys chinensis* Batal. or *Nardostachys jatamansi* DC. (family Valerianaceae). It is used as carminative for the treatment of gastro-intestinal distension with pain, and diarrhea.

檀香 [tán xiāng]

Sandal Wood; *Lignum Santali, Lignum Santali Albi*. The drug consists of the heart-wood of the Yellow Sandalwood Tree, *Santalum album* L. (family Santalaceae). It is used as carminative to warm up the *stomach* and to relieve pain for the treatment of gastro-intestinal distension with pain, and angina pectoris.

降香 [jiàngxiāng]

Dalbergia Wood; *Lignum Dalbergiae Odoriferae*. The drug consists of the dried heart-wood of *Dalbergia odorifera* T. Chen (family Leguminosae). It is used (1) as carminative and anodyne for the treatment of angina pectoris, gastro-intestinal distension with pain; (2) to promote the blood circulation and remove blood stasis for the treatment of various swellings and pains due to blood stasis.

沉香 [chénxiāng]

Eagle Wood; *Lignum Aquilariae Resinatum*. The drug consists of the resinous wood of *Aquilaris sinensis* (Lour.) Gilg. (family Thymelaeaceae). It is used as carminative and anodyne and anti-asthmatic by keeping the air or vital energy going downward for the treatment of thoraco-abdominal distension with pain, vomiting and hiccoughing, bronchitic asthma and pulmonary emphysema.

梭羅子 [suōluózǐ]

Horse-chestnut; *Semen Aesculi*. The drug consists of the dried seeds of *Aesculus chinensis* Bge. or *Aesculus wilsonii* Rehd. (family Hippocastanaceae). It is used as carminative for the treatment of gastro-intestinal distension with pain and stuffiness sensation, especially for gastralgia.

荔枝核 [lìzhīhé]

Litchi Seed, Lychee Seed, *Semen Litchi*. The drug consists of the dried seeds of *Litchi chinensis* Soon. (family Sapindaceae). It is used

187

as carminative and anodyne by dispersing cold for the treatment of lower abdominal distension with pain, swelling and pain of the testis.

梅花 [méihuā]; 綠萼梅 [lü'èméi]
Mume Flower; Japanese Apricot Flower; *Flos Mume.* The drug consists of the dried flowers of *Prunus mume* (Sieb.) Zieb. et Zucc. (family Rosaceae). It is used as carminative to restore the depressed *liver* for the treatment of stuffiness sensation in the chest, poor appetite and globus hystericus.

九香蟲 [jiuxiāngchóng]
Aspongopus, Stink-bug; *Aspongopus.* The drug consists of the dried body of *Aspongopus chinensis* Dallas (family Pentatomidae). It is used as carminative to regulate the flow of vital energy and restore the depressed *liver* and to relieve pain for the treatment of distension and pain at the sides of the chest.

柿蒂 [shìdì]
Kaki Calyx, Persimmon Calyx; *Calyx Kaki.* The drug consists of the dried, persistent calyx of *Diospyros kaki* L. f. (family Ebenaceae). It is used as carminative to stop hiccup.

川楝子 [chuānliànzi]
Sichuan Chinaberry; *Fructus Meliae Toosendan.* The drug consists of the dried fruit of *Melia toosendan* Sieb. et Zucc. (family Meliaceae). It is used as (1) carminative and anodyne for relieving pain at the sides of the chest, gastro-abdominal pain and pain in the lower abdominal region; (2) anthelmintic for ascariasis and enterobiasis.

理血藥
Drugs for Regulating Blood Conditions

止血藥 Hemostatics
仙鶴草 [xiānhècǎo]
Agrimony; *Herba Agrimoniae.* The drug consists of the dried aerial parts of Hairvein Agrimony, *Agrimonia pilosa* Ledeb. (family Rosaceae). It is used as an astringent hemostatic for the treatment of all kinds of bleeding.

三七 [sānqī]

Notoginseng; *Radix Notoginseng.* The drug consists of the dried root of *Panax notoginseng* (Burk.) F.H. Chen (family Araliaceae). It is used as hemostatic and anodyne by eliminating blood stasis and reducing swellings for the treatment of swellings with pain due to contused wounds and soft tissue injuries and all kinds of bleeding; also used for angina pectoris.

白及 [báijí]

Bletilla Tuber; *Rhizoma Bletillae.* The drug consists of the dried tuber of *Bletilla striata* (Thunb.) Reichb. f. (family Orchidaceae). It is used as hemostatic for the treatment of bleeding of the lung and stomach; to promote the recovery of wounds and relieve pain for the treatment of wounds, carbuncles, etc.

大薊 [dàjì]

Japanese Thistle; *Herba seu Radix Cirsii Japonici.* The drug consists of the dried aerial parts or root of *Cirsium japonicum* DC. (family Compositae). It is used as hemostatic for the treatment of vomiting blood and hematuria due to the presence of excessive heat in the blood; also used for skin infections and hypertension.

小薊 [xiǎojì]

Small Thistle; *Herba Cephalanoploris.* The drug consists of the dried aerial parts of *Cephalanoplos segetum* (Bge.) Kitam. or *Cephalanoplos setosum* (Willd.) Kitam. (family Compositae). It is used as hemostatic by removing evil heat from blood, chiefly for the treatment of bleeding of the urinary system; also used as antihypertensive.

茜草 [qiàncǎo]

Rubia Root, Madder Root; *Radix Rubiae.* The drug consists of the dried root and rhizome of Indian Madder, *Rubia cordifolia* L. (family Rubiaceae). It is used as hemostatic by eliminating blood stasis for the treatment of bleeding due to febrile diseases and functional bleeding of the uterus with symptom-complex of heat and blood-stasis.

地榆 [dì yú]

Sanguisorba Root, Burnet Root; *Radix Sanguisorbae.* The drug consists of the dried root of Garden Burnet. *Sanguisorba officinalis*

189

L. (family Rosaceae). It is used as astringent hemostatic and anti-diarrheal with the effect of eliminating evil heat from the blood for the treatment of bleeding due to peptic ulcers, hematuria, menorr-hagia, bloody stools, dysentery, etc.

槐花 [huáihuā]

Sophora Flower, Pagodatree Flower; *Flos Sophorae.* The drug consists of the dried flowers of Japanese Pagodatree, *Sophora japonica* L. (family Leguminosae). It is used as hemostatic by eliminating evil heat from blood, chiefly for the treatment of bleeding of hemorrhoids and bloody stools.

槐米 [huáimǐ]

Sophora Flower-bud, Pagodatree Flower-bud; *Flos Sophorae Immaturus.* The drug consists of the dried flower-bud of Japanese Pagodatree. *Sophora japonica* L. (family Leguminosae). It is used as 槐花 but nowadays it is chiefly used for the production of rutin.

槐角 [huáijiǎo]

Sophora Fruit, Pagodatree Fruit; *Fructus Sophorae.* The drug consists of the dried fruit of Japanese Pagodatree, *Sophora japonica* L. (family Leguminosae). It is used as 槐花 chiefly for the treatment of hemorrhoidal bleedings.

侧柏葉 [cèbǎiyè]

Biota Tops, Arborvitae Tops; *Cacumen Biotae.* The drug consists of the dried leafy twigs of *Biota orientalis* (L.) Endl. (family Cupressaceae). It is used as astringent hemostatic and to eliminate evil heat from blood for the treatment of spitting blood, nasal bleeding, bloody stool, hema-turia and functional bleeding of the uterus. It has also antimicrobial, antitussive, expectorant and anti-asthmatic effects for the treatment of chronic bronchitis.

白茅根 [báimáogēn]

Imperata Rhizome, Cogongrass Rhizome; *Rhizoma Imperatae.* The drug consists of the dried rhizomes of *Imperata cylindrica* Beauv. var. *major* (Nees) C. E. Hubb. (family Graminae). It is used as hemostatic and diuretic by eliminating evil heat from blood mainly for the treat-ment of nasal bleeding, hematuria and edema due to acute nephritis.

苧麻根 [zhùmágēn]

Boehmeria Root, Ramie Root; *Radix Boehmeriae*. The drug consists of the dried root of *Boehmeria nivea* (L.) Gaud. (family Urticaceae). It is used as hemostatic and to prevent miscarriage for the treatment of bleeding of threatened abortion and menorrhagia.

血餘炭 [xuèyútàn]

Carbonized Hair; *Crinis Carbonisatus*. It is used as hemostatic and to eliminate blood stasis for the treatment of all kinds of bleeding.

棕櫚炭 [zōnglǔtàn]

Carbonised Petiole of Windmill-palm; *Petiolus Trachycarpi Carbonisatus*. The drug consists of the carbonised petiole of Fortunes Windmill-palm, *Trachycarpus fortunei* H. Wendl. (family Palmae). It is used as astringent hemostatic, mainly for the treatment of blood sputum, nasal bleeding, bloody stool and menorrhagia.

花蕊石 [huāruìshí]

Ophicalcite; *Ophicalcitum*. The drug consists of a marble containing green serpentine. It is used as hemostatic and to eliminate blood stasis mainly for the treatment of blood sputum and vomiting blood. Powdered drug is used externally as hemostatic for incised wounds.

黃藥子 [huángyàozǐ]

Airpotato Yam; *Rhizoma Dioscoreae bulbiferae*. The drug consists of the dried rhizome of *Dioscorea bulbifera* L. (family Dioscoreaceae). It is used as hemostatic and to eliminate evil heat from blood and as a detoxicant for the treatment of various kinds of bleeding, boils and carbuncles, but nowadays mainly used for the treatment of tumors and goitres.

薺菜 [jìcài]

Capsella, Shepherd's Purse; *Herba Capsellae*. The drug consists of the dried entire plants of *Capsella bursa-pastoris* (L.) Medic. (family Cruciferae). It is used (1) as hemostatic and to eliminate evil heat from blood for the treatment of menorrhagia, post-partum hemorrhage and hematuria; (2) as antihypertensive and diuretic for the treatment of hypertension and nephritic edema.

瓦松 [wǎsōng]

Orostachys, Roof Stonecrop; *Herba Orostachyos*. The drug consists of the dried aerial parts of *Orostachys fimbriatus* (Turcz.) Berg. (family

Crassalaceae). It is used as hemostatic, mainly for bloody stool and vomiting blood; used externally for skin ulcers.

藕節 [ǒujié]

Lotus Node; *Nodus Nelumbinis Rhizomatis*. The drug consists of the dried nodes of the rhizomes of Hindu Lotus, *Nelumbo nucifera* Gaertn. (family Nymphaeaceae). It is used as hemostatic by eliminating evil heat from blood and to remove blood stasis for the treatment of nasal bleeding, hemoptysis, hematuria and functional bleeding of the uterus.

旱蓮草 [hànliáncǎo]; 墨旱蓮 [mòhànlián]

Eclipta; *Herba Ecliptae*. The drug consists of the aerial parts of *Eclipta prostrata* L. (family Compositae). It is used (1) as hemostatic by eliminating evil heat from blood for the treatment of bleeding due to the presence of excessive heat in blood; (2) as a tonic to nourish the *liver* and *kidney* for the treatment of diseases or symptoms due to the deficiency of vital essence of these organs such as tinnitus, prematurely greying hair and neurosis.

牛西西 [niúxīxī]

Patient Rumex Root; *Radix Rumecis Patientiae*. The drug consists of the dried root of *Rumex patientia* L. (family Polygonaceae). It is used as hemostatic by eliminating evil heat from blood and as a detoxicant for the treatment of thrombocytopenia, and all kinds of bleeding due to excessive heat in the blood.

活血化瘀藥 **Drugs for Invigorating Blood Circulation and Eliminating Blood-stasis**

川芎 [chuānxiōng]

Chuanxiong Rhizome; *Rhizoma Ligustici Chuanxiong*. The drug consists of the dried rhizome of *Ligusticum chuanxiong* Hort. (family Umbelliferae). It is used (1) to invigorate blood circulation and promote the flow of vital energy for the treatment of abnormal menstruation, dysmenorrhea, amenorrhea and coronary heart diseases; (2) to relieve pain for the treatment of headache and pain of the body due to wind and cold, and headache due to concussion of the brain.

赤芍 [chìsháo]

Red Peony Root; *Radix Paeoniae Rubra*. The drug consists of the dried root of *Paeonia lactiflora* Pall. *Paeonia obavata* Maxim. or *Paeonia veitchii* Lynch (family Ranunculaceae). It is used to remove stagnated blood and eliminate evil heat from blood for the treatment of pains due to blood-stasis, menorrhalgia, amenorrhea and acute inflammation with red swellings and pain.

紅花 [hónghuā]

Safflower; *Flos Carthami*. The drug consists of the dried flowers of *Carthamus tinctorius* L. (family Compositae). It is used to stimulate blood flow and relieve pain by removing stagnated blood for the treatment of amenorrhea, chest and abdominal pain, painful swellings due to bloodstasis, hepatomegaly and splenomegaly; also used for pain of traumatic wounds.

番紅花 [fānhónghuā]; 藏紅花 [zànghónghuā]

Saffron; *Stigma Croci, Crocus*. The drug consists of the dried stigmas and the top of the style of the saffron Crocus, *Crocus sativus* L. (family Iridaceae). It is used as 紅花 with stronger action.

桃仁 [táorén]

Peach Kernel, Peach Seed; *Semen Persicae*. The drug consists of the seeds of *Prunus persica* (L.) Batsch or *Prunus davidiana* (Carr.) Franch. (family Rosaceae). It is used (1) to eliminate blood stagnation for the treatment of amenorrhea with abdominal pain and traumatic pain due to blood stasis; (2) as aperient for the treatment of constipation of the aged and debilitated patients.

川牛膝 [chuānniúxī]

Cyathula Root; *Radix Cyathulae*. The drug consists of the dried root of *Cyathula officinalis* Kuan (family Amaranthaceae). It is used to promote the blood circulation by eliminating blood-stasis and facilitate the joints for the treatment of amenorrhea, hematuria and aching joints.

丹参 [dānshēn]

Red Sage Root; *Radix Salviae Miltiorrhizae*. The drug consists of the dried root and rhizome of *Salvia miltiorrhiza* Bge. (family Labiatae). It is used to promote blood circulation and to remove blood stasis for the treatment of dysmenorrhea, amenorrhea, abdominal masses due to stagnation of blood, carbuncles and ulcers; also used as a tranquilizer. It is now frequently used for the treatment of coronary heart disease.

鬱金 [yùjīn]

Curcuma Root; *Radix Curcumae.* The drug consists of the dried tuberous root of Aromatic Turmeric, *Curcuma aromatica* Salisb., Kwangsi Turmeric, *Curcuma kwangsiensis* S. Lee et C. F. Liang, Common Turmeric, *Curcuma longa* L. or Zedoary Turmeric, *Curcuma zedoaria* Rosc. (family Zingiberaceae). It is used (1) to relieve pain by regulating the circulation of vital energy for the treatment of pains in chest, abdomen or costal regions due to stagnation of vital energy and blood, such as the pain of liver area due to hepatitis ; (2) as a cholagogue for the treatment of hepatogenic jaundice.

薑黃 [jiānghuáng]

Turmeric; *Rhizoma Curcumae Longae.* The drug consists of the dried rhizomes of Common Turmeric, *Curcuma longa* L. (family Zingiberaceae). It is used to relieve pain by regulating the circulation of vital energy for the treatment of pains in the chest and abdomen and dysmenorrhea due to stagnation of vital energy and blood stasis.

鷄血藤 [jīxuèténg]

Spatholobus Stem; *Caulis Spatholobi.* The drug consists of the dried stems of *Spatholobus suberectus* Dunn (family Leguminosae). It is used to invigorate the blood circulation, to clear out the channels and collaterals and to nourish the blood for the treatment of abnormal menstruation due to deficiency of blood together with blood stasis, inflammation of peripheral blood vessels or thrombosis, numbness of the body and limbs. It is also effective for leucopenia induced by radiotherapy.

元胡 [yuánhú]; 延胡索 [yánhúsuǒ]

Corydalis Tuber; *Rhizoma Corydalis.* The drug consists of the dried tubers of *Corydalis turtschaninovii* Bess. f. *yanhusuo* Y. H. Chow et C. C. Hsu (family Papaveraceae). It is used to relieve pain by invigorating blood circulation and regulating the circulation of vital energy, frequently used for the treatment of all kinds of pain in the chest and abdomen. This drug possesses the effects of elevating the threshold of pain and relieving spastic pain; there is also a sedative effect.

五靈脂 [wǔlíngzhǐ]
Trogopterus Dung; *Faeces Trogopterorum.* The drug consists of the dried faeces of *Trogopterus xanthipes* Milne-Edwards (family Petauristidae). It is used to relieve pain by eliminating blood stasis mainly for the treatment of gastric and abdominal pain due to spasms of the smooth muscles and dysmenorrhea.

蒲黃 [pǔhuáng]
Cat-tail Pollen; *Pollen Typhae.* The drug consists of the pollen of *Typha angustifolia* L. or *Typha orientalis* Presl. (family Typhaceae). It is used to promote the circulation of blood and relieve pain by eliminating blood-stasis for the treatment of dysmenorrhea, postpartum abdominal pain and gastralgia due to blood-stasis. The carbonized drug is used as hemostatic for all kinds of bleeding.

穿山甲 [chuānshānjiǎ]
Pangolin Scales; *Squama Manitis.* The drug consists of the scales of the anteater, *Manis pentadactyla* L. (family Manidae). It is used (1) as emmenagogue and galactagogue for the treatment of amenorrhea and deficiency of lactation; (2) to reduce inflammation and dispel pus for the treatment of acute purulent inflammations.

皂角刺 [zàojiǎocì]
Honeylocust Thorn; *Spina Gleditsiae.* The drug consists of the thorns of Chinese Honeylocust, *Gleditsia sinensis* Lam. (family Leguminosae). It is used (1) to reduce inflammation and dispel pus for the treatment of acute purulent inflammations with the effect of promoting local rupture; (2) as antipruritic for the treatment of dermatopathies.

王不留行 [wángbùliúxíng]
Vaccaria Seed; Cow Soapwort Seed; *Semen Vaccariae.* The drug consists of the seeds of Cow-Soapwort (Cow Basil), *Vaccaria segetalis* (Neck.) Garcke (family Caryophyllaceae). It is used as emmenagogue and galactagogue for the treatment of amenorrhea and deficiency of lactation after child-birth. It is also used for the treatment of calculus formation in the urinary system.

水蛭 [shuǐzhì]
Leech; *Hirudo.* The drug consists of the dried body of *Whitmania pigra* Whitman, *Whitmania acranulata* Whitman or *Hirudo nipponica*

Whitman (family Hirudinidae). It is used to remove stagnated blood and to disperse swellings for the treatment of severe cases of blood-stasis, such as severe abdominal pain, amenorrhea and masses in abdomen, contused wounds, etc.

虻蟲 [méngchóng]

Gadfly; *Tabanus*. The drug consists of the dried female insect of *Tabanus bivittatus* Matsum. (family Tabanidae). It is used to remove stagnated blood and to disperse swellings for the treatment of severe cases of blood-stasis, such as amenorrhea and masses in abdomen.

土鱉蟲 [tǔbiēchóng]

Cockroach; *Eupolyphaga seu Steleophaga*. The drug consists of the dried body of *Eupolyphaga sinensis* Walk. or *Steleophaga plancyi* (Bol.) (family Corydiidae). It is used to relieve pain by removing stagnated blood for the treatment of hypochondriac pain due to hepatomegaly or splenomegaly, lumbago and sprain. It is also used for the treatment of amenorrhea, masses in abdomen, contused wounds, etc.

劉寄奴 [liújìnú]

Siphonostegia; *Herba Siphonostegiae*. The drug consists of the aerial parts of *Siphonostegia chinensts* Benth.(family Scrophulariaceae). It is used to relieve pain by removing stagnated blood for the treatment of abdominal pain due to blood-stasis and for painful swellings due to injury.

蘇木 [sūmù]

Sappan Wood; *Lignum Sappan*. The drug consists of the heart wood of *Caesalpinia sappan* L. (family Leguminosae). It is used to relieve pain by removing stagnated blood, mainly for the treatment of contused wounds and amenorrhea with abdominal pain.

益母草 [yìmǔcǎo]; 坤草 [kūncǎo]

Motherwort; *Herba Leonuri*. The drug consists of the dried aerial parts of *Leonurus heterophyllus* Sweet (family Labiatae). It is used to invigorate the blood circulation and to regulate the menstrual flow for the treatment of abnormal menstruation; it is also used as a diuretic for nephritic edema.

馬鞭草 [mǎbiāncǎo]

196

Vervain; *Herba Verbenae*. The drug consists of the dried aerial parts of Common Verbena (Vervain), *Verbena officinalis* L. (family Verbenaceae). It is used (1) to invigorate the blood circulation and to promote menstrual flow for the treatment of amenorrhea and dysmenorrhea; (2) as an antimalarial for the treatment of malarial splenomegaly; (3) as antipyretic and detoxicating agent for influenza.

鸭跖草 [yāzhícǎo]
Common Day-flower; *Herba Commelinae*. The drug consists of the dried aerial parts of *Commelina communis* L. (family Commelinaceae). It is used for relieving morbid thirst in febrile conditions, acute tonsillitis, sore-throat, enteritis, dysentery, furuncles and carbuncles. It is also used as a diuretic for relieving the edema due to nephritis or heart diseases.

三棱 [sānléng]
Burreed Tuber, *Rhizoma Sparganii*. The drug consists of the dried tubers of *Sparganium stoloniferum* Buch.-Ham.(family Sparganiaceae). It is used to remove stagnated blood and disintegrate mass for the treatment of dysmenorrhea, amenorrhea and masses in the abdomen.

莪术 [ézhú]
Zodoary; *Rhizoma Zedoariae*. The drug consists of the dried rhizome of Zedoary Turmeric, *Curcuma zedoaria* Rosc., Aromatic Turmeric, *Curcuma aromatica* Salisb. or Kwangsi Turmeric, *Curcuma kwangsiensis* S. Lee et C.F. Liang (family Zingiberaceae). It is used to relieve pain and invigorate blood circulation by removing bloodstasis for the treatment of chest pain, abdominal pain and masses, amenorrhea, etc. in severe cases of stagnation of vital energy and blood, also used as anticancer agent especially for cervical cancer of the uterus.

澤蘭 [zélán]
Bugleweed; *Herba Lycopi*. The drug consists of the dried aerial parts of *Lycopus lucidus* Turcz. var. *hirtus* Regel (family Labiatae). It is used to invigorate blood circulation and promote the menstrual flow for the treatment of abnormal menstruation and postpartum abdominal pain.

毛冬青 [máodōngqīng]

Pubescent Holly Root; *Radix Ilicis Pubescentis.* The drug consists of the dried root of Pubescent Holly, *Ilex pubescens* Hook. et Arn. (family Aquifoliaceae). It is used to invigorate blood circulation and clear the channels and collaterals for the treatment of Buerger's disease (presenile spontaneous gangrene), angina pectoris; (2) as antifebrile, detoxicant and anti-inflammatory agent for acute tonsillitis; (3) as antitussive and expectorant for acute bronchitis. It has a distinct effect of dilating coronary arteries.

乳香 ﹝rǔxiāng﹞

Frankincense; *Olibanum; Resina Olibani.* The drug consists of a gum-resin obtained from *Boswellia carterii* Birdwood and possibly other species of *Boswellia* (family Burseraceae). It is used to relieve pain and swelling by invigorating blood circulation for the treatment of pains due to blood-stasis, such as traumatic pain.

没藥 ﹝mòyào﹞

Myrrh; *Myrrha, Resina* Myrrhae. The drug consists of a gum-resin obtained from the stem of *Commphora molmol* Engler and probably other species (family Burseraceae). It is used to relieve pain and swelling for pains due to blood-stasis, such as traumatic pains.

自然銅 ﹝zìrántóng﹞

Pyrite; *Pyritum.* The drug consists of a brassy yellow mineral, iron disulphide, crystallising in the cubic system. It is used to set fractures and relieve pain by dispersing stagnated blood for the treatment of traumatic fracture and pain due to blood-stasis.

芳香開竅藥
Aromatic Stimulants

冰片 ﹝bīngpiàn﹞

Borneol; *Borneolum.* The drug consists of a crystalline organic compound, borneol, obtained synthetically or from natural sources. It is used (1) as an aromatic stimulant for the treatment of loss of consciousness and convulsions due to high fever; (2) as antifebrile and anodyne used externally for pharyngitis, tonsillitis, laryngitis, stomatitis, etc.

198

牛黄 [niúhuáng]

Ox Gallstone; *Calculus Bovis.* The drug is the gallstone of the Ox, *Bos taurus domesticus* Gmelin (family Bovidae). It is used as an antifebrile, detoxicant and anticonvulsive for the treatment of loss of consciousness, delirium, convulsions in acute febrile diseases, acute inflammation of the pharynx, larynx and mouth, and purulent inflammations of the skin.

石菖蒲 [shíchāngpǔ]

Grass-leaved Sweetflag Rhizome; *Rhizoma Acori Graminei.* The drug consists of the dried rhizomes of Grass-leaved Sweetflag, *Acorus gramineus* Soland. (family Araceae). It is used (1) as an aromatic stimulant and to remove the windphlegm for impaired consciousness, insanity, melancholia; (2) as a stomachic and carminative for poor appetite and gastro-intestinal distension.

蘇合香 [sūhéxiāng]

Storax; *Styrax, Styrax Liquidus.* The drug consists of a balsam obtained from the trunk of *Liquidamber orientalis* Miller (family Hamamelidaceae). It is used as an aromatic stimulant and to remove the wind-phlegm for loss of consciousness due to apoplexy. It is also used for angina pectoris.

麝香 [shèxiāng]

Musk; *Moschus.* The drug consists of the dried secretion obtained from the musk gland of the musk deers, *Muschus berezovskii* Flerov, *Moschus sifanicus* Przewalski or *Moschus moschiferus* L. (family Cervidae). It is used as a central nervous stimulant for the treatment of loss of consciousness due to high fever in acute infectious disease and apoplexy; (2) to invigorate the blood circulation and reduce inflammation for the treatment of painful swellings of boils, furuncles and carbuncles and Buerger's disease (presenile spontaneous gangrene).

安息香 [ānxīxiāng]

Benzoin; *Benzoinum.* The drug consists of the resin obtained from Tokin Snowbell, *Styrax tonkinensis* Pierre or *Styrax hypoglaucus* Perk. (family Styracaceae). It is used as an aromatic stimulant and to promote the circulation of vital energy and blood for the treatment of impaired consciousness due to apoplexy and for pains of the chest and abdomen.

安神藥
Sedatives and Tranquilizers

朱砂 [zhūshā]

Cinnabar; *Cinnabaris.* The drug consists of a mineral composed of red mercuric sulphide. It is used (1) as sedative and tranquilizer for the treatment of palpitation, insomnia, infantile convulsion due to high fever, epilepsy; (2) as a detoxicant for the treatment of boils, furuncles and carbuncles.

琥珀 [hǔpò]

Amber; *Succinum.* The drug consists of a yellowish or brownish fossil resin. It is used as sedative and tranquilizer for the treatment of insomnia, dreamfulness, palpitation and convulsion; (2) as a diuretic and hemostatic for urodynia and hematuria due to acute infection of the urinary system or calculus formation of the urinary tract.

磁石 [císhí]

Magnetite; *Magnetitum.* The drug consists of a kind of magnetic iron ore (Fe_3O_4); the form which exhibits polarity, called lode-stone, is preferred. It is used as sedative, tranquilizer and antiasthmatic for the treatment of tinnitus, headache, palpitation, insomnia, epilepsy and mania due to exuberance of vital function of the *liver* or the *heart*, and also used for chronic asthma.

酸棗仁 [suānzǎorén]

Wild (Spiny) Jujuba Seed; *Semen Ziziphi Spinosae.* The drug consists of the dried seeds of *Ziziphus spinosa* Hu(family Rhamnaceae). It is used (1) as a sedative and tranquilizer for the treatment of fidget, insomnia, and palpitation; (2) as anhidrotic for spontaneous perspiration and night sweat.

遠志 [yuǎnzhì]

Polygala Root; *Radix Polygalae.* The drug consists of the dried roots of *Polygala* tenuifolia Willd. or *Polygala sibirica* L. (family Polygalaceae). It is used (1) as a sedative for neurasthenia, palpitation and insomnia; (2) as expectorant for acute or chronic bronchitis and bronchiectasis.

合歡皮 [héhuānpí]

Albizia Bark; *Cortex Albiziae.* The drug consists of the dried bark of *Albizia julibrissin* Durazz. or *Albizia kalkora* (Roxb.) Prain (family Leguminosae). It is used (1) as a sedative for the treatment of palpitation and insomnia due to anxiety; (2) to relieve pain by invigorating blood circulation for the treatment of painful swellings due to injuries or furuncles and carbuncles.

合歡花 [héhuānhuā]

Albizia Flower; *Flos Albiziae.* The drug consists of the dried flower-heads of *Albizia julibrissin* Durazz. (family Leguminosae). It is used as sedative and tranquilizer for the treatment of fidget and insomnia.

首烏藤 [shǒuwūténg]; 夜交藤 [yèjiāoténg]

Fleece-flower Stem; *Caulis Polygoni Multiflori.* The drug consists of the dried stem of *Polygonum multiflorum* Thunb. (family Polygonaceae). It is used (1) as a sedative for neurasthenia, insomnia and dreamfulness; (2) to activate blood circulation in collaterals for the treatment of aching limbs.

靈芝 [língzhī]

Lucid Ganoderma; *Ganoderma Lucidum.* The drug consists of the dried fructifications of the fungus, *Ganoderma lucidum* (Leyss. ex Fr.) Karst. (family Polyporaceae).It is usually administered in the form of a liquid extract or tablets made of extract. It is used (1) as a sedative and tranquilizer for dizziness and insomnia due to neurasthenia and hypertension; (2) as a tonic for symptoms of weakness or debility. It is also used for chronic bronchitis and asthmatic conditions.

纈草 [xiécǎo]

Valerian Rhizome; *Rhizoma Valerianae.* The drug consists of the dried rhizome and roots of *Valeriana officinalis* L. (family Valerianaceae). It is used as a sedative and carminative for insomnia due to neurasthenia, hysteria and gastro-intestinal distension with pain.

珍珠 [zhēnzhū]

Pearl; *Margarita.* Pearls are lustrous concretions found in certain shell fish, e.g., *Pteria martensii* (Dunker) (family Pteriidae), *Hyriopsis* *cumingii* (Lea), *Cristaria plicata* (Leach) or *Anodonta woodiana* (Lea) (family Unionidae). It is used (1) as sedative and anticonvulsive agent for the treatment of convulsion due to high fever, infantile convulsion; (2) used externally to hasten the healing of wounds.

珍珠母 ［zhēnzhūmǔ］

Mother-of-pearl; Nacre; *Concha Margaritifera Usta.* The drug consists of the ignited shell of certain pearl-yielding shell fish, as *Hyriopsis cumingii* (Lea), *Schistodesmus lampreyanus* (Baird et Adams). *Anadonta woodiana* (Lea), *Cristaria plicata* (Leach), *Lamprotula leai* (Griffith et Pidgeon) (family Unionidae) or *Pteria martensii* (Dunker) (family Pteriidae). It is used (1) as a sedative and tranquilizer for the treatment of palpitation, insomnia, insanity or mania; (2) for treating headache and dizziness due to hypertension.

柏子仁 ［bǎizǐrén］

Arborvitae Seed; *Semen Biotae.* The drug consists of the dried seeds of *Biota orientalis* (L.) Endl. (family Cupressaceae). It is used (1) to nourish the *heart* and relieve mental strain for the treatment of palpitation and insomnia due to deficiency of blood in the *heart*; (2) as an aperient for constipation of debilitated patients.

茯神 ［fúshén］

Fu-shen; *Poria cum Radice Pino.* The drug consists of Fu-ling (cf. p.228) with a piece of Pine root embedded. It is used as a sedative for palpitation and insomnia.

紫貝齒 ［zǐbèichǐ］

Purple Cowrie, Purple Cowry Shells; *Concha Mauritiae.* The drug consists of the dried shells of *Mauritia (Arabica) arabica* (L.) (family Cypaeidae). It is used as a sedative and tranquilizer for the treatment of palpitation and infantile febrile convulsions.

龍骨 ［lónggǔ］

Dragon's Bone; *Os Draconis.* The drug consists of the fossil bone of ancient large mammals, such as *Stegodon orientalis* and *Rhinocerus sinensis.* It is used as a sedative and tranquilizer for the treatment of palpitation, insomnia, dreamfulness due to neurasthenia and hypertension.

龍齒 ［lóngchǐ］

Dragon's Teeth; *Dens Draconis*. The drug consists of the fossil teeth of ancient large mammals, such as *Stegodon orientalis* and *Rhinocerus sinensis*. It is used similarly as 龍骨 with a stronger action.

牡蠣 [mǔlì]

Oyster Shell; *Concha Ostreae*. The drug consists of the shells of oyster, *Ostrea gigas* Thunb., *Ostrea talienwhanensis* Crosse or *Ostrea rivularis* Gould (family Ostreidae). It is used (1) as a sedative and tranquilizer for the treatment of headache, dizziness, palpitation and insomnia; (2) to soften and disperse hard lumps in the body for the treatment of scrofula.

平肝熄風藥
Anticonvulsives or Drugs for Subduing the Hyperactivity of the Liver and the Endogenous Wind

天麻 [tiānmá]

Gastrodia Tuber; *Rhizoma Gastrodiae*. The drug consists of the dried tuber of *Gastrodia elata* Bl. (family Orchidaceae). It is used as an antihypertensive and anticonvulsive agent for the treatment of headache, vertigo and numbness of limbs induced by hypertension and the premonitory symptoms of apoplexy.

鈎藤 [gōuténg]

Uncaria Stem with Hooks; *Ramulus Uncariae cum Uncis*. It consists of the dried stem with hooks of *Uncaria rhynchophylla* (Miq.) Jack., *Uncaria macrphylla* Wall., *Uncaria hirsuta* Havil., *Uncaria sessilifructus* Roxb. or *Uncaria sinensis* (Oliv.) Havil. (family Rubiaceae). It is used as an antipyretic and anticonvulsive agent for the treatment of convulsions with high fever, hypertensive headache, vertigo and nervous headache.

全蝎 [quánxiē]; 全蟲 [quánchóng]

Scorpion, *Scorpio*. The drug consists of the dried body of *Buthus martensii* Karsch (family Buthidae). It is used to subdue the endogenous wind and convulsions for the treatment of various kinds of tics, convulsions, tetanus and sequelae of cerebrovascular accidents.

蜈蚣 [wúgōng]

Centipede; *Scolopendra*. The drug consists of the dried body of centipede, *Scolopendra subspinipes mutilans* L. Koch (family Scolopendridae). It is used (1) to subdue the endogenous wind and convulsions for the treatment of various kinds of tics, convulsions and tetanus; (2) as a detoxicant for joint tuberculosis and bone tuberculosis.

僵蚕 [jiāngcán]; 白僵蚕 [bái jiāng cán]

Batryticated Silkworm, White-stiff Silkworm; *Bombyx Batryticatus.* The drug consists of the dried larva of silkworm, *Bombyx mori* L., dead and stiffened due to the infection of *Beauveria bassiana* (Bals.) Vuill. (family Moniliaceae). It is used (1) to subdue the endogenous wind and convulsions for the treatment of headache, vertigo, tic and skin prurigo; (2) to resolve nodulation for the treatment of scrofula, tonsillitis, parotitis and purpura.

羚羊角 [língyángjiǎo]

Antelope's Horn; *Cornu Antelopis.* The drug consists of the horn of *Saiga tatarica* L. (family Bovidae). It is used to eliminate heat, subdue convulsions and endogenous wind for the treatment of impaired consciousness, delirium and convulsions with high fever, and acute conjunctivitis.

地龍 [dìlóng]

Earthworm; *Lumbricus.* The drug consists of the dried earthworm, *Pheretima aspergillum* (Perrier) or *Allolobophora liginosaca* (Savigny) *trapezoides* (Ant. Degés) (family Megascolecidae). It is used (1) to eliminate heat and subdue convulsions for the treatment of tics with high fever; (2) to clear the channels and subdue asthma for treating rheumatic pain, hemiplegia and asthma; (3) externally for ulcers in lower limbs (ulcus cruris), eczema, erysipelas and burns.

赭石 [zhéshī]

Hematite; *Haematitum.* A red coloured iron ore composed of ferric oxide. It is used to depress the retrograde motion of energy for the treatment of belch, nausea, vomiting and asthma; (2) to subdue the hyperactivity of the *liver* for the treatment of headache, vertigo and tinnitus; (3) as hemostatic for the treatment of spitting blood and nose bleeding due to heat in the blood.

石决明 [shíjuémíng]

Sea-ear Shell; *Concha Haliotidis.* The drug consists of the shell of sea-ear, *Haliotis diversicolor* Reeve, *Haliotis gigantea discus* Reeve or *Haliotis ovina* Chemnitz (family Haliotidae). It is used (1) to subdue the hyperactivity of the Yang of the *liver* for the treatment of headache and vertigo with hypertension, and convulsions of the limbs; (2) for the treatment of glaucoma and cataract.

蒺藜 [jílí]

Tribulus Fruit, Puncture-vine Fruit; *Fructus Tribuli.* The drug consists of the dried fruits of Puncture-vine, *Tribulus terrestris* L. (family Zygophylaceae). It is used to restore the depressed *liver* for the treatment of fullness in the chest and mastitis; (2) to dispel the wind and clear the eyes for the treatment of acute conjunctivitis, headache and vertigo.

玳瑁 [dàimào]

Hawksbill Shell; *Carapax Eretmochelydis.* The drug consists of the carapaces of the hawksbill turtle, *Eretmochelys imbricata* (L.) (family Chelonidae). It is used to subdue the endogenous wind and heat, and as anticonvulsive, antifebrile and detoxicant for the treatment of impaired consciousness, delirium and convulsions in febrile diseases.

熊膽 [xióngdǎn]

Bear Gall; *Fel Ursi.* The drug consists of the dried gall-bladder of the bear, *Selenarctos thibetanus* Cuvier or *Ursus arctos* L. (family Ursidae). It is used to eliminate heat, subdue the hyperactivity of the *liver* and clear the eye for the treatment of convulsions and tic; externally for acute conjunctivitis and sore-throat.

補養藥

Tonics

補氣藥 Drugs for Replenishing the Vital Energy

人參 [rénshēn]

Ginseng; *Radix Ginseng.* The drug consists of the dried roots of Asiatic Genseng, *Panax ginseng* C.A. Mey. (family Araliaceae). It is used to replenish the vital energy and to promote the secretion

of body fluids for the treatment of shock, prostration, etc. It has
been shown to possess the effects of stimulating the central nervous
system, cardiotonic, antifatigue and stimulating the mechanism of
bood formation.

党参 [dǎngshēn]

Pilose Asiabell Root; *Radix Codonopsis Pilosulae.* The drug consists of the dried root of *Codonopsis pilosula* (Franch.) Nannf. (family
Campanulaceae). It is used to invigorate the function of *spleen* and
stomach and to replenish the vital energy for the treatment of palpitation, short of breath, weakness of limbs, poor appetite and loose
bowel.

孩兒参 [háiérshēn]; 太子参 [tàizǐshēn]

Pseudostellaria Root; *Radix Pseudostellariae.* The drug consists
of the dried tuberous root of *Pseudostellaria heterophylla* (Miq.)
Pax ex Pax et Hoffm. (family Caryophyllaceae). It is used similarly
as 党参, but is less active as a tonic, more active in promoting the
secretion of body fluids.

黄芪 [huángqí]

Astraglus Root; *Radix Astragali.* The drug consists of the root of
Astragalus membranaceus (Fisch.) Bge. or *Astragalus membranaceus*
Bge. var. *mongholicus* (Bge.) Hsiao (family Leguminosae). It is used
(1) to replenish the vital energy and to stop perspiration (anhidrotic)
for the treatment of spontaneous perspiration, night sweat, prolapse
of uterus and anus; (2) to dispel pus and accelerating the healing of
wounds for the treatment of chronic ulcers; (3) as a diuretic for chronic
nephritis with edema and proteinuria.

红芪 [hóngqí]

Hedysarum Root, Red Sweetvetch Root; *Radix Hedysari.* The
drug consists of the root of *Hedysarum polybotrys* Hand. -Mazz.
(family Leguminosae). It is used as a substitute for 黄芪 [huángqí].

甘草 [gāncǎo]

Liquorice; Licorice Root; *Radix Glycyrrhizae.* The drug consists
of the dried root and rhizome of *Glycyrrhiza uralensis* Fisch., *Glycyrrhiza inflata* Bat. or *Glycyrrhiza glabra* L. (family Leguminosae). It
is used (1) to invigorate the functions of the *heart* and *spleen* for the

206

treatment of symptoms due to deficiency of vital energy of these viscera; (2) as spasmolytic and antitussive for peptic ulcers and cough; (3) as antiphlogistic for sore throat, boils and carbuncles; (4) as antitoxicant for drug poisoning.

白术 [báizhú]

White Atractylodes Rhizome; *Rhizoma Atractylodis Macrocephalae.* The drug consists of the dried rhizome of *Atractylodes macrocephala* Koidz. (family Compositae). It is used to invigorate the functions of the *spleen* and *stomach* for the treatment of poor appetite, dyspepsia and chronic diarrhea.

山药 [shānyào]

Chinese Yam, *Rhizoma Dioscoreae.* The drug consists of the dried rhizomes of *Dioscorea opposita* Thunb. (family Dioscoreaceae). It is used (1) to invigorate the functions of *spleen* and *stomach* for the treatment of poor appetite and chronic diarrhea; (2) to replenish the *lung* and *kidney* for dry cough, diabetes, noctural emmision and leukorrhagia.

大枣 [dàzǎo]

Jujube; Chinese Date; *Fructus Ziziphi Jujubae.* The drug consists of the dried fruit of *Ziziphus jujuba* Mill. (family Rhamnaceae). It is used to replenish the vital energy of *spleen* and *stomach* for the treatment of symptoms due to deficiency of vital energy of these organs. It is also used to moderate the actions of drug.

黄精 [huángjīng]

Siberian Solomonseal Rhizome; *Rhizoma Polygonati.* The drug consists of the dried rhizomes of *Polygonatum sibiricum* Red., *Polygonatum kingianum* Coll. et Hemsl. or *Polygonatum cyrtonema* Hua (family Liliaceae). It is used (1) to replenish the *spleen* and *stomach* for the treatment of fatiguability, poor appetite; (2) to nourish the vital essence of the *lung* for the treatment of dry cough due to chronic bronchitis and pulmonary tuberculosis.

饴糖 [yítáng]

Malt Extract; *Extractum Malti.* The drug is an amber or yellowish brown, viscous liquid, with an agreeable odour and a sweet taste, prepared from sound, malted grains of barley, *Hordeum vulgare* L. or a mixture of this and sound, malted grains of wheat, *Triticum aestivum* L., by digestion with water at a suitable temperature and by evaporation of the strained liquid at a temperature not exceeding 55°C, until a viscous product is obtained. It has nutritive properties and is used as a tonic to replenish vital energy of the *spleen* and *stomach* for general weakness and abdominal pain due to chronic diseases of the digestive tract. It is also used as an antitussive for chronic bronchitis and tuberculosis.

補血藥　Blood Tonics or Drugs for Nourishing the Blood

當歸 [dāngguī]

Chinese Angelica Root; *Radix Angelicae Sinensis.* The drug consists of the dried root of Chinese Angelica, *Angelica sinensis* (Oliv.) Diels (family Umbelliferae). It is used (1) to nourish the blood and to invigorate the blood circulation for the treatment of menstrual disorders, and (2) as an emollient and laxative for chronic constipation of the aged and debilitated.

白芍 [báisháo]

White Peony Root; *Radix Paeoniae Alba.* The drug consists of the dried peeled root of *Paeonia lacitflora* Pall. (family Ranunculaceae). It is used to nourish the blood and to regulate the menstrual flow for the treatment of menstrual disorders; (2) as a spasmolytic and pain-relieving agent for headache, abdominal pain, spasm of the calf muscles, etc.

阿膠 [ējiāo]; 驢皮膠 [lú pí jiāo]

Donkey-hide Gelatin; Ass-hide Glue; *Colla Corii Asini.* The drug consists of the glue prepared from the skin of Ass, *Equus asinus* L. (family Equidae). It is used (1) to nourish the blood and to stop bleeding for symptoms of deficiency of blood and all kinds of bleeding; (2) to nourish the vital essence and to soothe the *lung* for the treatment of insomnia, dry cough and bloody sputum (e.g. in pulmonary tuberculosis).

紫河車 [zǐhéchē]

Human Placenta; *Placenta Hominis.* The drug consists of the dried human placenta. It is used to replenish the vital energy, to nourish the blood and essence for general weakness, anemia and neurasthenia.

208

龍眼肉 [lóngyǎnròu]

Longan Aril; *Arillus Longan.* The drug consists of the dried aril of Longan, *Euphoria longan* (Lour.) Steud. (family Sapindaceae). It is used to nourish the blood and as a sedative for the treatment of palpitation, dizziness and insomnia.

熟地黃 [shúdìhuáng]

Prepared Rehmannia Root; *Radix Rehmanniae Praeparata.* The drug consists of the steamed and dried tuberous root of *Rehmannia glutinosa* Libosch. (family Scrophulariaceae). It is used to replenish the vital essence of the *kidney,* to nourish the blood and to regulate the menstrual flow for the treatment of chronic tidal fever, night sweat, dry mouth, lumbago, noctural emission, dizziness and palpitation, and menstrual disorder due to blood deficiency.

補陰藥 **Drugs for Replenishing the Vital Essence**

西洋參 [xīyángshēn]

American Ginseng; *Radix Panacis Quinquefolii; Radix Ginseng Americana.* The drug consists of the root of *Panax quinquefolium* L. (family Araliaceae). It is used to replenish the vital essence, to reduce the internal heat and to promote the secretion of body fluids for the treatment of low fever (usually in the afternoon), spontaneous or night sweating, fatigue due to chronic consumptive diseases.

石斛 [shíhú]

Dendrobium; *Herba Dendrobii.* The drug consists of the stem of *Dendrobium loddigesii* Rolfe., *Dendrobium chrysanthum* Wall., *Dendrobium fimbriatum* Hook. var. *oculatum* Hook., *Dendrobium nobile* Lindl. or *Dendrobium candidum* Wall. ex Lindl. (family Orchidaceae). It is used to replenish the vital essence of the *lung* and *stomach*, to clear up the excessive heat and to promote the secretion of body fluids for the treatment of febrile diseases with thirst and dry mouth, vomiturition, dry cough and chronic tidal fever.

玉竹 [yùzhú]

Fragrant Solomonseal Rhizome; *Rhizoma Polygonati Odorati.* The drug consists of the dried rhizomes of *Polygonatum odoratum* (Will.) Druce (family Liliaceae). It is used to replenish the vital essence and promote the secretion of body fluids for the treatment of dipsosis, dry throat, dry cough, etc. which are due to diabetes or pulmonary disease.

麥冬 [màidōng]; 麥門冬 [màiméndōng]

Ophiopogon Root, Lilyturf Root; *Radix Ophiopogonis.* The drug consists of the tuberous root of Dwarf Lilyturf, *Ophiopogon japonicus* (Thunb.) Ker.-Gawl. (family Liliaceae). It is used (1) to replenish the vital essence and to promote the secretion of body fluids, to stop coughing by soothing the *lung* for the treatment of dipsosis, dry throat, dry cough and bloody sputum, (2) to nourish the *heart* for the treatment of palpitation and fearfulness.

天冬 [tiāndōng]; 天門冬 [tiānméndōng]

Asparagus Root; *Radix Asparagi.* The drug consists of the dried tuberous roots of *Asparagus cochinchinensis* (Lour.) Merr. (family Liliaceae). It is used to replenish the vital essence and to promote the secretion of body fluids for the treatment of dipsosis, dry throat, cough with sticky phlegm, bloody sputum and constipation.

北沙參 [běishāshēn]

Glehnia Root; *Radix Glehniae.* The drug consists of the dried root of *Glehnia littoralis* Fr. Schmidt ex Miq. (family Umbelliferae). It is used to replenish the vital essence of *lung and stomach* and to promote the secretion of body fluids for the treatment of dipsosis, dry throat and dry cough. (cf. 南沙參)

玄參 [xuánshēn]; 元參 [yuánshēn]

Scrophularia Root, Figwort Root; *Radix Scrophulariae.* The drug consists of the dried root of *Scrophularia ningpoensis* Hemsl. (family Scrophulariaceae). It is used (1) to replenish the vital essence and to relieve pyogenic inflammation for the treatment of dipsosis and erythematous eruption due to acute infectious diseases, acute swelling and pain in the throat, boils and carbuncles; (2) to resolve hard lumps in the body for the treatment of scrofula.

枸杞子 [gǒuqízǐ]

Wolfberry Fruit; *Fructus Lycii.* The drug consists of the dried fruit of *Lycium barbarum* L. (family Solanaceae). It is used to replenish the vital essence of the *liver* and *kidney* and to improve the eyesight for the treatment of aching back and legs, impotence and noc-

210

turnal emission, vertigo and decreased eye-sight.

山茱萸［shānzhūyú］; 山萸肉［shānyúròu］

Dogwood Fruit; *Fructus Corni.* The drug consists of the dried sarcocarp of Medicinal Dogwood, *Cornus officinalis* Sieb. et Zucc. (family Cornaceae). It is used to replenish the vital essence of the *liver* and *kidney* and to stop sweating for the treatment of aching back and knees, vertigo, frequent micturition, nocturnal emission and spontaneous perspiration.

首烏［shǒuwū］; 何首烏［héshǒuwū］

Fleeceflower Root; *Radix Polygoni Multiflori.* The drug consists of the dried tuberous roots of *Polygonum multiflorum* Thunb. (family Polygonaceae). The prepared drug is made by boiling with a decoction of black beans until the decoction is entirely absorbed into the drug. The prepared drug is used to replenish the vital essence of the *liver* and *kidney* and to nourish the blood for the treatment of anemia, early greying of hair, aching back and knees, neurasthenia and hypercholesteremia. The raw drug is used as a laxative for constipation and also as detoxicant for boils.

牛膝［niúxī］; 懷牛膝［huáiniúxī］

Achyranthes Root; *Radix Achyranthis Bidentatae.* The drug consists of the dried roots of *Achyranthes bidentata* Bl. (family Amaranthaceae). It is used to nourish the *liver* and *kidney* and to strengthen the sinews and bones for the treatment of aching back and knees, asthenia of the lower limbs, and hypertension.

沙苑子［shāyuánzǐ］; 潼蒺藜［tóngjílí］

Flattened Milkvetch Seed; *Semen Astragali Complanati.* The drug consists of the seeds of *Astragalus complanatus* R.Br. (family Leguminosae). It is used to replenish the vital essence of the *liver* and *kidney* for the treatment of spontaneous seminal emission, frequent micturition, urorrhea and vertigo.

女貞子［nǚzhēnzǐ］

Lucid Ligustrum Fruit, Grossy Privet Fruit; *Fructus Ligustri Lucidi.* The drug consists of the dried fruit of Grossy Privet, *Ligustrum lucidum* Ait. (family Oleaceae). If is used to replenish the vital essence of *liver* and *kidney*, to darken the hair and to improve the eyesight for the treatment of early greying of the hair, dim eyesight, lumbago and neurasthenia.

桑寄生 [sāngjìshēng]

Mulberry Mistletoe, *Ramulus Loranthi.* The drug consists of the dried foliferous stem and branch of *Loranthus parasiticus* (L.) Merr. (family Loranthaceae). It is used (1) to replenish the vital energy of the *liver* and *kidney,* to strengthen the sinews and bones and as an antirheumatic agent for the treatment of aching back and limbs, rheumatism; (2) to nourish the blood and to prevent miscarriage for the treatment of menorrhea and threatened abortion.

鹿銜草 [lùxiáncǎo]

Pyrola; *Herba Pyrolae.* The drug consists of the dried entire plant of *Pyrola decorata* H. Andres, *Pyrola rotundifolia* L. subsp. *chinensis* H. Andres or *Pyrola rotundifolia* L. (family Pyrolaceae). It is used to replenish the vital essence of the *kidney,* to strengthen the sinews and bones, and as an antirheumatic and hemostatic agent for the treatment of lumbago, neurasthenia, rheumatism, menorrhea, bloody sputum and epistaxis.

龜板 [guībǎn]

Tortoise Plastron; *Plastrum Testudinis.* The drug consists of the plastron of fresh-water tortoise, *Chinemys reevesii* (Gray) (family Testudinidae). It is used to replenish the vital essence and to check the exuberance of the vital function of the *liver,* and to nourish the *kidney* for the treatment of vertigo, chronic tidal fever, night sweat, dry mouth and throat, aching back and knees with asthenia, osteomalacia and rickets.

鱉甲 [biējiǎ]

Turtle Shell; *Carapax Trionycis.* The drug consists of the carapace of the soft shelled turtle, *Trionyx sinensis* Wiegmann (family Trionychidae). It is used to replenish the vital essence and eliminate pathogenic heat, to soften and resolve hard lumps in the body for the treatment of chronic tidal fever, night sweat, abdominal masses such as hepatomegaly and splenomegaly.

桑椹 [sāngshèn]

Mulberry; *Fructus Mori.* The drug consists of the dried fruit-spike of White Mulberry, *Morus alba* L. (family Moraceae). It is used to replenish the vital essence and nourish the blood for the treatment of dizziness, tinnitus, polydipsia, etc. due to anemia, neurasthenia hypertension and diabetes.

補陽藥 **Drugs for Reinforcing the Vital Function**

鹿茸 [lùróng]

Pilose Antler; Pilose Deerhorn, *Cornu Cervi Pantotrichum*. The drug consists of the hairy, young horn of male deer or stag, *Cervus nippon* Temminck or *Cervus elaphus* L. (family Cervidae). It is used to reinforce the vital function of the *kidney* and to strengthen the bones and muscles for the treatment of intolerance of cold, loss of strength, impotence, spontaneous seminal emission, leukorrhea and other symptoms due to deficiency of vital function in chronic diseases.

鹿角 [lùjiǎo]

Antler; Deerhorn; *Cornu Cervi*. The drug consists of the ossified horn of the male deer or stag, *Cervus elaphus* L. (family Cervidae). It is used similarly as 鹿茸 [lùróng] but is less active. It is also used to remove blood-stasis for the treatment of traumatic wounds.

鹿角膠 [lùjiǎojiāo]

Antler Glue; Antler Gelatin; *Colla Cornus Cervi*. Its action of nourishing the *kidney* is superior to that of 鹿角 [lùjiǎo] with additional effects of nourishing the blood and stopping bleeding.

鹿角霜 [lùjiǎoshuāng]

Deglued Antler Powder; *Cornu Cervi Degelatinatum*. Its action is similar to but inferior to that of 鹿角

肉蓯蓉 [ròucōngróng]; 大芸 [dàyún]

Cistanche; *Herba Cistanchis*. The drug consists of the dried fleshy stem of *Cistanche deserticola* V.C. Ma (family Orobanchaceae). It is used (1) to reinforce the vital function of the *kidney* especially that of the sexual organs for the treatment of impotence and premature ejaculation; (2) as a mild laxative for chronic constipation of the aged.

仙茅 [xiānmáo]

Curculigo Rhizome; *Rhizoma Curculiginis*. The drug consists of the dried rhizomes of *Curculigo orchioides* Gaertn. (family Amaryllidaceae). It is used to warm up the *kidney* and to reinforce the vital function of sexual organ for the treatment of aching back and knees with intolerance of cold, impotence, urorrhea and climacteric hypertension.

淫羊藿 [yínyánghuò]; 仙靈脾 [xiānlíngpí]

Epimedium; *Herba Epimedii.* The drug consists of the dried aerial parts of *Epimedium brevicornum* Maxim., *Epimedium koreanum* Nakai or *Epimedium sagittatum* (Sieb. et Zucc.) Maxim. (family Berberidaceae). It is used (1) to replenish the vital function of the *kidney* especially that of sexual organs for the treatment of sexual neurasthenia; (2) as an antirheumatic agent for rheumatic pains.

鎖陽 [suǒyáng]

Cynomorium; *Herba Cynomorii.* The drug consists of the dried fleshy stem of *Cynomorium songaricum* Rúpr. (family Cynomoriaceae). It is used (1) to reinforce the vital function of the *kidney* for the treatment of impotence, seminal emissions, and (2) as a mild laxative for chronic constipation of the aged.

巴戟天 [bājǐtiān]

Morinda Root; *Radix Morindae Officinalis.* The drug consists of the dried root of *Morinda officinalis* How (family Rubiaceae). It is used to reinforce the vital function of the *kidney* especially that of the sexual organs for the treatment of impotence and premature ejaculation in men, and infertility in women.

葫蘆巴 [húlúbā]

Fenugreek Seed; *Semen Trigonellae.* The drug consists of the dried seeds of *Trigonella foenum-graecum* L. (family Leguminosae). It is used to warm up the *kidney*, to disperse cold and relieve pain for the treatment of cold pain in the testis, abdominal pain due to gastro-intestinal spasm.

補骨脂 [bǔgǔzhī]

Psoralea Fruit; *Fructus Psoraleae.* The drug consists of the dried fruits of *Psoralea corylifolia* L. (family Leguminosae). It is used to warm up the *kidney* and to reinforce the vital function of the sexual organs for the treatment of impotence, nocturnal emission, urorrhea and "fifth-watch diarrhea" (diarrhea occurring daily just before dawn).

菟絲子 [tùsīzǐ]

Dodder Seed; *Semen Cuscutae*. The drug consists of the seeds of Chinese Dodder, *Cuscuta chinensis* Lam. (family Convolvulaceae). It is used to replenish the *liver* and *kidney*, to improve eyesight and prevent miscarriage for the treatment of nocturnal emission, urorrhea, vertigo, decreased eyesight and threatened abortion.

杜仲 [dùzhòng]

Eucommia Bark; *Cortex Eucommiae*. The drug consists of the dried bark of *Eucommia ulmoides* Oliv. (family Eucommiaceae). It is used to replenish the *liver* and *kidney* and to strengthen the bones and muscles for the treatment of aching back and knees, threatened abortion and hypertension.

狗脊 [gǒujǐ]

Cibot Rhizome; *Rhizoma Cibotii*. The drug consists of the dried rhizome of *Cibotium barometz* (L.) J.Sm. (family Dicksoniaceae). It is used to replenish the *liver* and *kidney*, to strengthen the back and knees and as an antirheumatic agent for the treatment of aching back and knees, rheumatic pain in the back and strain of lumbar muscles.

續斷 [xùduàn]

Dipsacus Root, Teasel Root; *Radix Dipsaci*. The drug consists of the dried root of Himalaya Teasel, *Dipsacus asper* Wall. (family Dipsacaceae). It is used (1) to replenish the *liver* and *kidney* for the treatment of aching back and joints, rheumatic pain of the lumbar region; (2) to improve the healing of fractures; (3) to stop bleeding and prevent miscarriage for the functional uterine bleeding and threatened abortion.

冬蟲夏草 [dōngchóngxiàcǎo]

Cordyceps; Chinese Caterpillar Fungus; *Cordyceps*. The drug consists of the dried fungus, *Cordyceps sinensis* (Berk.) Sacc. growing on the larva of caterpillar. It is used to replenish the *kidney* and soothe the *lung* for the treatment of impotence, nocturnal emission, night sweat, chronic cough with hemoptysis (e.g. in pulmonary tuberculosis).

蛤蚧 [géjiè]

Gecko; *Gecko*. The drug consists of the dried lizard, *Gekko gecko* L (family Geckonidae). It is used to replenish the *lung* and *kidney* for the treatment of chronic asthma.

海馬 [hǎimǎ]

Sea Horse; *Hippocampus.* The drug consists of the dried body of *Hippocampus kelloggi* Jordan et Snyder, *H. histrix* Kaup, *H. kuda* Bleeker, *H. trimaculatus* Leach or *H. japonicus* Kaup. (family Syngnathidae). It is used to replenish the vital function of the *kidney* especially that of sexual organs for the treatment of impotence, swellings in the abdomen, scrofula, traumatic wounds, and is also used externally for the treatment of carbuncles and furuncles.

固澀藥

Astringents and Haemostatics

浮小麥 [fúxiǎomài]

Light Wheat; *Fructus Tritici Levis.* The drug consists of the dried light grains of *Triticum aestivum* L. (family Graminae). It is used as an antihidrotic agent for spontaneous or night sweating.

麻黃根 [máhuánggēn]

Ephedra Root; *Radix Ephedrae.* The drug consists of the dried roots of Chinese Ephedra, *Ephedra sinica* Stapf. or *Ephedra intermedia* Schrenk et C.A.Mey. (family Ephedraceae). It is used as an anhidrotic agent for the treatment of spontaneous perspiration and night sweat.

五倍子 [wǔbèizǐ]

Chinese Gall; *Galla Chinensis.* The drug consists of the excrescences produced by an insect on the leaf of Chinese Sumac, *Rhus chinensis* Mill., Potanin Sumac, *Rhus potaninii* Maxim., Punjab Sumac, *Rhus punjabensis* Stew. var. *sinica* (Diels) Rehd. et Wils. (family Anacardiaceae). It is used as an astringent agent for the treatment of persistent cough, night sweating, chronic diarrhea, bloody stool, urorrhea; used externally for burns, bleeding due to traumatic injuries, hemorrhoids and ulcers in mouth.

訶子 [hēzǐ]

Chebula Fruit; *Fructus Chebulae.* The drug consists of the dried fruit of *Terminalia chebula* Retz. or *Terminalia chebula* var. *tomentella* Kurt. (family Combretaceae). It is used as an antidiarrhetic and antitussive agent for the treatment of chronic diarrhea or dysentery, persistent cough and hoarse voice.

石榴皮 [shíliúpí]

Pomegranate Rind; *Pericarpium Granati.* The drug consists of the dried pericarp of Common Pomegranate, *Punica granatum* L. (family Punicaceae). It is used as an antidiarrhetic agent for the treatment of chronic diarrhea or dysentery; also used as an anthelmintic for intestinal taeniasis and ascariasis.

赤石脂 [chìshízhī]

Red Halloysite; *Halloysitum Rubrum.* The drug consists of a mineral, hydrated aluminium silicate, in red colour due to the presence of iron oxides. It is used as an antidiarrhetic and hemostatic agent for the treatment of chronic diarrhea, menorrhagia and leukorrhagia.

蓮子 [liánzǐ]

Lotus Seed, *Semen Nelumbinis.* The drug consists of the dried seeds of Lotus, *Nelumbo nucifera* Gaertn. (family Nymphaeaceae). It is used as an astringent for the treatment of chronic diarrhea, spontaneous emission and leukorrhagia.

蓮鬚 [liánxū]

Lotus Stamen; *Stamen Nelumbinis.* The drug consists of the dried stamens of Lotus, *Nelumbo nucifera* Gaertn. (family Nymphaeaceae). It is used as an astringent to consolidate the vital energy of the *kidney* for the treatment of seminal emission and leucorrhagia.

芡實 [qiànshí]

Euryale Seed; *Semen Euryales.* The drug consists of the dried seed of Gordon Euryale, *Euryale ferox* Salisb. (family Nymphaeaceae). It is used as an astringent for the treatment of chronic diarrhea, spontaneous emission, urorrhea and leukorrhagia.

禹餘糧 [yǔyúliáng]; 禹糧石 [yǔliángshí]

Limonite; *Limonitum.* The drug consists of a kind of iron ore, mainly composed of ferric oxide. It is used as an astringent for the treatment of chronic diarrhea or dysentery, menorrhagia and leukorrhagia.

伏龍肝 [fúlónggān]

Ignited Yellow Earth; *Terra Flava Usta.* The drug consists of

217

ignited yellow earth in small lumps. It is used as (1) anti-emetic for the treatment of nausea and vomiting due to chronic gastric diseases or pregnancy, (2) antidiarrhetic and hemostatic agent for chronic diarrhea, uterine bleeding and chronic bleeding of the gastro-intestinal tract due to failure of the *spleen* to keep the blood circulating within the vessels.

乌梅 [wūméi]

Black Plum; Mume; *Fructus Mume.* The drug consists of the dried fruits of Japanese Apricot, *Prunus mume* (Sieb.) Sieb. et Zucc. (family Rosaceae). It is used as an antidiarrhetic, antitussive, antidiptic and anthelmintic agent for chronic diarrhea, persistent cough, morbid thirst and ascariasis.

肉豆蔻 [ròudòukòu]; 肉果 [ròuguǒ]

Nutmeg; *Semen Myristicae.* The drug consists of the seeds of **Myristica fragrans** Houtt. (family Myristicaceae). It is used as an anti-diarrhetic agent by warming up the *spleen* and *stomach* for the treatment of chronic diarrhea.

罂粟殼 [yīngsúqiào]; 米殼 [mǐqiào]

Poppy Capsule; *Pericarpium Papaveris.* The drug consists of the dried capsule of Opium Poppy, *Papaver somniferum* L. (family Papaveraceae). It is used as an antidiarrhetic, antitussive and analgesic agent for the treatment of chronic diarrhea, persistent asthma and abdominal pain.

五味子 [wǔwèizǐ]

Schisandra Fruit, Magnoliavine Fruit; *Fructus* **Schisandrae.** The drug consists of the dried fruit of Chinese Magnoliavine, *Schisandra chinensis* (Turcz.) Baill. or Orange Magnoliavine, *Schisandra sphenanthera* Rehd. et Wils. (family Magnoliaceae). It is used as an astringent for the treatment of dry cough, asthma, night sweating, seminal emission and chronic diarrhea; also used as tonic for neurasthenia.

桑螵蛸 [sāngpiāoxiāo]

Mantis Egg-case, *Oötheca Mantidis.* The drug consists of the steamed and dried egg-case of praying mantis, *Tenodera sinensis* Saussure, *Statilia maculata* (Thunb.) or *Hierodula patellifera* (Serrille) (family Mantidae). It is used as an astringent for the treatment of

218

frequent micturition, urorrhea, seminal emission and leukorrhagia.

海螵蛸 [hǎipiāoxiāo]; 乌贼骨 [wūzéigǔ]

Cuttlefish Bone; *Os Sepiae.* The drug consists of the dried interanl shell of the cuttlefish, *Sepiella maindroni* de Rochebrune or *Sepia esculenta* Hoyle (family Sepiadae). It is used as a hemostatic and antacid agent for the treatment of hematemesis, bloody stool, menorrhagia, gastric hyperacidity and leukorrhagia.

瓦楞子 [wǎléngzǐ]

Ark Shell; *Concha Arcae.* The drug consists of the shells of *Arca subcrenata* Lischke, *Arca granosa* L. or *Arca inflata* Reeve (family Arcidae). It is used as an antacid agent and to resolve hard lumps for the treatment of gastric hyperacidity and nodular swellings.

煅龙骨 [duànlónggǔ]

Ignited Dragon's Bone; *Os Draconis Ustum.* The drug consists of the ignited fossil bone of ancient large mammals, such as *Stegodon orientalis* and *Rhinocerus sinensis.* It is used as an astringent for the treatment of seminal emission, night sweating, leukorrhagia and uterine bleeding.

煅牡蛎 [duànmǔlì]

Ignited Oyster Shell; *Concha Ostreae Usta.* The drug consists of the ignited shells of oyster, *Ostrea gigas* Thunb., *Ostrea talienwhanensis* Crosse or *Ostrea rivularis* Gould (family Ostreidae). It is used as an astringent and antacid for the treatment of excessive sweating, seminal emission, leukorrhagia and gastric hyperacidity.

金樱子 [jīnyīngzǐ]

Cherokee Rose-Hip; *Fructus Rosae Laevigatae.* The drug consists of the fruit of Cherokee Rose, *Rosa laevigata* Michx. (family Rosaceae). It is used as an astringent for the treatment of seminal emission, urorrhea, frequent micturition and chronic diarrhea.

覆盆子 [fùpénzǐ]

Raspberry Fruit; *Fructus Rubi.* The drug consists of the dried fruit of *Rubus chingii* Hu (family Rosaceae). It is used as an astringent for the treatment of frequent micturition, urorrhea and seminal emission.

白果 [báiguǒ]; 银杏 [yínxìng]

Ginkgo Seed; *Semen Ginkgo*. The drug consists of the seed of Maidenhair tree, *Ginkgo biloba* L. (family Ginkgoaceae). It is used as an astringent for the treatment of persistent cough and asthma, urorrhea and leukorrhea.

消導藥
Digestives and Evacuants

山楂 [shānzhā]

Hawthorn Fruit, *Fructus Crataegi*. The drug consists of the dried fruit of Large Chinese Hawthorn, *Crataegus pinnatifida* Bge. var. *major* N.E.Br., Chinese Hawthorn, *Crataegus pinnatifida* Bge. or Nippon Hawthorn, *Crataegus cuneata* Sieb. et Zucc. (family Rosaceae). It is used to improve digestion and eliminate the stagnated food for the treatment of dyspepsia and stagnation of fatty food. The charred drug is usually preferred for the above purpose. The raw drug is used to improve blood circulation for amenorrhea and postpartum abdominal pain due to blood-stasis.

麥芽 [màiyá]

Germinated Barley; *Frutcus Hordei Germinatus*. The drug consists of the dried, germinated fruits of Barley, *Hordeum vulgare* L. (family Graminae). The charred drug is used to improve digestion for the treatment of dyspepsia induced by cereal food and infantile lacto-dyspepsia. The raw drug is also used as a carminative.

稻芽 [dàoyá]

Germinated Rice; *Fructus Oryzae Germinatus*. The drug consists of the dried germinated fruits of Rice, *Oryza sativa* L. (family Graminae). It is called 穀芽 [gǔyá] in South China and used to improve digestion for the treatment of poor appetite and dyspepsia.

穀芽 [gǔyá]

Germinated Millet; *Fructus Setariae Germinatus*. The drug consists of the dried, germinated fruits of Millet, *Setaria italica* (L.) Beauv. (family Graminae). It is used as same as 稻芽 [dào yá] to improve digestion for the treatment of poor appetite and dyspepsia.

神麴 [shénqū]

220

Medicated Leaven; *Massa Fermentata Medicinalis*. The drug consists of a dried mass of a fermented mixture of wheat flour, fresh aerial parts of *Artemisia annua, Xanthium sibiricum, Polygonum hydropiper*, etc. It is used to improve digestion for the treatment of dyspepsia and abdominal distension due to food stagnation.

焦三仙 [jiāosānxiān]

Charred Triplet. A mixture consists of equal parts of the following drugs: Charred Medicated Leaven, Charred Crataegus Fruit and Charred Germinated Barley. This combination has a stronger effect for improving digestion.

鷄内金 [jīnèijīn]

Chicken's Gizzard-skin; *Endothelium Corneum Gigeriae Galli*. The drug consists of the dried lining membrane of the gizzard of Common Fowl, *Gallus gallus domesticus* Briss. (family Phasianidae). The roasted drug is used to improve appetite and digestion for the treatment of poor appetite and dyspepsia. The raw drug is used to eliminate stagnated food and calculi of all kinds.

萊菔子 [láifúzǐ]

Radish Seed, *Semen Raphani*. The drug consists of the dried seeds of Garden Radish, *Raphanus sativus* L. (family Cruciferae). The roasted drug is used to improve digestion and as a carminative for the treatment of gastro-intestinal distension and pain due to stagnation of food, and rectal tenesmus. The raw drug is used as an expectorant for chronic bronchitis.

瀉下藥

Purgatives

蜂蜜 [fēngmì]

Honey; *Mel*. The drug consists of the saccharine fluid made by the hive-bee, *Apis cerana* Fabr. or *Apis mellifera* L. (family *Apidae*). It is used as antitussive and aperient for the treatment of dry cough, sore-throat and dry stool of the aged.

郁李仁 [yùlǐrén]

Bush-cherry Seed; *Semen Pruni*. The drug consists of the dried seeds of Bush Cherry; *Prunus humilis* Bge. or *Prunus japonica* Thunb. (family Rosaceae). It is used as aperient and diuretic for the treatment of constipation and edema.

火麻仁 ［huǒmárén］
Hemp Seed; *Fructus Cannabis*. The drug consists of the dried fruits of Common Hemp, *Cannabis sativa* L. (family Moraceae). It is used as aperient for the treatment of constipation of the debilitated or aged.

大黄 ［dàhuáng］
Rhubarb; *Radix et Rhizoma Rhei*. The drug consists of the dried root and rhizome of Palmate Rhubarb, *Rheum palmatum* L., Tangut Rhubarb, *Rheum tanguticum* Maxim. ex Balf. or Medicinal Rhubarb, *Rheum officinale* Baill. (*family* Polygonaceae). It is used as an purgative and detoxicant and to eliminate evil heat, stagnated food and blood stasis for the treatment of fever with constipation and fullness in the abdomen, acute jaundice, acute appendicitis, incomplete intestinal obstruction, amenorrhea due to blood stasis, hematemesis and epistaxis associated with excessive heat in the blood; used externally for burns, suppurative skin diseases, carbuncles and furuncles.

番瀉葉 ［fānxièyè］
Senna Leaf; *Folium Sennae*. The drug consists of the dried leaflets of *Cassia angustifolia* Vahl or *Cassia acutifolia* Delile (family Leguminosae). It is used as a purgative for the treatment of constipation, especially habitual constipation.

芒硝 ［mángxiāo］
Mirabilite; Glauber's Salt, Sodium Sulphate; *Natrii Sulfas*. The drug consists of the crystalline sodium sulphate, usually made from natural sources. It is used as a purgative for the treatment of constipation; used externally for acute mastitis.

玄明粉 ［xuánmíngfěn］
Dried Glauber's Salt, Exiccated Sodium Sulfate; *Natrii Sulfas Exsiccatus*. The drug consists of a white powder composed of sodium sulphate. It is used as a purgative for the treatment of constipation.

蘆薈 ［lúhuì］
Aloes; *Aloe*. The drug consists of the dried leaf juice of *Aloe vera*

L. var. *chinensis* (Haw.) Berger or related species (family Liliaceae). It is used as a purgative for the treatment of constipation, amenorrhea and malnutrition of child.

驅蟲藥
Anthelmintics

苦棟皮 [kǔliànpí]; 苦棟根皮 [kǔliàngēnpí]

Chinaberry Bark; *Cortex Meliae.* The drug consists of the dried stem- or root - bark of *Melia toosendan* Sieb. et Zucc. or *Melia azedarach* L. (family Meliaceae). It is used as anthelmintic for the treatment of ascariasis.

使君子 [shǐjūnzǐ]

Quisqualis Fruit, Rangoon Creeper Fruit; *Fructus Quisqualis.* The drug consists of the dried fruit of Rangoon Creeper, *Quisqualis indica* L. (family Combretaceae). It is used as anthelmintic for the treatment of ascariasis, enterobiasis and malnutrition of child.

檳榔 [bīngláng]

Areca Seed, Betel Nut; *Semen Arecae.* The drug consists of the dried seeds of Betel Palm, *Areca catechu* L. (family Palmae). It is used as anthelmintic for the treatment of taeniasis, ascariasis (of the bile duct), fasciolopsiasis; also used as an evacuant for abdominal distension and constipation due to stagnation of food, and as a diuretic for edema.

南瓜子 [nānguāzǐ]

Pumpkin Seed; *Semen Cucurbitae.* The drug consists of the dried seeds of *Cucurbita moschata* Duch. (family Cucurbitaceae). It is used as anthelmintic for the treatment of taeniasis, schistosomiasis and clonorchiasis.

榧子 [fěizǐ]

Torrya Seed; *Semen Torreyae.* The drug consists of the seed of Chinese Torreya, *Torreya grandis* Fort. (family Taxaceae). It is used as an anthelmintic and laxative for the treatment of taeniasis, enterobiasis, ancylostomiasis, ascariasis and fasciolopsiasis.

雷丸 [léiwán]

Omphalia; *Omphalia.* The drug consists of the dried sclerotium of *Omphalia lapidescens* Schroet. (family Polyporaceae). It is used as an anthelmintic for the treatment of taeniasis and ancylostomiasis.

鶴虱 [hèshī]

Carpesium Fruit; *Fructus Carpesii.* The drug consists of the dried fruit of *Carpesium abrotanoides* L. (family Compositae). It is used as an anthelmintic for the treatment of ascariasis, enterobiasis and taeniasis.

南鶴虱 [nánhèshī]

Carrot Fruit; *Fructus Dauci Carotae.* The drug consists of the dried fruits of Wild Carrot, *Daucus carota* L. (family Umbelliferae). In South China, this drug is usually used as 鶴虱.

鶴草芽 [hècǎoyá]

Agrimonia Bud; *Gemma Agrimoniae.* The drug consists of the dried buds, with a short piece of rhizome attached, of *Agrimonia pilosa* Ledeb. (family Rosaceae). It is used as an anthelmintic for the treatment of taeniasis. Purified extract or preparations of the active principle (Agrimopholum) is preferred for this purpose.

外用藥
Drugs for External Use

硫磺 [liúhuáng]

Sulphur; *Sulfur.* It is used (1) externally as antiparasitic for scabies; (2) internally to reinforce the vital function for the treatment of impotence and chronic asthma.

雄黃 [xiónghuáng]

Realgar; *Realgar.* The drug consists of a mineral composed of arsenic disulfide. It is used externally as a detoxicant and antiparasitic agent for snake and insect bites, boils, scabies, etc.

信石 [xìnshí]; 白砒 [báipī]

Arsenic Trioxide; *Arsenicum Trioxidum.* It is used (1) externally as a caustic to remove dead tissue for the treatment of furuncles, carbuncles, ulcers, scrofula and hemorrhoids; (2) internally in minute quantities as an expectorant and anti-asthmatic agent for the treatment of asthmatic condition with cold phlegm.

輕粉 [qīngfěn]; 甘汞 [gāngǒng]

Calomel, *Calomelas.* The drug consists of a crystalline mercurous chloride. It is used (1) externally as antiparasitic for scabies, tinea, neurodermatitis and eczematous conditions; (2) internally in small quantities as expectorant for persistent phlegm.

白礬 [báifán]; 明礬 [míngfán]

Alum, *Alumen.* The drug consists of a crystalline mineral salt, potassium aluminium sulphate. The calcined drug called 枯礬 [kūfán] is used (1) externally as an antiparasitic and antipruritic agent for scabies, tinea, neurodermatitis and eczematous conditions; (2) internally as an astringent for chronic diarrhea and bloody stool. The raw drug taken internally is used for epilepsy.

爐甘石 [lúgānshí]

Calamine; *Calamina.* The drug consists of a kind of ore (Smithsonite), mainly composed of zinc carbonate. Before use, it must be calcined and elutriated to form a very fine powder with a pink tint due to the presence of small amounts of ferric oxide. It is used externally as an astringent for chronic ulcers, eczema, conjunctivitis and keratitis.

血竭 [xuèjié]

Dragon's Blood; *Sanguis Draconis.* The drug consists of a red resin secreted from the fruit of *Daemonorops draco* Bl. (family Palmae). It is used to eliminate blood-stasis, to relieve pains and to promote the healing of wounds for the treatment of traumatic wounds and bleedings.

硇砂 [náoshā]

when this is prescribed, either 白硇砂 or 紫硇砂 may be supplied. Both are used externally for nebula and pterygium and internally for cancer of the oesophagus.

紫硇砂 [zǐnáoshā]

Purple Rocksalt; *Sal Purpureum.* The drug consists of a purple-coloured rocksalt.

白硇砂 [báináoshā]

Sal Ammoniac; *Sal Ammoniac.* The drug consists of a crystalline mineral, ammonium carbonate.

硼砂 ［péngshā］

Borax, *Borax.* The drug consists of a crystalline mineral salt, hydrated sodium tetraborate. It is used externally as gargles for ulcers of the mouth and acute tonsilitis; internally as an expectorant.

蛇床子 ［shéchuángzǐ］

Cnidium Fruit; *Fructus Cnidii.* The drug consists of the dried fruits of *Cnidium monnieri* (L.) Cuss. (family Umbelliferae). It is used (1) externally as an astringent and antiparasitic for eczema, pruritus and trichomonas vaginitis; (2) internally for the treatment of impotence.

斑蝥 ［bānmáo］

Mylabris, Chinese Blistering Beetle, Chinese Cantharides; *Mylabris.* The drug consists of the dried body of *Mylabris phalerata* Pall. or *Mylabris cichorii* L. (family Meloidae). It is used (1) externally as a rubefacient, irritant and caustic to promote local blood circulation, remove dead tissue and accelerate the healing of wounds for the treatment of psoriasis, neurodermatitis, chronic ulcers and scrofula; (2) internally in small quantities for the treatment of swellings of the lymph glands, and rabies.

蟾酥 ［chánsū］

Toad Venom; *Venenum Bufonis.* The drug consists of the dried secretion of the skin glands of the toad, *Bufo bufo gargarizans* Cantor or *Bufo melanostictus* Schneider (family Bufonidae). It is used as a detoxicant, discutient and anodyne, apllied externally and taken internally for the treatment of boils, carbuncles, ulcers, tumor, chronic osteomyelitis, and sore-throat.

蜂房 ［fēngfáng］

Wasp's Nest; *Nidus Vespae.* The drug consists of the nest of wasps or hornets, *Polistes olivaceus* (Deg.), *Polistes japonicus* Sauss. or *Parapolybia varia* Fabr. (family Vespidae). It is used externally for suppurative skin diseases; as gargles for pain and swelling of gums; internally for convulsions, urticaria, tumor and chronic cough.

兒茶 ［érchá］

Cutch, Black Catechu; *Catechu.* The drug is a dry extract prepared

226

from the stem and branches of *Acacia catechu* Willd. (family Leguminosae). It is used as an astringent for hemoptysis, diarrhea and cough with yellow, thick phlegm, used externally for suppurative infections, wounds and eczematous skin diseases.

IX Prescriptions

方 [fāng]; 方劑 [fāngjì]

prescription; recipe

單方 [dānfāng]

simple recipe consisting of one or two medical substances for treating a particular illness in uncomplicated condition

奇方 [jīfāng]

prescription with ingredients odd in number

偶方 [ǒufāng]

prescription with ingredients even in number

複方 [fùfāng]

compound prescription formed by (1) two or more set recipes; (2) one recipe with additional ingredients

成方 [chéngfāng]

set recipe

驗方 [yànfāng]

proved recipe

良方 [liángfāng]

well-tried recipe

秘方 [mìfāng]; 禁方 [jìnfāng]

secret recipe

祖傳秘方 [zǔchuán mìfāng]

secret recipe handed down from ancestors

偏方 [piānfāng]

special but irregular prescription

土方 [tǔfāng]

folk recipe; folk remedy

土方土法 [tǔfāngtǔfǎ]

folk recipes and treatment

經方 [jīngfāng]

classical prescriptions or recipes: (1) prescriptions recorded in Nei

Jing ("Internal Classic" or "Canon of Medicine") and in Zhang Zhong-jing's works; (2) prescriptions recorded in Zhang Zhong-jing's works only

時方 [shífāng]
contemporary prescriptions or recipes; prescriptions introduced by physicians after the great physician Zhang Zhong-jing

大方 [dàfāng]
major or heavy recipe: (1) a heavy recipe or prescription which consists of many ingredients with strong action; (2) large dosage of medicine to be taken at one time to give strong action; (3) recipes for the treatment of diseases ascribed to the lower part of the body cavity

小方 [xiǎofāng]
minor or mild recipe: (1) a mild recipe or prescription which consists of only a few ingredients for mild illness; (2) small dosage for the treatment of uncomplicated diseases or diseases ascribed to the upper part of the body cavity

緩方 [huǎnfāng]
slow-acting prescription or recipe, which is composed of ingredients that act slowly or counteract each other to moderate effect, and is indicated in the treatment of chronic debilitated cases

急方 [jífāng]
quick-acting prescription or recipe, which is employed for immediate effect in the treatment of emergency or critical cases

配方 [pèifāng]
to dispense a prescription or recipe

湯頭 [tāngtóu]
recipes of decoctions

湯頭歌 [tāngtóugē]
recipes put in rhyme to make them easier to memorize

方劑配伍 [fāngjìpèiwǔ]
combination of various ingredients in a prescription with the purpose of producing desired therapeutic effect in unison and reducing toxic or side effects

君臣佐使 [jūn chén zuǒ shǐ]; 主輔佐引 [zhǔ fǔ zuǒ yǐn]
the principal, adjuvant, auxiliary and conductant ingredients in a

229

prescription: the 君 (or 主) or principal ingredient provides the principal curative action, the 臣 (or 輔) or the adjuvant helps strengthen the principal action, the 佐 or auxiliary and correctant ingredient relieves secondary symptoms or tempers the action of the principal ingredient when the latter is too potent, while the 使 (or引) or conductant directs action to the affected channel or site

引經報使 [yǐnjīngbàoshǐ]

action in directing other ingredients to work on the affected channel or site. For instance, *Radix Bupleuri* is said to be able to conduct other drugs to the Minor Yang Channel, *Radix Platycodi* to the throat, *Radix Cyathulae* to the lower extremities, etc.

藥引子 [yào yǐng zǐ]

extra conductant ingredient in a prescription, used to strengthen the efficacy of the medicine

相須 [xiāng xū]

mutual reinforcement, two ingredients with similar properties used in combination to reinforce each other's action

相使 [xiāng shǐ]

assistance, two or more ingredients in a prescription used in combination, one being the principal substance while the rest play a subsidiary role to reinforce the action of the former

相畏 [xiāngwèi]

mutual restraint, the mutual restraining effect of different ingredients to weaken or neutralize each other's action

相惡 [xiāngwù]

counteraction, the property of one drug or ingredient to weaken the action of another drug or ingredient

相殺 [xiāngshā]

neutralization, the property of one drug or ingredient to neutralize the toxicity of another drug or ingredient

相反 [xiāngfǎn]

incompatibility, the property of not being suitable for combination or simultaneous administration. Severe side effects may result when two incompatible ingredients are used in combination.

十八反 [shíbāfǎn]

eighteen incompatible medicaments which, if given in combination, are believed to give rise to serious side effects: *Radix Glycyrrhizae* being incompatible with *Radix Euphorbiae Kansui, Radix Euphorbiae Pekinensis, Flos Genkwa* and *Sargassum; Radix Aconiti* incompatible with *Bulbus Fritillariae, Fructus Trichosanthis, Rhizoma Pinelliae, Radix Ampelopsis* and *Rhizoma Bletillae; Radix Veratri Nigri* incompatible with *Radix Ginseng, Radix Glehniae, Radix Salviae Miltiorrhizae, Radix Scrophulariae, Radix Sophorae Flavescentis, Herba Asari* and *Radix Paeoniae*

十九畏 ［shíjiǔwèi］

nineteen medicaments of mutual restraint which, if used in combination, may restrain or neutralize each other's action: sulfur restraining crude mirabilite; mercury restraining arsenic; *Radix Euphorbiae Ebracteolatae* restraining litharge; *Semen Crotonis* restraining *Semen Pharbitidis; Flos Caryophylli* restraining *Radix Curcumae;* crystallized mirabilite restraining *Rhizoma Sparganii; Radix Aconiti* and *Radix Aconiti Kuznezoffii* restraining *Cornu Rhinoceri; Radix Ginseng* restraining *Faeces Trogopterorum; Cortex Cinnamomi* restraining *Halloysitum Rubrum*

常用方劑
Commonly Used Recipes

解表劑 ［jiěbiǎojì］

diaphoretic recipes, recipes to dispel pathogenic factors from the exterior of the body for the treatment of exterior symptom-complex

麻黄湯 ［máhuáng tāng］

Decoction of Ephedra (麻黄 *Herba Ephedrae,* 桂枝 *Ramulus Cinnamomi,* 苦杏仁 *Semen Armeniacae Amarum,* 甘草 *Radix Glycyrrhizae*), used as a diaphoretic and antasthmatic for the treatment of affections by wind and cold with chills and fever, headache and general aching, dyspnea, hypohidrosis, floating and tense pulse

桂枝湯 ［guìzhītāng］

Decoction of Cinnamon Twigs (桂枝 *Ramulus Cinnamomi,*

白芍 Radix Paeoniae Alba, 生薑 Rhizoma Zingiberis Recens 甘草 Radix Glycyrrhizae, 大棗 Fructus Ziziphi Jujubae), used to expel exogenous pathogenic factors from the exterior of the body and rectify derangement of the constructive and defensive systems for the treatment of exterior symptom-complex with fever, headache, sweating and intolerance of wind; and also used in a variety of conditions other than exterior symptom-complex owing to its regulating effect

荊防敗毒散 [jīng fáng bàidú sǎn]

Antiphlogistic Powder of Schizonepeta and Ledebouriella (荊芥 Herba Schizonepetae, 防風 Radix Ledebouriellae, 羌活 Rhizoma seu Radix Notopterygii, 獨活 Radix Angelicae Pubescentis, 川芎 Rhizoma Ligustici Chuanxiong, 柴胡 Radix Bupleuri, 前胡 Radix Peucedani, 桔梗 Radix Platycodi, 枳殼 Fructus Aurantii,茯苓Poria, 甘草 Radix Glycyrrhizae, 薄荷 Herba Menthae), used to dispel wind, cold and dampness from the exterior of the body, for the treatment of influenza or common cold with chills and fever, headache, pains in muscles and joints, white greasy fur of the tongue and floating pulse; also for the early treatment of dysentery and boils with cold symptom-complex in the exterior of the body

銀翹散 [yín qiào sǎn]

Powder of Lonicera and Forsythia (金銀花 Flos Lonicerae, 連翹 Fructus Forsythiae, 牛蒡子 Fructus Arctii, 薄荷 Herba Menthae, 荊芥 Herba Schizonepetae,豆豉 Semen Sojae Praeparatum, 桔梗 Radix Platycodi, 甘草 Radix Glycyrrhizae, 淡竹葉 Herba Lophatheri, 蘆根 Rhizoma Phragmitis), used as a diaphoretic, febrifugal and detoxicant remedy for heat symptom-complex in the exterior of the body, such as the early stage of influenza, upper respiratory infections, pneumonia, measles, etc., with fever, headache, sore throat, cough, floating and rapid pulse

桑菊飲 [sāng jú yǐn]

Decoction of Morus and Chrysanthemum (桑葉 Folium Mori, 菊花 Flos Chrysanthemi, 薄荷 Herba Menthae, 苦杏仁 Semen Armeniacae Amarum, 桔梗 Radix Platycodi, 甘草 Radix Glycyrrhizae, 連翹 Fructus Forsythiae, 蘆根 Rhizoma Phragmitis), used as a febrifugal and antibechic remedy for the early treatment of upper respiratory infections with coughing, headache and mild fever

清热剂 [qīngrèjì]

febrifugal recipes, recipes which are composed of drugs cold or cool in nature and are used to relieve fever or other heat symptoms by clearing up heat in the interior of the body

白虎湯 [báihǔ tāng]

Baihu (White Tiger) Decoction (石膏 *Gypsum Fibrosum,* 知母 *Rhizoma Anemarrhenae,* 甘草 *Radix Glycyrrhizae,* 粳米 *Semen Oryzae Nongglutinosae**), used to clear up evil heat from the Qi (secondary defensive) system (the *lung* and the *stomach*) for high fever with dire thirst, sweating and full and gigantic pulse.

犀角地黃湯 [xījiǎo dìhuáng tāng]

Decoction of Rhinoceros Horn and Rehmannia (犀角 *Cornu Rhinoceri,* 生地黃 *Radix Rehmanniae,* 赤芍 *Radix Paeoniae Rubra,* 牡丹皮 *Cortex Moutan Radicis*), used to clear up toxic heat from the *heart* and blood, and is used for the treatment of fever with impaired consciousness, hemorrhagic exanthesis, etc.

黃連解毒湯 [huánglián jiědú tāng]

Detoxicant (Antiinfective) Decoction of Coptis (黃連 *Rhizoma Coptidis,* 黃芩 *Radix Scutellariae,* 黃柏 *Cortex Phellodendri,* 栀子 *Fructus Gardeniae*), used to cure various pyogenic infections, such as acute dysentery, acute infection of the urinary tract, pneumonia, septicemia, and carbuncle or furuncle with systemic symptoms

龍膽瀉肝湯 [lóngdǎn xiègān tāng]

Decoction of Gentiana to Purge the Liver(龍膽 *Radix Gentianae,* 黃芩 *Radix Scutellariae,* 栀子 *Fructus Gardeniae,* 澤瀉 *Rhizoma Alismatis,* 關木通 *Caulis Aristolochiae Manshuriensis,* 車前子 *Semen Plantaginis,* 當歸 *Radix Angelicae Sinensis,* 生地黃 *Radix Rehmanniae,* 柴胡 *Radix Bupleuri,* 甘草 *Radix Glycyrrhizae*), used to eliminate intense heat or fire and dampness from the *liver* and *gallbladder,* manifestations of which are pain in the head, ear and hypochondrium, redness of eyes, bitter taste in the mouth, ear swelling or pain, itching in perin-

---

*Semen Oryzae Nonglutinosae=Nonglutinous Rice

233

eum, yellow and thick leukorrhea, red borders of tongue, yellow fur and rapid taut pulse

茵陳蒿湯 [yīnchénhāo tāng]

Decoction of Artemisia Scoparia (茵陳 *Herba Artemisiae Scopariae*, 梔子 *Fructus Gardeniae*, 大黃 *Radix et Rhizoma Rhei*), used to clear up heat and dampness in the *liver* and *gallbladder* and is indicated in the treatment of acute jaundice

竹葉石膏湯 [zhúyè shígāo tāng]

Decoction of Bamboo Leaves and Gypsum (淡竹葉 *Herba Lophatheri*, 石膏 *Gypsum Fibrosum*, 麥冬 *Radix Ophiopogonis*, 半夏 *Rhizoma Pinelliae*, 人參 *Radix Ginseng* or 黨參 *Radix Codonopsis Pilosulae*, 粳米 *Semen Oryzae Nonglutinosae*, 甘草 *Radix Glycyrrhizae*), used to clear up evil heat, replenish vital energy, promote secretion of body fluid, and regulate the functioning of the *stomach*, and is used for the treatment of febrile diseases at the stage of restoration with lingering heat and impaired vital essence and energy marked by fidget and thirst, anorexia, nausea and vomiting, red furless tongue, and rapid and fine pulse

青蒿鱉甲湯 [qīnghāo biējiǎ tāng]

Decoction of Chinghao and Turtle Shell (青蒿 *Herba Artemisiae Chinghao*, 鱉甲 *Carapax Trionycis*, 生地黃 *Radix Rehmanniae*, 知母 *Rhizoma Anemarrhenae*, 牡丹皮 *Cortex Moutan Radicis*), used to replenish vital essence for relieving tidal fever due to deficiency of vital essence or persistent low fever as seen in chronic consumptive diseases

瀉下劑 [xièxiàjì]

purgative recipes, recipes used for relieving constipation and purging out various kinds of pathogenic factors from the interior of the body

大承氣湯 [dà chéngqì tāng]

Drastic Purgative Decoction (大黃 *Radix et Rhizoma Rhei*, 芒硝 *Natrii Sulfas*, 枳實 *Fructus Aurantii Immaturus*, 厚朴 *Cortex Magnoliae Officinalis*), used to purge the bowels of accumulated waste matter and internal heat, and is indicated in the treatment of Yangming Channel Syndrome with the bowels involved, marked by fever, constipation, abdominal pain with tenderness, yellow and thick fur of the tongue, slippery and full pulse, seen in acute febrile diseases and also in acute intestinal obstruction, acute cholecystitis and acute pancreatitis

和解劑〔héjiějì〕

mediation recipes, recipes which regulate the correlations of viscera, channels, vital energy and blood, so as to remove pathogenic factors and restore normal functions

小柴胡湯〔xiǎo cháihú tāng〕

Minor (Mild) Decoction of Bupleurum (柴胡 *Radix Bupleuri,* 黃芩 *Radix Scutellariae,* 大棗 *Fructus Ziziphi Jujubae,* 生薑 *Rhizoma Zingiberis Recens,* 制半夏 *Rhizoma Pinelliae Praeparata,* 甘草 *Radix Glycyrrhizae,* 黨參 *Radix Codonopsis Pilosulae*) used to strengthen the body resistance, remove pathogenic factors and reestablish normal correlation between the interior and exterior of the body, for the treatment of Syndrome of the Yang Minor Channel marked by alternate fever and chills, fullness and tightness in the chest and costal regions, fidget and nausea, dryness of throat and bitterness in the mouth, taut and rapid pulse, seen in infectious diseases such as infectious hepatitis, cholecystitis, malaria, colds in the period of menstruation, etc.

逍遙散〔xiāoyáo sǎn〕

Xiao-yao Powder; Ease Powder (柴胡 *Radix Bupleuri,* 當歸 *Radix Angelicae Sinensis,* 白芍 *Radix Paeoniae Alba,* 白朮 *Rhizoma Atractylodis Macrocephalae,* 茯苓 *Poria,* 甘草 *Radix Glycyrrhizae,* 煨生薑 *Rhizoma Zingiberis Praeparata,* 薄荷 *Herba Menthae*), used to coordinate the functioning of the *liver* and the *spleen* for the treatment of stagnancy of the vital energy of these two organs marked by costal pains, dizziness, lassitude, loss of appetite, dull mastalgia and menstrual complaints in women, taut and fine pulse, seen in cases of neurosis, menopathies and chronic disorders of liver and gall-bladder

祛寒劑〔qūhánjì〕

warming recipes, recipes used for dispelling cold, composed chiefly of drugs warm or hot in nature

理中湯〔lǐzhōng tāng〕

Lizhong Decoction, decoction to regulate the functioning of the Middle Burner, i.e., the *spleen* and *stomach* (黨參 *Radix Codonopsis Pilosulae,* 乾薑 *Rhizoma Zingiberis,* 白朮 *Rhizoma Atractylodis Macro-*

cephalae, 炙甘草 *Radix Glycyrrhizae Praeparata*), used to warm the *spleen* and *stomach*, dispel cold from them, and restore their normal functioning by replenishing vital energy, for the treatment of deficiency of vital function of the *spleen* and *stomach* marked by cold pains in the stomach, dyspepsia and chronic diarrhea, swollen tongue with white slippery coat, deep and slow pulse, such as seen in cases of chronic gastro-enteritis, peptic ulcer, chronic dysentery, etc.

小建中湯 [xiǎo jiànzhōng tāng]

Xiao Jianzhong Decoction, mild decoction for restoring the normal functioning of the Middle Burner (白芍 *Radix Paeoniae Alba*, 桂枝 *Ramulus Cinnamomi*, 炙甘草 *Radix Glycyrrhizae Praeparata*, 生薑 *Rhizoma Zingiberis Recens*, 大棗 *Fructus Ziziphi Jujubae*, 飴糖 malt extract), used to warm and tonify the *spleen* and *stomach* and relieve spasmodic pains for the treatment of abdominal pain caused by deficiency of vital energy and accumulation of cold in the *spleen* and *stomach*, as seen in cases of gastric and duodenal ulcer, gastric and intestinal spasm

四逆湯 [sìnì tāng]

Sini Decoction, decoction for treating vital prostration with cold limbs (制附子 *Radix Aconiti Praeparata*, 乾薑 *Rhizoma Zingiberis*, 炙甘草 *Radix Glycyrrhizae Praeparata*), used to restore vital function from collapse and shock with cold limbs

獨活寄生湯 [dúhuó jìshēng tāng]

Decoction of Pubescent Angelica and Loranthus (獨活 *Radix Angelicae Pubescentis*, 桑寄生 *Ramulus Loranthi*, 川芎 *Rhizoma Ligustici Chuanxiong*, 細辛 *Herba Asari*, 秦艽 *Radix Gentianae Macrophyllae*, 防風 *Radix Ledebouriellae*, 牛膝 *Radix Achyranthis Bidentatae*, 杜仲 *Cortex Eucommiae*, 當歸 *Radix Angelicae sinensis*, 白芍 *Radix Paeoniae Alba*, 熟地黃 *Radix Rehmanniae Praeparata*, 茯苓 *Poria*, 黨參 *Radix Codonopsis Pilosulae*, 桂枝 *Ramulus Cinnamomi*, 甘草 *Radix Glycyrrhizae*). It is used for treating rheumatic troubles and allied conditions such as rheumatoid arthritis, sciatica, strain of lumbar muscles, etc. by tonifying the *liver* and the *kidney*, replenishing vital energy and blood, and dispelling wind and dampness.

補益劑 [bǔyìjì]

tonifying recipes, recipes to reinforce vital function or replenish

236

vital essence, energy and blood in their deficiencies

四君子湯 [sìjūnzǐ tāng]

Sijunzi Decoction; Decoction of Four Noble Ingredients (人參 *Radix Ginseng* or 黨參 *Radix Codonopsis Pilosulae,* 茯苓 *Poria,* 白朮 *Rhizoma Atractylodis Macrocephalae,* 炙甘草 *Radix Glycyrrhizae Praeparata*), the basic tonifying recipe for treating deficiency of vital energy of the *spleen* and *stomach* manifested by debility, lassitude, anorexia, etc.

四物湯 [sìwù tāng]

Siwu Decoction; Decoction of Four Drugs(熟地黃 *Radix Rehmanniae Praeparata,* 白芍 *Radix Paeoniae Alba,* 當歸 *Radix Angelicae Sinensis,* 川芎 *Rhizoma Ligustici Chuanxiong*), used to replenish blood, promote circulation and normalize menstruation for the treatment of deficinecy of blood alone or with blood stasis, as seen in cases of menstrual disorders

當歸補血湯 [dāngguī bǔxuè tāng]

Blood Tonifying Decoction with Chinese Angelica (當歸 *Radix Angelicae Sinensis,* 黃芪 *Radix Astragali*), used to replenish vital energy and promote hematogenesis for deficiency of vital energy and blood (e.g., after profuse uterine bleeding or childbirth) marked by sallowness, lassitude and low-grade fever and weak pulse

六味地黃丸 [liùwèi dìhuáng wán]

Pills of Six Drugs with Rehmannia (熟地黃 *Radix Rehmanniae Praeparata,* 山茱萸 *Fructus Corni,* 山藥 *Rhizoma Dioscoreae,* 澤瀉 *Rhizoma Alismatis,* 茯苓 *Poria,* 牡丹皮 *Cortex Moutan Radicis*), used to replenish vital essence of both the *liver* and the *kidney* for the treatment of its deficiency in chronic diseases with symptoms of asthenic fire such as dizziness, tinnitus, sore throat, tidal fever, nocturnal emission, etc.

金匱腎氣丸 [jīnguì shènqì wán]

Jingui Shenqi Pills, pills for restoring vital energy and function of the *kidney* recommended by "Synopsis of Prescriptions of the Golden Chamber" (附子 *Radix Aconiti Praeparata,* 肉桂 *Cortex Cinnamomi,* 熟地黃 *Radix Rehmanniae Praeparata,* 山茱萸 *Fructus Corni,* 山藥 *Rhizoma Dioscoreae,* 澤瀉 *Rhizoma Alismatis,* 茯苓 *Poria,* 牡丹皮

Cortex Moutan Radicis), used for the treatment of cool sensation in the lower part of the body, dysuria, urorrhagia, nocturia, cough and asthma, edema, persistent diarrhea, etc., due to hypofunction of the *kidney*

消散剂〔xiāosànjì〕

discutient recipes, recipes to resolve stagnated food, tumors and masses, calculi, etc.

保和丸〔bǎohéwán〕

Baohe Pills, pills for keeping the functioning of the stomach in good condition (山楂 *Fructus Crataegi,* 神曲 *Massa Fermentata Medicinalis,* 萊服子 *Semen Raphani,* 茯苓 *Poria,* 陳皮 *Pericarpium Citri Reticulatae,* 半夏 *Rhizoma Pinelliae,* 連翹 *Fructus Forsythiae*), used to remove stagnated food by promoting digestive function for the treatment of food stagnation with resultant fullness and distention in gastric region, belching and hiccup, loss of appetite, constipation or diarrhea, yellow and slippery fur, slippery pulse, etc.

膽道排石湯〔dǎndào páishí tāng〕

Biliary Lithagogue Decoction (金錢草 *Herba Lysimachiae,* 茵陳 *Herba Artemisiae Scopariae,* 鬱金 *Radix Curcumae,* 枳殼 *Fructus Aurantii,* 木香 *Radix Aucklandiae,* 生大黃 *Radix et Rhizoma Rhei*), used for cholelithiasis to expel the calculi from the bile duct

理氣劑〔lǐqìjì〕

carminative recipes, recipes to regulate and normalize the flow of vital energy

四逆散〔sìnì sǎn〕

Sini Powder, powder for relieving depression with cold limbs (柴胡 *Radix Bupleuri,* 白芍 *Radix Paeoniae Alba,* 枳實 *Fructus Aurantii Immaturus,* 甘草 *Radix Glycyrrhizae*), the principal recipe for restoring the normal function of a depressed *liver* in which the flow of the vital energy is impeded by evil heat leading to stagnancy of vital energy in the interior of the body together with coldness in the extremities, accompanied with costal or abdominal pain and menstrual complaints

瓜蔞薤白半夏湯〔guālóu xièbái bànxià tāng〕

Decoction of Trichosanthes, Allium and Pinellia (瓜蔞 *Fructus*

Trichosanthis, 薤白 *Bulbus Allii Macrostemi,* 白酒 *Spiritus,* 半夏 *Rhizoma Pinelliae*), used for relieving chest pain due to obstruction in the flow of vital energy with phlegm marked by profuse expectoration, shortness of breathing, white slippery fur of the tongue, as seen in angina pectoris or chronic bronchitis, intercostal pain, etc.

旋複代赭湯 [xuánfù dàizhě tāng]
Decoction of Inula and Haematitum (旋複花 *Flos Inulae,* 赭石 *Haematitum,* 生薑 *Rhizoma Zingiberis Recens,* 制半夏 *Rhizoma Pinelliae Praeparata,* 炙甘草 *Radix Glycyrrhizae Praeparata,* 大棗 *Fructus Ziziphi Jujubae,* 黨參 *Radix Codonopsis Pilosulae*), used to relieve nausea and arrest vomiting due to dysfunction of the *stomach* as seen in gastritis, gastric neurosis, Ménière's syndrome and partial pyloric obstruction. It is also used for treating asthma with profuse sputum.

理血劑 [lǐxuèjì]
blood-regulating recipes, including blood-tonifying recipes, blood-activating or blood circulation-promoting recipes, hemostatic recipes

血府逐瘀湯 [xuèfǔ zhúyú tāng]
Xuefu Zhuyu Decoction, decoction for removing blood stasis in chest (當歸 *Radix Angelicae Sinensis,* 赤芍 *Radix Paeoniae Rubra,* 生地黃 *Radix Rehmanniae,* 川芎 *Rhizoma Ligustici Chuanxiong,* 桃仁 *Semen Persicae,* 紅花 *Flos Carthami,* 柴胡 *Radix Bupleuri,* 枳殼 *Fructus Aruantii,* 桔梗 *Radix Platycodi,* 甘草 *Radix Glycyrrhizae,* 牛膝 *Radix Achyranthis Bidentatae*), used to remove blood stasis by activating the blood and relieve pain by regulating the flow of vital energy for the treatment of chest pain, headache, palpitation, insomnia, etc. with manifestations of blood stasis, as seen in angina pectoris, neurosis and menorrhalgia

補陽還五湯 [bǔyáng huánwǔ tāng]
Buyang Huanwu Decoction, decoction for reinforcing vital function and restore normal functioning of Five Viscera (黃芪 *Radix Astragali,* 當歸 *Radix Angelicae Sinensis,* 赤芍 *Radix Paeoniae Rubra,* 川芎 *Rhizoma Ligustici Chuanxiong,* 桃仁 *Semen Persicae,* 紅花 *Flos Carthami,* 地龍 *Lumbricus*), used to promote blood circulation by replenishing vital energy and activate the collateral circulations by removing blood stasis for the treatment of apoplexy and hemiplegia as its sequela

生化湯 [shēnghuà tāng]

Shenghua Decoction, decoction for removing stagnant blood and promoting hemogenesis (當歸 *Radix Angelicae Sinensis,* 川芎 *Rhizoma Ligustici Chuanxiong,* 桃仁 *Semen Persicae,* 炮薑 *Rhizoma Zingiberis Praeparata,* 炙甘草 *Radix Glycyrrhizae Praeparata*), used to activate the blood circulation of the uterus for the treatment of retaining of lochia, and pain in the lower abdomen after childbirth

小薊飲子 [xiǎojì yǐnzí]

Decoction of Cephalanoplos (生地黄 *Radix Rehmanniae* 小薊 *Herba Cephalanoplosis,* 滑石 *Pulvis Talci,* 木通 *Caulis Aristolochiae Manshuriensis,* 炒蒲黄 *Pollen Typhae Carbonizatum,* 藕節 *Nodus Nelumbinis Rhizomatis,* 淡竹葉 *Herba Lophatheri,* 當歸 *Radix Angelicae Sinensis,* 梔子 *Fructus Gardeniae,* 甘草 *Radix Glycyrrhizae*), used for hematuria to check the blood in the urine by removing evil heat and promoting urination in acute infections of urinary tract and other urinary diseases with heat symptoms

祛痰劑 [qūtánjì]

phlegm-expelling recipes, recipes used for expelling or dissipating phlegm

二陳湯 [èrchén tāng]

Erchen Decoction, decoction of two old drugs (tangerine peel and pinellia tuber) (陳皮 *Pericarpium Citri Reticulatae* or 桔紅 *Exocarpium Citri Grandis,* 制半夏 *Rhizoma Pinelliae Praeparata,* 茯苓 *Poria,* 炙甘草 *Radix Glycyrrhizae Praeparata*), used to resolve phlegm by drying internal dampness and regulating the function of the *spleen* and the *stomach* for the treatment of symptom-complex caused by damp-phlegm marked by profuse watery foamy sputum, fullness over the epigastric region, nausea, dizziness, white greasy fur of the tongue and slippery pulse, as seen in cases of chronic bronchitis

小青龍湯 [xiǎoqīnglóng tāng]

Minor Decoction of Qinglong (Blue Dragon)(麻黄 *Herba Ephedrae,* 桂枝 *Ramulus Cinnamomi,* 細辛 *Herba Asari,* 乾薑 *Rhizoma Zingiberis,* 制半夏 *Rhizoma Pinelliae Praeparata,* 五味子 *Fructus Schisandrae,* 白芍 *Radix Paeoniae Alba,* 甘草 *Radix Glycyrrhizae*), used to disperse cold from the exterior of the body and remove excessive humor from the lung, for the treatment of acute attacks of chronic bronchitis and bronchial asthma with profuse, watery and foamy sputum, brought on by cold

祛濕劑 [qūshījì]

desiccating recipes, recipes used for expelling dampness from the body, through diuresis or by desiccation

藿香正氣散 [huòxiāng zhèngqì sǎn]

Huoxiang Zhengqi Powder, powder for dispelling turbidity with Agastache (藿香 *Herba Agastachis,* 紫蘇葉 *Folium Perillae,* 白芷 *Radix Angelicae Dahuricae,* 大腹皮 *Pericarpium Arecae,* 茯苓 *Poria,* 白朮 *Rhizoma Atractylodis Macrocephalae* or 蒼朮 *Rhizoma Atractylodis,* 陳皮 *Pericarpium Citri Reticulatae,* 半夏曲 *Massa Pinelliae Fermentata,* 厚朴 *Cortex Magnoliae Officinalis,* 桔梗 *Radix Platycodi,* 甘草 *Radix Glycyrrhizae*), used to resolve damp-turbidity and dispel pathogenic factors from the exterior of the body with aromatic drugs for the treatment of affection by wind and cold with accumulation of dampness in the interior, usually manifested by vomiting and diarrhea as seen in cases of cold in summer, acute gastro-enteritis and influenza with gastrointestinal symptoms

真武湯 [zhēnwǔ tāng]

Decoction of Zhenwu (the God who controls water) (茯苓 *Poria,* 白朮 *Rhizoma Atractylodis Macrocephalae,* 白芍 *Radix Paeoniae Alba,* 生薑 *Rhizoma Zingiberis Recens,* 制附子 *Radix Aconiti Praeparata*), used to relieve water retention by invigorating the vital function of the *kidney* and the *spleen.* It is indicated in the treatment of nephrotic and cardiac edema and prolonged diarrhea due to chronic enteritis or dysentery with symptoms brought on by deficiency of vital function of both the *kidney* and the *spleen.*

五苓散 [wǔlíng sǎn]

Powder of Five Drugs with Poria (茯苓 *Poria,* 豬苓 *Polypolus umbellatus,* 白朮 *Rhizoma Atractylodis Macrocephalae,* 澤瀉 *Rhizoma Alismatis,* 桂枝 *Ramulus Cinnamomi*), a recipe commonly used for diuresis. It can be used for various kinds of edema and is especially indicated in the treatment of symptom-complex due to affection by external cold and stagnation of humor in the interior marked by headache and fever, fidget and thirstiness, frequent vomiting and diarrhea, difficulty in urination, white dense fur, floating pulse, etc.

八正散 [bāzhèng sǎn]

Bazheng Powder (車前子 *Semen Plantaginis*, 關木通 *Caulis Aristolochiae Manshuriensis*, 瞿麥 *Herba Dianthi*, 萹蓄 *Herba Polygoni Avicularis*, 滑石 *Pulvis Talci*, 甘草 *Radix Glycyrrhizae*, 栀子 *Fructus Gardeniae*, 熟大黃 *Radix et Rhizoma Rhei Praeparata*, 燈芯草 *Medulla Junci*), used to clear up evil heat and dispel dampness by promoting urination, and is used for acute nephritis and acute urinary infections with accumulation of dampness and heat in the urinary bladder marked by fullness and distension of the lower abdomen, frequent, scanty and painful urination, yellow and red urine, etc.

固濇劑 [gùsèjì]

astringent recipes, recipes to arrest discharges, including excessive perspiration, persistent diarrhea, seminal emission, incontinence of urine, profuse uterine bleeding and leukorrhea, etc.

玉屏風散 [yùpíngfēng sǎn]

Yupingfeng Powder; Jade-Screen Powder (黃芪 *Radix Astragali,* 白朮 *Rhizoma Atractylodis Macrocephalae,* 防風 *Radix Ledebouriellae*), used to replenish vital energy so as to consolidate the superficial resistance of the body and check excessive spontaneous perspiration due to deficiency of vital energy which renders one susceptible to cold

四神丸 [sìshén wán]

Sishen Pills, pills of four miraculous drugs (補骨脂 *Fructus Psoraleae,* 五味子 *Fructus Schisandrae,* 肉豆蔻 *Semen Myristicae,* 吳茱萸 *Fructus Evodiae*), used to relieve diarrhea by invigorating functioning of the *spleen* and the *kidney* for the treatment of habitual diarrhea before dawn in chronic colitis, chronic dysentery, etc.

固精丸 [gùjīng wán]

Gujing Pills; Pills for Seminal Consolidation (潼蒺藜 *Semen Astragali Complanati,* 芡實 *Semen Euryales,* 蓮鬚 *Stamen Nelumbinis,* 煅龍骨 *Os Draconis Usta,* 煅牡蠣 *Concha Ostreae Usta*), used for nocturnal and spontaneous emission due to deficiency in the *kidney*

安神劑 [ānshénjì]

sedative or tranquilizing recipes

242

酸棗仁湯 [suānzǎorén tāng]

Decoction of Wild Jujube Seed (酸棗仁 *Semen Ziziphi Spinosae*, 知母 *Rhizoma Anemarrhenae*, 茯苓 *Poria*, 川芎 *Rhizoma Ligustici Chuanxiong*, 炙甘草 *Radix Glycyrrhizae Praeparata*), which has sedative effects by nourishing the blood of the *liver* and eliminating endogenous heat, and is used for fidget and insomnia

甘麥大棗湯 [gān mài dàzǎo tāng]

Decoction of Liquorice, Wheat and Jujube (炙甘草 *Radix Glycyrrhizae Praeparata*, 大棗 *Fructus Ziziphi Jujubae*, 浮小麥 *Fructus Tritici Levis*), used as a sedative for psychoneurosis, especially hysteria, marked by the lack of control over emotion

熄風劑 [xīfēngjì]

anticonvulsive recipes, recipes used for subduing endogenous wind

天麻鈎藤飲 [tiānmá gōuténg yǐn]

Decoction of Gastrodia and Uncaria (天麻 *Rhizoma Gastrodiae*, 鈎藤 *Ramulus Uncariae cum Uncis*, 生石決明 *Concha Haliotidis*, 桑寄生 *Ramulus Loranthi*, 杜仲 *Cortex Eucommiae*, 梔子 *Fructus Gardeniae*, 黃芩 *Radix Scutellariae*, 牛膝 *Radix Achyranthis Bidentatae* 益母草 *Herba Leonuri*, 茯神 *Lignum Pini Poriaferum*, 首烏藤 *Caulis Polygoni Multiflori*), used to subdue endogenous wind by checking the hyperactivity of the *liver* and nourishing its vital essence to treat hypertensive patients with symptoms of endogenous wind stirring in the *liver* due to exuberance of its vital function (cf. 肝陽上亢, 肝風內動)

成 藥
Patent Medicines

銀翹解毒丸(片) [yínqiào jiědú wán/piàn]

Yin Qiao Antipyretic Pills (Tablets); Febrifugal Pills (Tablets) of Lonicera and Forsythia (金銀花 *Flos Lonicerae*, 連翹 *Fructus Forsythiae*, 薄荷 *Herba Menthae*, 桔梗 *Radix Platycodi*, 牛蒡子 *Fructus Arctii*, 荆芥 *Herba Schizonepetae, etc.*), used to expel toxic heat from the exterior of the body, to cure affections by wind and heat with chills and fever, headache, and sore throat, such as seen in influenza

小活络丹 [xiǎo huóluò dān]

Xiao Huo Luo Pills, pills for activating circulation in collateral channels (mild recipe) (附子 *Radix Aconiti Praeparata,* 制草乌 *Radix Aconiti Kusnezoffii Praeparata,* 当归 *Radix Angelicae Sinensis,* 乳香 *Olibanum,* 没药 *Myrrha,* 地龙 *Lumbricus, etc.*), used to relieve rheumatic pain, numbness and difficulty in movement of joints by dispelling wind and dampness, and invigorating blood flow in collaterals

大活络丸(丹) [dà huóluò wán/dān]

Da Huo Luo Pills, pills for activating circulation in collateral channels (heavy recipe)(蕲蛇 *Agkistrodon,* 乌梢蛇 *Zaocys,* 天麻 *Rhizoma Gastrodiae,* 人参 *Radix Ginseng,* 牛黄 *Calculus Bovis,* 麝香 *Moschus,* 犀角 *Corni Rhinoceri,* 地龙 *Lumbricus,* 天南星 *Rhizoma Arisaematis,* 威灵仙 *Radix Clematidis,* 血竭 *Sanguis Draconis, etc.*), used to dispel wind and dampness, activate blood flow in collateral channels, and relax the muscles and joints for treating arthritis with pain, stiffiness or contracture of limbs, and apoplectic hemiplegia

金不换膏 [jīnbùhuàn gāo]

Jin Bu Huan Plaster, plaster not exchangeable for gold (大黄 *Radix et Rhizoma Rhei,* 没药 *Myrrha,* 血竭 *Sanguis Draconis,* 穿山甲 *Squama Manitis,* 麻黄 *Herba Ephedrae,* 草乌 *Radix Aconiti Kusnezoffii,* etc.), used to relieve pain by expelling wind and cold and promoting blood circulation, and for the treatment of pains of muscles and joints due to cold, sprain and other injuries

牛黄上清丸 [niúhuáng shàngqīng wán]

Niu Huang Shang Qing Pills, Bezoar pills for clearing up heat of the upper part of the body (牛黄 *Calculus Bovis,* 黄连 *Rhizoma Coptidis,* 大黄 *Radix et Rhizoma Rhei,* 黄芩 *Radix Scutellariae,* 连翘 *Fructus Forsythiae,* 栀子 *Fructus Gardeniae,* 生石膏 *Gypsum Fibrosum,* 菊花 *Flos Chrysanthemi,* etc.), used to clear up toxic heat, and to cure affections of the upper part of the body with symptoms such as headache, dizziness, redness of eyes, tinnitus, ulceration of the mouth and tongue, swelling and pain of the gum, constipation, etc.

牛黄解毒丸(片) [niúhuáng jiědú wán/piàn]

Bezoar Antipyretic Pills (Tablets) (黃芩 *Radix Scutellariae*, 黃連 *Rhizoma Coptidis*, 黃柏 *Cortex Phellodendri*, 大黃 *Radix et Rhizoma Rhei*, 連翹 *Fructus Forsythiae*, 金銀花 *Flos Lonicerae*, 牛黃 *Calculus Bovis, etc.*), used to clear up toxic heat for the treatment of symptoms due to intense heat or fire in the *liver* and *stomach*, including headache and dizziness, red eyes and tinnitus, oral ulcers and periodontitis, and constipation; also used for curing boil or furuncle

牛黃清心丸(片) [niúhuáng qīngxīn wán/piàn]

Bezoar Sedative Pills (Tablets) (牛黃 *Calculus Bovis*, 麝香 *Moschus*, 犀角 *Corni Rhinoceri*, 羚羊角 *Corni Antelopis*, 朱砂 *Cinnabaris*, etc.), used to clear up evil heat from the *heart* and induce sedation, for the treatment of excessive heat in the Heart Channel marked by vertigo, irritability, delirium, convulsion, etc.

防風通聖丸 [fángfēng tōng shèn wán]

Fang Feng Tong Shen Pills, pills of Ledebouriella with magical therapeutic effects (防風 *Radix Ledebouriellae*, 連翹 *Fructus Forsythiae*, 麻黃 *Herba Ephedrae*, 栀子 *Fructus Gardeniae*, 大黃 *Radix et Rhizoma Rhei*, 石膏 *Gypsum Fibrosum*, 黃芩 *Radix Scutellariae*, 白芍 *Radix Paeoniae Alba*, 川芎 *Rhizoma Ligustici Chuanxiong*, etc.), used to clear up intense heat or fire in both the exterior and interior of the body for the treatment of affections by wind and heat marked by headache, sore throat, fullness in the chest, constipation, skin ruption or ulcers, etc.

腦立清 [nǎo lì qīng]

Nao Li Qing; Head-Clearing Pills (赭石 *Haematitum*, 半夏 *Rhizoma Pinelliea*, 牛膝 *Radix Achyranthis Bidentatae*, 珍珠母 *Concha Margaritifera Usta*, etc.), used to quench the fire in the *liver* for treating hypertension due to deficiency of Yin (vital essence) of the *liver* with exuberance of its Yang (vital function) marked by dizziness, tinnitus, insomnia, etc.

麻仁滋脾丸 [márén zī pí wán]

Laxative Pills with Cannabis Seed (火麻仁 *Semen Cannabis*, 大黃 *Radix et Rhizoma Rhei*, 苦杏仁 *Semen Armeniacae Amarum*, 厚朴 *Cortex Magnoliae Officinalis*, 枳實 *Fructus Aruantii Immaturus*, etc.), used to relieve constipation due to deficiency of fluids in the *spleen*

and constipation of the aged and debilitated.

通宣理肺丸(片) [tōng xuān lǐfèi wán/piàn]

Tong Xuan Li Fei Pills; Lung-ventilating Pills (Tablets) (紫蘇葉 *Folium Perillae*, 麻黃 *Herba Ephedrae*, 苦杏仁 *Semen Armeniacae Amarum*, 前胡 *Radix Peucedani*, 桔梗 *Radix Platycodi*, 黃芩 *Radix Scutellariae*, 陳皮 *Pericarpium Citri Reticulatae*, 半夏 *Rhizoma Pinelliae*, etc.), used to cure cough, stuffed nose and headache due to affections by wind and cold

二母寧嗽丸(片) [èr mǔ níngsòu wán/piàn]

Cough Pills (Tablets) with Anemarrhena and Fritillary, (知母 *Rhizoma Anemarrhenae*, 川貝母 *Bulbus Fritillariae Cirrhosae*, 桑白皮 *Cortex Mori Radicis*, 瓜蔞仁 *Semen Trichosanthis*, 石膏 *Gypsum Fibrosum*, 栀子 *Fructus Gardeniae*, 陳皮 *Pericarpium Citri Reticulatae*, 茯苓 *Poria*, etc.), used to relieve cough with yellow sputum by clearing up pathogenic heat in the *lung*

複方川貝精片 [fùfāng chuānbèijīng piàn]

Compound Tablets of Fritillary Extract (川貝母 *Bulbus Fritillariae Cirrhosae*, 麻黃 *Herba Ephedrae*, 甘草 *Radix Glycyrrhizae*, 五味子 *Fructus Schisandrae*, 陳皮 *Pericarpium Citri Reticulatae*, etc.), used for cough and asthma due to affections by wind and cold

橘紅丸(片) [júhóng wán/piàn]

Cough Pills (Tablets) with Pummelo Peel (桔紅 *Exocarpium Citri Grandis*, 款冬花 *Flos Farfarae*, 茯苓 *Poria*, 紫菀 *Radix Asteris*, 瓜蔞皮 *Pericarpium Trichosanthis*, 生石膏 *Gypsum Fibrosum*, etc.), used to remove pathogenic heat from the *lung* and resolve phlegm to relieve cough and dyspnea with sticky or yellow sputum seen in cases of acute or chronic bronchitis

定喘丸 [dìngchuǎn wán]

Antasthmatic Pills (紫蘇子 *Fructus Perillae*, 苦杏仁 *Semen Armeniacae Amarum*, 川貝母 *Bulbus Fritillariae Cirrhosae*, 黃芪 *Radix Astragali*, 阿膠 *Colla Corii Asini*, 款冬花 *Flos Farfarae*, etc.), used to relieve cough and asthma in chronic cases by replenishing and regulating the vital energy of the *lung*

補心丹 [bǔxīn dān]

Bu Xin Pills, Mind-easing Tonic Pills (茯苓 *Poria*, 人參 *Radix Gin-*

seng, 麥冬 *Radix Ophiopogonis*, 酸棗仁 *Semen Zizyphi Spinosae*, 柏子仁 *Semen Boitae*, 遠志 *Radix Polygalae*, 當歸 *Radix Angelica Sinensis*, etc.), used to calm the nerves by nourishing the blood of the *heart*, for the treatment of neurasthenia with restlessness, insomnia, forgetfulness, etc.

朱砂安神丸 [zhūshā ānshén wán]

Cinnabar Sedative Pills (朱砂 *Cinnabaris*, 龍齒 *Dens Draconis*, 當歸 *Radix Angelicae Sinensis*, 黃連 *Rhizoma Coptidis*, 酸棗仁 *Semen Zizyphi Spinosae*, 熟地黃 *Radix Rehmanniae Praeparata*, etc.), used to calm the nerves for the treatment of fidget and insomnia, forgetfulness, palpitation and shortness of breath due to deficiency of vital energy and blood in the *heart* as seen in cases of neurosis

再造丸 [zàizào wán]; 人參再造丸 [rénshēn zàizào wán]

Ginseng Restorative Pills (人參 *Radix Ginseng*, 三七 *Radix Pseudoginseng*, 威灵仙 *Radix et Rhizoma Clematidis*, 牛黃 *Calculus Bovis*, 朱砂 *Cinnabaris*, 犀角 *Cornu Rhinoceri*, 蕲蛇 *Agkistrodon*, etc.), used for apoplectic coma and hemiplegia by dispelling windphlegm and promoting blood circulation.

舒肝丸 [shūgān wán]

Shu Gan Pills; Liver-soothing pills (厚朴 *Cortex Manoliae Officinalis*, 薑黃 *Rhizoma Curcumae Longae*, 沉香 *Lignum Aquilariae Resinatum*, 紅豆蔻 *Fructus Galangae*, 柴胡 *Radix Bupleuri*, 元胡 *Rhizoma Corydalis*, etc.), used for removing stagnancy of vital energy of the *liver* manifested by depression, pain and fullness over the costal and epigastric regions, eructation, acid regurgitation, etc.

木香順氣丸 [mùxiāng shùnqì wán]

Aucklandia Carminative Pills (木香 *Radix Aucklandiae*, 青皮 *Pericarpium Citri Reticulatae Viride*, 厚朴 *Cortex Magnoliae Officinalis*, 烏藥 *Radix Linderae*, 大黃 *Radix et Rhizoma Rhei*, 牽牛子 *Semen Pharbitidis*, etc.), used to relieve stagnancy of food and gas for the treatment of indigestion with flatulence and constipation

香砂養胃丸 [xiāng shā yǎngwèi wán]

Stomachic Pills with Cyperus and Amomum (香附 *Rhizoma Cypri*, 砂仁 *Fructus Amomi*, 木香 *Radix Aucklandiae*, 白朮 *Rhizoma Atractylodis Macrocephalae*, 陳皮 *Pericarpium Citri Reticulatae*, 厚朴 *Cortex*

Magnoliae Officinalis, etc.), used for dyspepsia due to weakness of the stomach marked by epigastric distension, vomiting, belching and acid regurgitation

参苓白术丸 [shēn líng bái zhú wán]

Pills of Codonopsis, Poria and Atractylodes (黨參 *Radix Codonopsis Pilosulae*, 茯苓 *Poria*, 白术 *Rhizoma Atractylodis Macrocephalae*, 蓮子 *Semen Nelumbinis*, 砂仁 *Fructus Amomi*, etc.), used to reinforce the function of the *spleen* and the *stomach* for the treatment of weakness of these organs marked by loss of appetite, abdominal distension, diarrhea, lassitude, etc.

八珍丸 [bāzhēn wán]

Ba Zhen Pills, pills of eight precious ingredients (人參 *Radix Ginseng*, 白术 *Rhizoma Atractylodis Macrocephalae*, 當歸 *Radix Angelicae Sinensis*, 熟地黃 *Rhizoma Rehmanniae Praeparata*, etc.), used to improve the function of the *spleen* and *stomach*, reinforce the vital energy and nourish the blood for treating general debility, loss of appetite, lassitude, etc.

十全大補丸 [shìquán dàbǔ wán]

Far-Reaching Tonic Pills, general tonic pills of ten ingredients (人參 *Radix Ginseng*, 熟地黃 *Rhizoma Rehmanniae Praeparata*, 當歸 *Radix Angelicae Sinensis*, 白术 *Rhizoma Atractylodis Macrocephalae*, 肉桂 *Cortex Cinnamomi*, 白芍 *Radix Paeoniae Alba*, 茯苓 *Poria*, 黃芪 *Radix Astragali*, etc.), used to replenish both vital energy and blood for general debility after illness

補中益氣丸 [bǔzhōng yìqì wán]

Bu Zhong Yi Qi Pills, pills for reinforcing the Middle Burner and replenishing the vital energy (人參 *Radix Ginseng*, 黃芪 *Radix Astragali*, 陳皮 *Pericarpium Citri Reticulatae*, 甘草 *Radix Glycyrrhizae*, 白术 *Rhizoma Atractylodis Macrocephalae*, 升麻 *Rhizoma Cimicifugae*, 柴胡 *Radix Bupleuri*), used to reinforce the vital energy of the *spleen* for the treatment of general debility, lassitude and somnolence, prolonged diarrhea, uterine bleeding, etc.

河車大造丸 [héchē dà zào wán]

Placenta Compound Restorative Pills, pills with placenta for general restoration (紫河車 *Placenta Hominis*, 麥冬 *Radix Ophiopogonis*,

248

天冬 *Radix Asparagi*, 杜仲 *Cortex Eucommiae*, 龜板 *Plastrum Testudinis*, 熟地黃 *Rhizoma Rehmannia Praeparata*, etc.), used to nourish vital essence of the *kidney* for the treatment of general debility, night sweat, nocturnal emission, lassitude, tidal fever and maldevelopment.

龜齡集 [guīlíng jí]

Gui Ling Ji; Elixir (Granules) (鹿茸 *Cornu Cervi Pantotrichum*, 海馬 *Hippocampus*, 淫羊藿 *Herba Epimedi*, 人參 *Radix Ginseng*, etc.), used to invigorate vital function of the *kidney* for impotence, sterility, amnesia, mental delibity due to old age, etc.

全鹿丸 [quánlù wán]

Deer Tonic Pills (人參 *Radix Ginseng*, 鹿茸 *Cornu Cervi Pantotrichum*, 鎖陽 *Herba Cynomorii*, 巴戟天 *Radix Morindae Officinalis*, 當歸 *Radix Angelicae Sinensis*, 沉香 *Lignum Aquilariae Resinatum*, 熟地黃 *Radix Rehmanniae Praeparata*, etc.), used as tonics for deficiency in the *kidney* marked by asthenia lassitude, amnesia, insomnia, night sweat and spontaneous emission, or metrorrhagia, leukorrhea and miscarriage

當歸丸 [dānggūi wán]

Pills of Chinese Angelica (當歸 *Radix Angelicae Sinensis*), used to cure menstrual disturbance such as infrequent menstruation, menorrhalgia, morbid leukorrhea, by activating and tonifying blood

神經衰弱丸 [shénjīng shuāiruò wán]

Anti-Neurasthenia Pills (磁石 *Magnetitum*, 首烏藤 *Caulis Polygoni Multiflori*, 黃精 *Rhizoma Polygonati*, 丹參 *Radix Salviae Miltiorrhizae*, 酸棗仁 *Semen Zizyphi Spinosae*, 當歸 *Radix Angelicae Sinensis*, 遠志 *Radix Polygalae*, 五味子 *Fructus Schisandrae*, etc.), used to nourish the *heart* and calm the nerves for neurasthesia with insomnia, palpitation, headache, dizziness, etc.

紫雪丹 [zǐxuě dān]

Zi Xue Powder; Purple Snowy Powder (犀角 *Cornu Rhinoceri*, 羚羊角 *Cornu Antelopis*, 麝香 *Moschus*, 沉香 *Lignum Aquilariae Resinatum*, etc.), used to clear up evil heat and induce sedation, for delirium, restlessness and infantile convulsion due to high fever in acute infectious diseases

249

安宮牛黃丸 [āngōng niúhuáng wán]

Bezoar Resurrection Pills (牛黃 *Calculus Bovis*, 犀角 *Cornu Rhinoceri*, 珍珠 *Margarita*, 麝香 *Moschus*, 梔子 *Fructus Gardeniae*, etc.), used to eliminate toxic heat and bring the patient back to consciousness from coma and relieve convulsions due to high fever (e.g., in encephalitis) or cerebral hemorrhage

氣管炎丸 [qìguǎnyán wán]

Anti-Bronchitis Pills (麻黃 *Herba Ephedrae*, 款冬花 *Flos Farfarae*, 苦杏仁 *Semen Armeniacae Amarum*, 川貝母 *Bulbus Fritillariae Cirrhosae*, etc.), used to expel phlegm and relieve cough and asthma to treat chronic bronchitis

燕窩秋梨膏 [yànwō qiūlí gāo]

Pear Syrup with Edible Bird's Nest, used to relieve coughs, resolve phlegm, and improve appetite for patients with chronic bronchitis suffering from poor appetite and general weakness

七厘散 [qīlí sǎn]

Anti-bruises Powder (血竭 *Sanguis Draconis*, 紅花 *Flos Carthami*, 乳香 *Olibanum*, 沒藥 *Myrrha*, 兒茶 *Catechu seu Gambir*, etc.), used to promote blood circulation and relieve pain for traumatic wounds with local ecchymosis

烏鷄白鳳丸 [wūjī báifèng wán]

White Phoenix Pills (烏鷄 white-feathered chicken with dark skin, 人參 *Radix Ginseng*, 當歸 *Radix Angelicae Sinensis*, 香附 *Rhizoma Cyperi*, 地黃 *Radix Rehmanniae*, 黃芪 *Radix Astragali*, 鹿角膠 *Colla Cornus Cervi*, etc.), used for menstrual disturbances and morbid leukorrhea due to deficiency of vital energy and blood

參茸衛生丸 [shēn róng wèishēng wán]

Ginseng and Pilose Antler Life-Preserving Pills (人參 *Radix Ginseng*, 鹿茸 *Cornu Cervi Pantotrichum*, 蓮子 *Semen Nelumbinis*, 酸棗仁 *Semen Zizyphi Spinosae*, 鎖陽 *Herba Cynomorii*, 巴戟天 *Radix Morindae Officinalis*, 枸杞子 *Fructus Lycii*, etc.), used to replenish vital energy and blood, nourish essence of both the *liver* and the *kidney*, and invigorate the function of the *spleen* and *stomach*, for the treatment of deficiency of vital energy and blood and lowered functioning of the *kidney* with lassitude, fatigue, poor appetite, spermatorrhea, anemia, early graying of the hair, etc.

人參健脾丸 ［rénshēn jiànpí wán］

Ginseng stomachic Pills (人參 *Radix Ginseng,* 茯苓*Poria,* 山藥*Rhizoma Dioscoreae,* 黃芪 *Radix Astragali,* 白朮 *Rhizoma Atractylodis Macrocephalae,* 陳皮 *Pericarpium Citri Reticulatae,* etc.), used to strengthen the functioning of the *spleen* and *stomach* and regulate the flow of vital energy, for the treatment of weakness of the *spleen* and *stomach* with symptoms such as emaciation, feeble limbs, loss of appetite, alternate diarrhea and constipation

人參鹿茸丸 ［rénshēn lùróng wán］

Ginseng Antler Pills (人參*Radix Ginseng,* 鹿茸*Cornu Cervi Pantotrichum,* 杜仲*Cortex Eucommiae,* 當歸 *Radix Angelicae Sinensis,*巴戟天 *Radix Morindae Officinalis,* 牛膝*Radix Achyranthis Bidentatae,* 龍眼肉 *Arillus Longan,* etc.), used as an analeptic for the treatment of deficiency of vital energy and blood and hypofunctioning of the *kidney* function with general debility, anemia, seminal emission, lassitude of loins and legs

小金丹 ［xiǎo jīn dān］

Xiao Jin Pills; Antiphlogistic Pills (麝香 *Moschus,* 乳香*Olibanum,* 當歸 *Radix Angelicae Sinensis,* 草烏 *Radix Aconiti Kusnezoffii,* etc.), used to cure traumatic wounds by promoting blood circulation, removing blood stasis and reducing swelling, also for the treatment of scrofula, carbuncle, cutaneous abscess and ulcer

柏子養心丸 ［bǎizǐ yǎngxīn wán］

Bai Zi Yang Xin Pills, mind-easing tonic pills with the seed of arborvitae (柏子仁 *Semen Biotae,* 人參 *Radix Ginseng,* 黃芪 *Radix Astragali,* 酸棗仁 *Semen Zizyphi Spinosae,* 當歸 *Radix Angelicae Sinensis,* 五味子 *Fructus Schizandrae,* 遠志 *Radix Polygalae,* etc.) used to relieve anxiety and mental strain, also for palpitation, insomnia and amnesia

六神丸 ［liùshén wán］

Liu Shen Pills, pills of six ingredients with magical effects (牛黃 *Calculus Bovis,* 珍珠*Margarita,* 冰片 *Borneol,* 樟腦*Camphora,* 蟾酥*Venenum Bufonis,* 雄黃 *Realgar,* 麝香 *Moschus*), used as an antiphlogistic for acute tonsillitis, sore throat, boils, etc.

251

婦科十味片 [fùkē shíwèi piàn]

Fu Ke Shi Wei Tablets, tablets with ten ingredients for women's diseases (黨參 *Radix Codonopsis Pilosulae,* 白朮 *Rhizoma Atractylodis Macrocephalae,* 當歸 *Radix Angelicae Sinensis,* 地黃 *Radix Rehmanniae,* 大棗 *Fructus Zizyphi Jujubae,* 香附 *Rhizoma Cyperi,* 茯苓 *Poria,* 川芎 *Rhizoma Ligustici Chuanxiong,* 白芍 *Radix Paeoniae Alba,* 甘草 *Radix Glycyrrhizae*), used to regulate menstrual disturbances by replenishing vital energy and blood

傷濕止痛膏 [shāngshī zhǐtòng gāo]

Plasters for Rheumatic Pains (乳香 *Olibanum,* 没藥 *Myrrha,* 肉桂 *Cortex Cinnamomi,* 丁香 *Flos Caryophylli,* 薄荷 *Herba Menthae,* 細辛 *Herba Asari cum Radice,* etc.), used externally for rheumatic pains, sprain and injuries

X Acupuncture and Moxibustion, Channels and Points

針 法
Acupuncture

針灸 [zhēnjiǔ]
acupuncture and moxibustion
針灸科 [zhēnjiǔ kē]
department of acupuncture and moxibustion
針灸醫生 [zhēnjiǔ yīshēng]
acupuncturist
針柄 [zhēnbǐng]
the handle (holder) of the acupuncture needle
針根 [zhēngēn]
the root of the acupuncture needle, the junction between the handle and the body of the needle
針體 [zhēntǐ]
the body of the acupuncture needle
針尖 [zhēnjiān]
the tip or point of the acupuncture needle
同身寸 [tóngshēn cùn]
identical unit or proportional unit of the body, a length unit for measurement in locating points. A certain part of the patient's limbs is divided into certain parts of equal length taken as unit for measurement in locating points.
指寸法 [zhǐcùn fǎ]
finger-length measurement. The patient's finger is divided into certain parts of equal length taken as unit for measurement in locating points.
中指同身寸 [zhōngzhǐ tóngshēn cùn]
middle finger identical unit. The length between the twisted

folds at the two ends of the second segment of the patient's middle finger when bent is taken as one *cun*, a unit of measurement. (Fig.1)

拇指同身寸 [mǔzhǐ tóngshēn cùn]

thumb identical unit. The width of the phalangeal joint of the patient's thumb is taken as one *cun*, a unit of measurement.

一夫法 [yīfū fǎ]

measurement by the transverse width of the patient's four fingers (namely, the point finger, middle finger, ring finger and small finger). The maximal width of the four fingers (at the level of the juncture of the 1st and 2nd segment of the middle finger) held together with the hand open, is taken as a unit of measurement for 3 *cun*. (Fig.2)

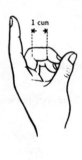
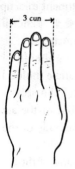

fig. 1   fig. 2

解剖標誌法 [jiěpōu biāozhì fǎ]

locating points using anatomical structures for reference, such as the five sense organs, hairline, vertebral processes, nipples, umbilicus, joints and ankles

骨度法 [gǔdù fǎ]

bone-length measurement. The length of a certain part of the patient's body is divided into several equal parts, each taken as a unit of measurement for locating points, e.g., the length between the two nipples is divided into eight parts or *cun*. (Fig.3)

毫針 [háo zhēn]

filiform needle, a most commonly used acupuncture needle,

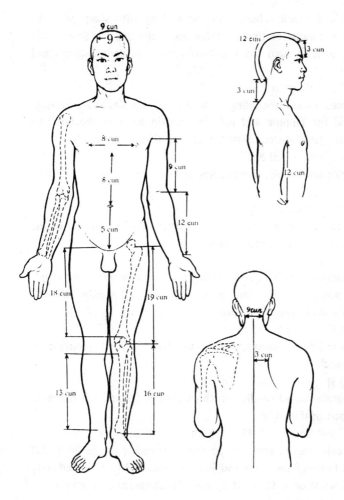

fig. 3

with length ranging from 0.5 to 5.0 inches, calibre ranging from gauge 26 to gauge 32

三棱針 [sānléng zhēn]
three-edged needle, about two inches long with sharp point to make surface venous section to cause small bleeding for therapeutic purpose in treating such cases as fevers, impaired consciousness and sore throat

皮膚針 [pífū zhēn]
cutaneous needle including plumblossom needle and seven-star needle, used for tapping and pricking certain areas of the body to treat neurosis, gastro-enteric disturbances and skin diseases

梅花針 [méihuā zhēn]
plum-blossom needle, five needles tied on one end of a rod about a foot long

七星針 [qīxīng zhēn]
seven-star needle, a disc fixed with seven needles attached to the end of a handle about 5-6 inches long

皮内針 [pínèi zhēn]
subcutaneous needle, needle embedded subcutaneously for therapeutic purpose, including two different shapes of needle: thumb-nail-shaped and wheat-grain-shaped

圖釘型針 [túdīngxíng zhēn]; 鍬針 [xiān zhēn]
thumb-nail-shaped needle, which is usually embedded subcutaneously in the auricle

麥粒型針 [màilìxíng zhēn]
wheat-grain-shaped needle, which may be embedded subcutaneously at any part of the body

火針 [huǒ zhēn]; 燔針 [fán zhēn]; 燒針 [shāo zhēn]
fire needle; burnt needle, an acupuncture needle (gauge 20 or 22) heated red hot and then inserted into the diseased part immediately and withdrawn at once, for treating scrofula, abscess and rheumatism

砭石 [biānshí]
stone needle used in acupuncture and surgical operations in ancient times

九針 [jiǔ zhēn]

256

nine kinds of needles used for acupuncture in ancient times,
namely, 鑱針 [chán zhēn] the arrow-headed needle, 圓針 [yuán
zhēn] the round needle, 鍉針 [chí zhēn] the blunt needle, 鋒針
[fēng zhēn] the sharp three-edged needle, 鈹針 [fēi zhēn] or
鈹針 [pí zhēn] the sword-like needle, 圓利針 [yuān lì zhēn] the
sharp round needle,毫針 [háo zhēn]the filiform needle,長針 [cháng
zhēn] the long needle and 大針 [dà zhēn] the large needle

針灸銅人 [zhēnjiǔ tóngrén]
bronze figure marked with acupuncture points used for teaching
purpose, originated in the Song Dynasty

提插 [tíchā]
lifting and thrusting of the acupuncture needle—a manipulation
of acupuncture

捻轉 [niǎnzhuàn]
twisting and rotating of the needle—a manipulation of acupuncture

震顫 [zhènchàn]
vibrating the needle, i.e., rapidly but slightly lifting and thrusting,
twisting and rotating the needle to enhance the effect

點刺 [diǎncì]
prompt prick, a fast pricking method in acupuncture

透刺 [tòucì]
joined puncture, puncture two or more adjoining points in one
insertion of the needle

直刺 [zhícì]
perpendicular inserting, 90 degree insertion, used for most of
the points

斜刺 [xiécì]
oblique inserting, 45 degree insertion, used for points on thin
layer of muscles or with important internal organs underlying below
the area

平刺 [píngcì]
horizontal inserting, 15 to 25 degrees to the surface, used for
points where the muscle layer is quite thin

進針 [jìnzhēn]
inserting the needle, usually with the needle in the right hand

to be inserted into the body rapidly with the cooperation of the left hand in order to reduce the pain to the minimum

指切進針法 [zhǐqiē jìnzhēn fǎ]

insertion of the needle with the help of finger pressure, pressing the thumb of the left hand near the point and inserting the needle into the point against the thumb nail—a method of insertion for short filiforms

挾持進針法 [jiāchí jìnzhēn fǎ]

inserting the needle by holding it with the thumb and point finger of the left hand (now usually with a sterilized cotton ball) — a method used for inserting long filiforms

舒張進針 [shūzhāng jìnzhēn]

inserting needle with fingers stretching the skin. Stretch the skin around the point with the thumb and the index finger of the left hand and insert the needle rapidly into the point with the right hand. This method is indicated where the skin is loose, such as points Tianshu (St. 25) and Guanyuan (Ren 4) on the abdomen.

撮捏進針 [cuōniē jìnzhēn]

inserting the needle by pinching up the skin. Pinch up the skin around the point with the thumb and index finger of the left hand, and insert the needle rapidly into the point with the right hand. This method is suitable for locations where the muscle is thin, such as points Yintang (Extra. 1) and Dicang (St. 4) on the face.

行針 [xíngzhēn]

manipulating the needle after insertion to produce desired effect

留針 [liúzhēn]

retaining the needle in the point for a time to maintain and prolong the effect

出針 [chūzhēn]; 引針 [yǐnzhēn]; 拔針 [bázhēn]

withdrawing the needle with the right hand while the left hand pressing the point (now usually with a piece of sterilized cotton ball)

得氣 [déqì]

getting the Qi or the feeling of acupuncture, with soreness, heaviness, numbness and distension felt by the patient and tightness of the needle by the doctor, which are normal sensations of successful acup-

258

uncture

補瀉法 [bǔxièfǎ]

method of reinforcement and reduction. Reinforcement means to activate and restore hypofunction to normal, while reduction method means to expel pathogenic factors and thus to restore hyperfunction to normal.

提插補瀉 [tíchā bǔxiè]

reinforcing or reducing by lifting and thrusting the needle. After getting the feeling of acupuncture reinforcement may be attained by lifting the needle with little force and slowly and thrusting it with great force and rapidly, reduction may be attained just in the opposite way.

捻轉補瀉 [niǎnzhuàn bǔxiè]

reinforcing or reducing by twisting and rotating the needle. After getting the feeling of acupuncture the needle is twisted and rotated in small amplitude and slowly for reinforcement. Reduction can be attained with the needle twisted and rotated in large amplitude and swiftly.

呼吸補瀉 [hūxī bǔxiè]

reinforcing or reducing by timing the insertion and withdrawal of the needle according to the phases of the patient's respiration. Reinforcement is achieved by inserting the needle when the patient exhales and withdrawing the needle while the patient has inhaled to the fullest capacity. Reduction is effected if insertion is made during the patient's inspiration and withdrawal at the end of expiration process.

迎隨補瀉 [yíngsuí bǔxiè]

reinforcing or reducing by inserting the needle in the same direction as the channel runs (reinforcement) or in the opposite direction (reduction).

開闔補瀉 [kāihé bǔxiè]

reinforcing or reducing by closing or enlarging the acupuncture hole. Reinforcement is achieved by closing the acupuncture hole after withdrawing the needle with slight finger pressure and massage so as to prevent the vital energy of the channel from escaping. Reduction is effected by enlarging the hole and leaving it open to let the pathogenic factor out.

平補平瀉 [píngbǔ píngxiè]

normal reinforcement and normal reduction by lifting and thrusting or twisting and twirling the needle evenly, causing mild sensations, and withdrawing the needle with moderate speed. This method is employed when the case is not so distinct as an excessive or insufficient one.

行氣法 [xíngqì fǎ]

method of conducting the Qi or feeling of acupuncture

指壓行氣法 [zhǐyā xíngqì fǎ]

conducting the Qi or feeling of acupuncture by finger pressure. If one wishes to have the feeling go proximally, one must apply finger pressure at the distal side of the point, and vice versa.

針向行氣法 [zhēnxiàng xíngqì fǎ]

conducting the Qi or feeling of acupuncture by direction of insertion, which must be in the same direction as that of Qi desired

經絡感傳現象 [jīngluò gǎnchuán xiǎnxiàng]

transmission of acupuncture feeling by the channels

經絡現象 [jīngluò xiǎnxiàng]

transmission by the channels, including transmission of the acupuncture feeling by the channels, spasmodic pains by the channels, appearance of red line, white line or papules along the channels

暈針 [yūnzhēn]

fainting spell during acupuncture treatment, with dizziness, pallor, cold sweat, nausea, palpitation, shortness of breath, cold limbs, etc. (an accident in acupuncture)

滯針 [zhìzhēn]

sticking of the needle, impossible to rotate, lift and thrust, or even to withdraw the needle after it is inserted

彎針 [wānzhēn]

bending of the needle after it is inserted into the point

折針 [zhézhēn]

breaking of the needle within the patient's body while insertion is being made (an accident in acupuncture)

經絡和俞穴
Channels and Points

經絡學説 [jīngluò xuéshuō]

theory of the channels, an important component part of the
theories of traditional Chinese medicine, which deals with physiological and pathological changes of the human body, serving as guiding
principle of diagnosis and treatment, the core of the theory of acupuncture and moxibustion. According to this theory, there exists
within the human body a system of channels through which the vital
energy and blood circulate, and by which the internal organs are
connected with superficial organs and tissues, and the body is made
an organic whole. The points on the body surface are the particular
spots where the vital energy of the internal organs reaches. When one
is ill, the physician can regulate his flow of vital energy and blood by
puncturing certain points on his body surface and thus cure the illness
of the associated internal organs.

經絡 [jīng luò]

(1) channels and collaterals; (2) conduits through which vital
energy and blood circulate and by which the internal organs are related
with superficial organs and tissues, making the body an organic whole

經脈 [jīngmài]

channels; meridians, cardinal conduits of vital energy and blood
coursing vertically, composed of the Twelve Channels and the Eight
Extra Channels

絡脈 [luòmài]

collaterals; reticular conduits, the branches of the channels,
broadly speaking, they consist of the Fifteen Collaterals, reticular
branch conduits and reticular conduits of the third generation (the
latter is called 孫絡 [sūnluò]). But in a narrow sense, they consist of
the Fifteen Collaterals and their branches all over the body. The function of the collaterals is to help the channels in connecting the tissues
of the body and conveying vital energy and blood.

十二經脈 [shíèr jīngmài]; 十二經 [shíèr jīng]; 正經 [zhèng

jīng〕

　　the Twelve Channels, known as the Regular Channels, each being connected with a particular internal organ and each possessing an exterior-interior relation. They are:

(1)　the Lung Channel of Hand Taiyin (Lu.C.);

(2)　the Large Intestine Channel of Hand Yangming (L.I.C.);

(3)　the Stomach Channel of Foot Yangming (St. C.);

(4)　the Spleen Channel of Foot Taiyin (Sp.C.);

(5)　the Heart Channel of Hand Shaoyin (H.C.);

(6)　the Small Intestine Channel of Hand Taiyang (S.I.C.);

(7)　the Urinary Bladder Channel of Foot Taiyang (U.B.C.);

(8)　the Kidney Channel of Foot Shaoyin (K.C.);

(9)　the Pericardium Channel of Hand Jueyin (P.C.);

(10)　the Triple Burners Channel of Hand Shaoyang (T.B.C.);

(11)　the Gallbladder Channel of Foot Shaoyang (G.B.C.);

(12)　the Liver Channel of Foot Jueyin (Liv.C.).

手三陰經〔shǒu sānyīnjīng〕

　　the Three Yin Channels of the Hand, running through the anterior side of the upper limbs from the chest to the hands. They are the Lung Channel of Hand Taiyin, the Heart Channel of Hand Shaoyin, and the Pericardium Channel of Hand Jueyin

手三陽經〔shǒu sānyángjīng〕

　　the Three Yang Channels of the Hand, running through the posterior side of the upper limbs from the hands to the head. They are the Large Intestine Channel of Hand Yangming, the Small Intestine Channel of Hand Taiyang, and the Triple Burners Channel of Hand Shaoyang

足三陽經〔zú sānyánjīng〕

　　the Three Yang Channels of the Foot, running from the head through the trunk downward to the feet. They are the Stomach Channel of Foot Yangming, the Urinary Bladder Channel of Taiyang, and the Gallbadder Channel of Foot Shaoyang.

足三陰經〔zú sānyīnjīng〕

　　the Three Yin Channels of the Foot, running through the inner side of the lower limbs from the feet to the abdomen and the chest. They are: the Spleen Channel of Foot Taiyin, the Kidney Channel

262

of Foot Shaoyin, and the Liver Channel of Foot Jueyin

六經 [liùjīng]

the Six Channels, the Taiyang Channel, the Yangming Channel, the Shaoyang Channel, the Taiyin Channel, the Shaoyin Channel, and the Jueyin Channel, which, in conformity with the twelve Channels, may be subdivided into the Six Channels of the Hand and the Six Channels of the Foot

陽經 [yángjīng]

the Yang Channels, including the Three Yang Channels of the Hand and the Foot, the Back Middleline Channel, the Regulating Channel of Yang and the Motility Channel of Yang

陰經 [yīnjīng]

the Yin Channels, including the Three Yin Channels of the Hand and the Foot, the Front Middleline Channel, the Chong (Vital) Channel, the Regulating Channel of Yin and the Motility Channel of Yin

三陰 [sānyīn]

(1) the Three Yin, a collective name for the Three Yin Channels of both the Hand and Foot, six in all; (2) "the Third Yin", i.e., the Taiyin Channel, with the Shaoyin Channel called 二陰 [èr yīn] "the Second Yin" and the Jueyin Channel called 一陰 [yī yīn] "the First Yin"

三陽 [sānyáng]

(1) the Three Yang, a collective name for the Three Yang Channels of both the Hand and the Foot, six in all; (2) "the Third Yang" i.e., the Taiyang Channel, with the Yangming Channel as 二陽 [èr yáng] "the Second Yang", and the Shaoyang Channel as 一陽 [yī yáng], "the First Yang"

十四經 [shísìjīng]

the Fourteen Channels, the Twelve Channels Plus the Front and Back Middle Channels

手太陰肺經 [shǒu tàiyīn fèijīng]

the Lung Channel of Hand Taiyin (Lu. C.) or the Hand Yin Maximum Lung Meridian, or simply the Lung Meridian which originates in point 中府 Zhongfu (Lu. 1) in the chest and ends in 少商 Shaoshang (Lu. 11), a point near the thumbnail, with 11 points on either side

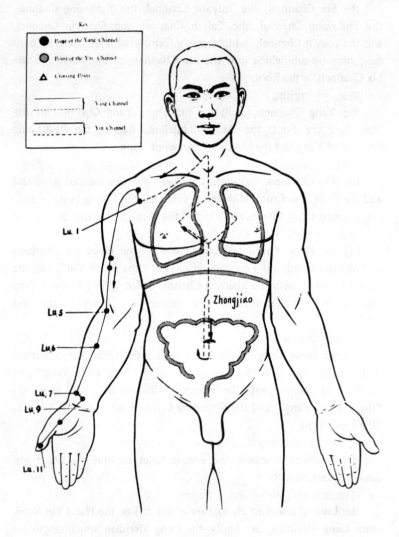

Key

● Point of the Yang Channel

● Point of the Yin Channel

△ Crossing Point

Yang Channel

Yin Channel

Lu 1

Zhongjiao

Lu 5

Lu 6

Lu 7

Lu 9

Lu 11

fig. 4

(Fig.4). This channel pertains to the *lung* and connects with the *large intestine*. Indications are cough, hemoptysis, asthma, tightness in the chest, sore throat, chest pains, pains or numbness of the shoulder and the forearm where this channel passes.

The most commonly used points of this channel and their indications are given below:

Points	Indications
中府 Zhongfu (Lu.1)	cough, asthma, pain in the chest, shoulder and back
尺澤 Chize (Lu.5)	cough, asthma, sore throat, pain in the elbow and arm
孔最 Kongzui (Lu.6)	the same as above
列缺 Lieque (Lu.7)	headache, stiff neck, cough, asthma, sore throat and facial paralysis
太淵 Taiyuan (Lu.9)	cough, asthma, hemoptysis, sore throat, chest pain, pain in the back and shoulder
少商 Shaoshang (Lu.11)	cough, sore throat, coma, apoplexy, febrile diseases

手陽明大腸經 [shǒu yángmíng dàchángjīng]
the large Intestine Channel of Hand Yangming (L.I.C.); the Hand Yang in Equilibrium Large Intestine Meridian; or simply the Large Intestine Meridian, which originates in 商陽 Shangyang (L.I.1) near the nail of the point finger and ends in 迎香 Yingxiang (L.I.20), a point just on the outer border of the nasal ala, with 20 points on either side (Fig.5). This channel pertains to the *large intestine* and connects with the *lung*. Indications are abdominal pain, borborygmi, diarrhea, dysentery, sore throat, toothache, pain and paralysis of the shoulder or the arm along the channel.

The most commonly used points of this channel and their indications are given below:

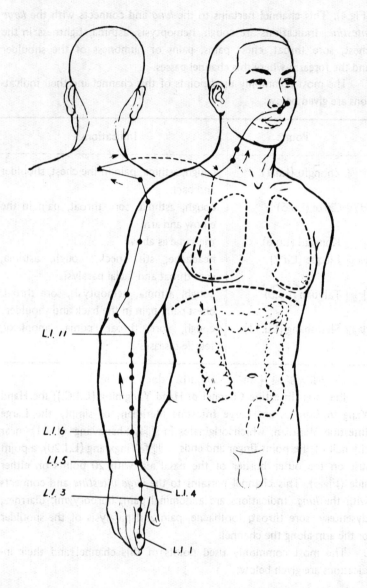

fig. 5

Points	Indications
商陽Shangyang (L.I.1)	coma, apoplexy, sore throat, toothache, febrile diseases
三間Sanjian (L.I.3)	ache of lower teeth, sore throat
合谷 Hegu (H.I.4)	febrile diseases, toothache, sore throat, facial paralysis
陽溪Yangxi (L.I.5)	headache, toothache, pharyngitis, pain in wrist and hand
偏厲 Pianli (L.I.6)	epistaxis, sore throat, edema
曲池Quchi (L.I.11)	febrile diseases, hypertension, sore throat, abdominal pain, diarrhea, paralysis of upper extremities

足陽明胃經 [zú yángmíng wèijīng]
the Stomach Channel of Foot Yangming (St.C.); the Foot Yang Equilibrium Stomach Meridian, or simply the Stomach Meridian, which runs from 承泣 Chengqi (St. 1), a point just below the eye, downward to 厲兑 Lidui (St.45), a point on the lateral side of the tip of the second toe, through the trunk and the lower limb with 45 points on either side (Fig.6). This channel pertains to the *stomach* and connects with the *spleen*. Indications are borborygami, abdominal distension, edema, gastralgia, vomiting, facial paralysis, sore throat, fever, mania.

The most commonly used points of this channel and their indications are given below:

Points	Indications
承泣 Chengqi (St.1)	optic neuritis, optic atrophy, myopia, conjunctivitis
地倉 Dicang (St.4)	facial paralysis, salivation
頰車 Jiache (St.6)	facial paralysis, toothache, parotitis
下關 Xiaguan (St.7)	facial paralysis, toothache
頭維 Touwei (St.8)	headache, ophthalmalgia, lacrimation

梁門 Liangmen (St.21)	gastralgia, poor appetite
天樞 Tianshu (St.25)	diarrhea in children and infants, abdominal pain
犢鼻 Dubi (St.35)	arthritis of the knee joint
足三里 Zusanli (St.36)	gastralgia, vomiting, abdominal distension, general weakness
豐隆 Fenglong (St.40)	cough, profuse sputum, vertigo, paralysis of the lower limbs
厲兌 Lidui (St.45)	febrile diseases, epilepsy

足太陰脾經 [zú tàiyīn píjīng]

the **Spleen Channel of Foot** Taiyin **(Sp.C.); the Foot Yin Maximum Spleen Meridian,** or simply **the Spleen Meridian,** running from 隱白 Yinbai **(Sp. 1).** a point in the medial side of the great toe, to 大包 Dabao (Sp. 21), a point on the midaxillary line, in the 6th intercostal space, through the lower limbs and abdomen, with 21 points (Fig 7). This channel pertains to the *spleen* and connects with the *stomach.* Indications are belching, vomiting, gastralgia, abdominal distension, diarrhea, edema, lassitude, jaundice, and swelling and pain in the inner side of the lower limbs. The most commonly used points of this channel and their indications are given below:

Points	Indications
隱白 Yinbai (Sp.1)	abdominal distension, irregular menstruation, dreamfulness and insomnia, mental disorder
太白 Taibai (Sp.3)	gastralgia, abdominal distension, vomiting, diarrhea
公孫 Gongsun (Sp.4)	gastralgia, vomiting, diarrhea, poor appetite
三陰交 Sanyinjiao (Sp.6)	irregular menstruation, impotence, enuresis, pollution
血海 Xuehai (Sp. 10)	irregular menstruation, urticaria
大橫 Daheng (Sp. 15)	dysentery, abdominal pain

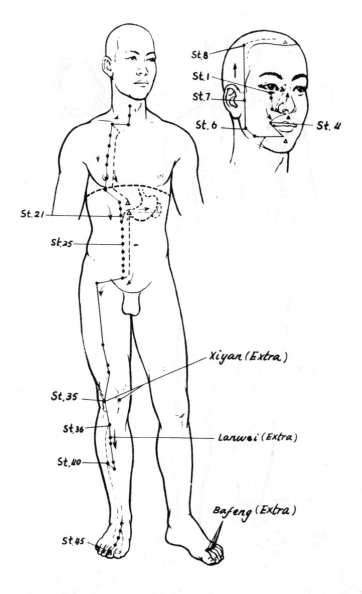

St.8
St.1
St.7
St.6
St. 4

St.21
St.25

Xiyan (Extra)

St.35

St.36

Lanwei (Extra)

St.40

Bafeng (Extra)

St.45

fig. 6

269

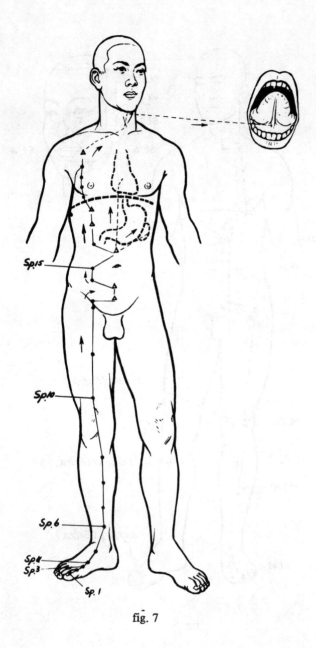

Sp.15

Sp.10

Sp.6

Sp.4
Sp.3

Sp.1

fig. 7

270

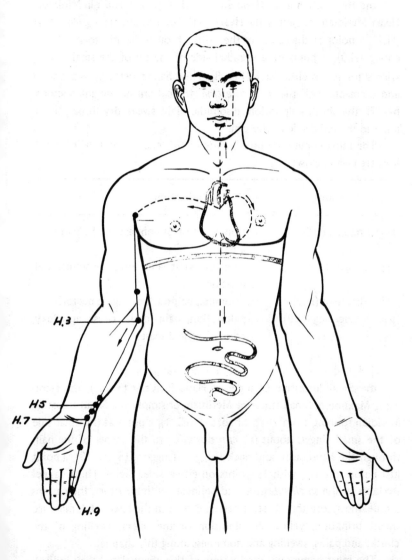

fig. 8

手少陰心經 [shǒu shàoyīn xīnjīng]
the Heart Channel of Hand Shaoyin (H.C.), the Hand Yin Minimum
Heart Meridian, or simply the Heart Meridian, running from 極泉 Jiquan
(H.1), a point at the center of the axilla, through the arm to 少沖 Shaochong (H.9), a point on the radial side of the tip of the small finger,
with 9 points on either side (Fig. 8). This channel pertains to the *heart*
and connects with the *small intestine*. Indications are angina pectoris,
pain in the chest, palpitation, insomnia, night sweat, dry throat, thirst,
pains in the inner side of the arm.

The most commonly used points of this channel and their indications are given below:

Points	Indications
少海 Shaohai (H.3)	pain in chest, numbness of the hand and arm
通裏 Tongli (H.5)	pain in wrist and arm, insomnia, pal- pitation
神門 Shenmen (H.7)	insomnia, palpitation, angina pectoris
少沖 Shaochong (H.9)	palpitation, pain in the chest, apoplexy, coma, febrile diseases

手太陽小腸經 [shǒu tàiyáng xiǎochángjīng]
the Small Intestine Channel of Hand Taiyang (S.I.C.), the Hand
Yang Maximum, Small Intestine Meridian, or simply the Small Intestine
Meridian, running from 少澤 Shaoze (S.I.C. 1), a point at the ulnar side
of the small finger, about 0.1 *cun* posterior to the corner of the nail,
through the hand, arm, and neck to 聽宮 Tinggong (S.I.C. 19), a point
just before the ear, with 19 points on either side (Fig. 9) This Channel
pertains to the *small intestine* and connects with the *heart*. Indications
are deafness, sore throat, stuffiness and pain in the lower abdomen, frequent urination, yellow discoloration of the sclera, swelling of the
cheek, and pains, swelling and numbness along this channel.

The most commonly used points of this channel and their indications are given below:

272

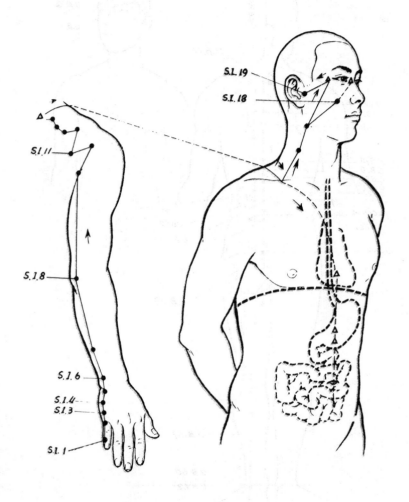

S.I. 19

S.I. 18

S.I. 11

S.1.8

S.1.6

S.1.4

S.I.3

S.I. 1

fig. 9

273

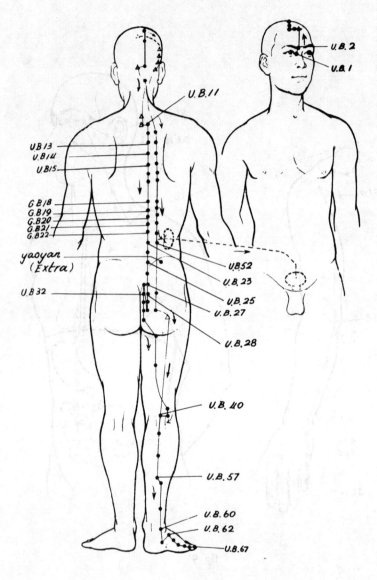

U.B. 2
U.B. 1
U.B. 11
U.B 13
v.B 14
U.B 15
G B 18
G.B 19
G.B 20
G.B 21
G.B 22
yaoyan
(Extra)
U.B 32
U.B 52
U.B. 23
U.B. 25
U.B. 27
U.B. 28
U.B. 40
U.B. 57
U.B. 60
U.B. 62
U.B. 67

fig. 10

Points	Indications
少澤 Shaoze (S.I.1)	febrile diseases, headache, mastitis, deficient lactation
後溪 Houxi (S.I. 3)	occipital headache, rigidity of the neck
手腕骨 Hand-Wangu (S.I.4)	headache, tinnitus, arthritis of wrist and finger joints
養老 Yanglao (S.I.6)	blurring of vision, pain in the shoulder, back, elbow and arm
小海 Xiaohai (S.I. 8)	pain in the small finger, elbow joint, shoulder and back
天宗 Tianzong (S.I.11)	pain in the shoulder
顴髎 Quanliao (S.I.18)	facial paralysis, toothache, neuralgia of trigeminal nerve
聽宮 Tinggong (S.I.19)	deafness, tinnitus, otalgia

足太陽膀胱經 [zú tàiyáng pángguāngjīng]
the. Urinary Bladder Channel of Foot Taiyang (U.B.C.), the Foot
Yang Maximum Urinary Bladder Meridian, or simply the Urinary Bladder Meridian, running from the face upward to the top of the head, and
then to the posterior side of the head, neck, and trunk, and then the
back of the foot to the tip of the small toe, originating from 睛明 Jing-
ming (U.B.1), a point 0.1 *cun* lateral and superior to the inner canthus
and terminating at 至陰 Zhiyin (U.B.67), a point on the lateral side of
the tip of the small toe, with 67 points on either side (Fig.10). This
channel pertains to the *urinary bladder* and connects with the *kidney*.
Indications are rigidity and pain in the head and neck, pain in the back
and lumbar region, eye diseases, dysuresis, enuresis, mania, pain in the
gastrocnemius muscles and in the small toe.

The most commonly used points of this channel and their indications are given below:

Points	Indications
睛明 Jingming (U.B.1)	eye diseases
攢竹 Zanzhu (U.B.2)	pain in the superciliary arch, eye diseases facial paralysis
大杼 Dashu (U.B.11)	cough, fever, pain in the shoulder joint
次髎 Ciliao (U.B.32)	lumbago, irregular menstruation
委中 Weizhong (U.B.40)	lumbago, pain and swelling of the knee, paralysis of the lower extremities
志室 Zhishi (U.B.52)	spermatorrhea, impotence, pain in the back and lumbar region
承山 Chengshan (U.B.57)	spasm of the gastrocnemius muscles, lumbago
昆侖 Kunlun (U.B. 60)	headache, rigidity of the neck, lumbago, pain in the heel
申脈 Shenmai (U.B. 62)	epilepsy, headache, dizziness and vertigo
至陰 Zhiyin (U.B. 67)	malposition of fetus (moxibustion), headache

足少陰腎經 [zú shàoyīn shènjīng]
the Kidney Channel of Foot Shaoyin (K.C.), the Foot Yin Minimum Kidney Meridian, or simply the Kidney Meridian, running from 湧泉 Yongquan (K.C.1), a point in the center of the sole, through the inner side of the lower limb, abdomen and chest, up to 俞府 Shufu (K.C.27), a point in the depression between the first rib and the lower border of the clavicle, with 27 points on either side (Fig.11). This channel pertains to the *Kidney* and connects with the *urinary bladder*. Indications are enuresis, spermatorrhea, frequent urination, impotence, menstruous complaints, asthma, sore throat, edema, lumbago, weakness of the lower limbs.

The most commonly used points of this channel and their indications are given below:

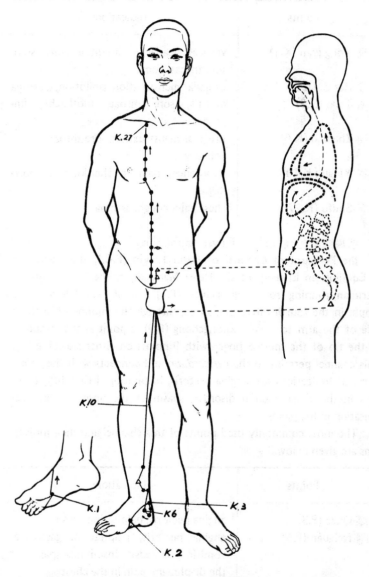

fig. 11

277

Points	Indications
湧泉 Yongquan (K.1)	vertical headache, infantile convulsion, sore throat, coma
然谷 Rangu (K.2)	irregular menstruation, pollution, diarrhea
太溪 Taixi (K.3)	cystitis, sore throat, toothache, impotence
照海 Zhaohai (K.6)	irregular menstruation, sore throat, epilepsy
陰谷 Yingu (K.10)	impotence, pain in the knee, menorrhagia
俞府 Shufu (K.27)	chest pain, cough, asthma

手厥陰心包經 [shǒu juéyīn xīnbāojīng]

the Pericardium Channel of Hand Jueyin (P.C.), the Hand Yin in Equilibrium Envelop of the Heart Meridian, or the Circulation-sex Meridian, running from 天池 Tianchi (P.1), a point 1 *cun* lateral to the nipple in the fourth intercostal space, through the midline of anterior side of the arm to 中冲 Zhongchong (P.9), a point at the midpoint of the tip of the middle finger with 9 points on either side (Fig.12). This channel pertains to the *pericardium* and connects with the *Triple Burners*. Indications are angina pectoris, palpitation, irritability, tightness in the chest, mental disorder, spasm of the upper limbs, heat sensation in the palms.

The most commonly used points of this channel and their indications are given below:

Points	Indications
曲澤 Quze (P.3)	angina pectoris, palpitation, fever
內關 Neiguan (P.6)	angina pectoris, palpitation, gastralgia, vomiting, epilepsy, insomnia, spasm of the diaphragm, pain in the chest
大陵 Daling (P.7)	angina pectoris, palpitation, epilepsy,

	gastralgia, pain in the chest
中冲 Zhongchong (P.9)	apoplexy, coma, sunstroke, febrile diseases

手少陽三焦經 [shǒu shàoyáng sānjiāojīng]
the Sanjiao (Triple Burners) Channel of Hand Shaoyang (T.B.C. or S.J.C.), the Hand Yang Minimum Triple Burners Meridian, or simply the Sanjiao or the Triple Burners Meridian, running from 關冲 Guanchong (S.J.1), a point at the ulnar side of the ring finger, to 絲竹空 Siz-

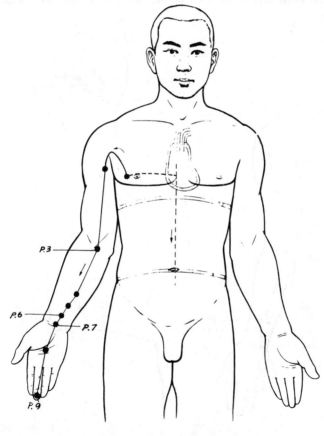

fig. 12

279

hųkong (S.J.23), a point on the lateral border of the orbit at the lateral tip of the eyebrow, along the midline of the posterior side of the arm and through the regions of the shoulder, neck, ear and eye, with 23 points on either side (Fig. 13). This channel pertains to Sanjiao (the Triple Burners) and connects with the *pericardium*. Indications are deafness, sore throat, abdominal distension, edema, swelling and pain behind the ear, in the shoulder, arm, or elbow or in areas along this channel.

The most commonly used points and their indications are given below:

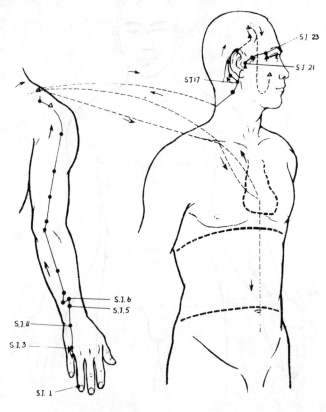

fig. 13

Points	Indications
關冲 Guanchong (S.J.1)	headache, sore throat, febrile diseases
中渚 Zhongzhu (S.J.3)	deafness, headache, sore throat
陽池 Yangchi (S.J.4)	pain in the wrist joint, malaria, deafness
外關 Waiguan (S.J.5)	fever, headache,thoracocostal pain, paralysis of the upper extremities
支溝 Zhigou (S.J.6)	deafness, tinnitus, sore throat, vomiting
翳風 Yifeng (S.J.17)	facial paralysis, tinnitus, deafness
耳門 Ermen (S.J.21)	deafness, tinnitus, toothache
絲竹空 Sizhukong (S.J.23)	headache, eye diseases

足少陽膽經 [zú shàoyáng dǎnjīng]
the Gallbladder Channel of Foot Shaoyang (G.B.C.), the Foot Yang Minimum Gallbladder Meridian, or simply the Gallbladder Meridian, running from 瞳子髎 Tongziliao (G.B.1), a point 0.5 *cun* lateral to the outer canthus, through the regions of the eye, temple, ear, neck, shoulder, flank, and the outer side of the lower limb, terminating at 足竅陰 Foot-Qiaoyin (G.B.44), a point on the lateral side of the tip of the 4th toe, 0.1 *cun* posterior to the corner of the nail, with 44 points on either side (Fig. 14). This channel pertains to the *gallbladder* and connects with the *liver*. Indications are migraine, vertigo, bitterness in the mouth, malaria, pain in the costal regions, pain in the abdomen and lateral side of the lower limbs.

The most commonly used points and their indications are given below:

Points	Indications
瞳子髎 Tongziliao (G. B.1)	headache, eye diseases
聽會 Tinghui (G.B.2)	deafness, tinnitus, toothache
率谷 Shuaigu (G.B.8)	migraine
陽白 Yangbai (G.B.14)	frontal headache, facial paralysis, eye diseases

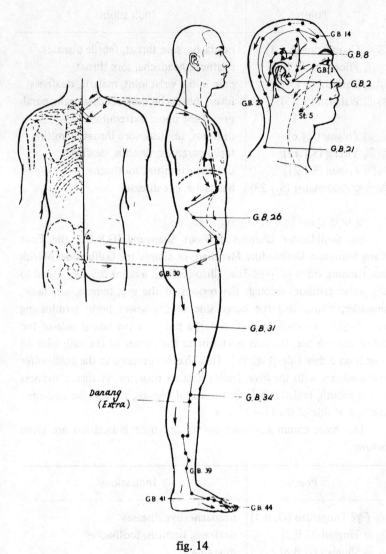

GB 14
G.B. 8
GB 1
G.B. 2
GB 20
St. 5
G.B. 21
G.B. 26
G.B. 30
G.B. 31
G.B. 34

Danang
(Extra)

G.B. 39
GB 41
GB 44

fig. 14

風池 Fengchi (G.B.20)	common cold, headache, rigidity of the neck, hypertension, febrile diseases
肩井 Jianjing (G.B.21)	pain in shoulder and back, rigidity, mastitis
帶脈 Daimai (G.B.26)	irregular menstruation, lumbago, costal and back pain
環跳 Huantiao (G.B.30)	ischialgia, paralysis of lower extremities
風市 Fengshi (G.B.31)	pain or paralysis of the lower limbs
陽陵泉 Yanglingquan (G.B.34)	diseases of the gallbladder, hemiplegia, pain in the knee joint
懸鐘 Xuanzhong (G.B.39)	pain and swelling of ankle joint, paralysis of lower extremities
足竅陰 Foot-Qiaoyin (G.B.44)	migraine, costalgia, febrile diseases

足厥陰肝經 [zú juéyīn gānjīng]

the Liver Channel of Foot Jueyin (Liv.C.), the Foot Yin in Equilibrium Liver Meridian, or simply the Liver Meridian, running from 大敦 Dadun (Liv.1), a point on the big toe just behind the nail, through the inner side of the lower limb, external genitalia and abdomen, to 期門 Qimen, a point about 2 *cun* below the nipple, with 14 points on either side (Fig.15). This channel pertains to the *liver* and connects with the *gallbladder*. Indications are stuffiness and pain in the costal regions, stuffiness in the chest, pain in the lower abdomen, hernia, pain in the top of the head.

The most commonly used points and their indications are given below:

Points	Indications
大敦 Dadun (Liv.1)	menorrhagia, enuresis, hernia
行間 Xingjian (Liv.2)	menorrhagia, enuresis, costalgia, redness and swelling of the eye
太冲 Taichong (Liv.3)	menorrhagia, convulsion in children and infants, hypertension

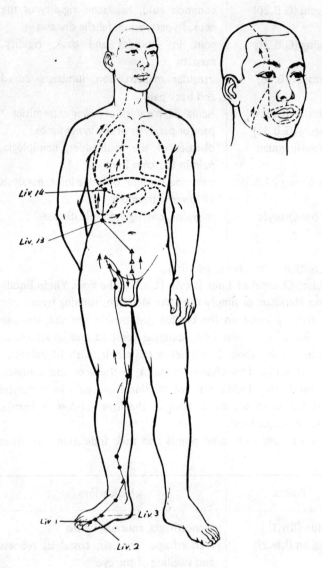

Liv. 14

Liv. 13

Liv 1

Liv 3

Liv. 2

fig. 15

284

章門 Zhangmen (Liv.13)	vomiting, diarrhea, abdominal distension, costalgia
期門 Qimen (Liv.14)	chest pain, abdominal distension, pain in the hypochondriac region

奇經八脈 [jījīng bāmài]

The Eight Extra Channels; the Eight Odd Conduits: the Front Middle Channel, the Back Middle Channel, the Vital Channel, the Belt Channel, the Motility Channel of Yin, the Motility Channel of Yang, the Regulating Channel of Yin, the Regulating Channel of Yang. They are different from the Twelve Regular Channels in that they are not directly connected with the internal organs. Their physiological function is to help regulate and keep in reserve the vital

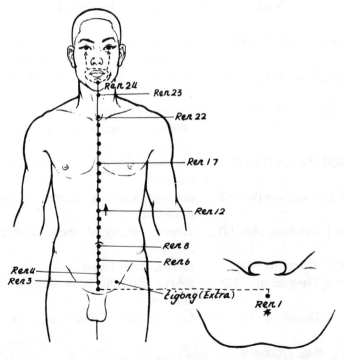

fig. 16

285

energy and blood circulating in the Twelve Channels.

任脈 [rènmài]

the Ren (Front Middle) Channel, or the Conception Meridian, running from the perineum along the midline of the abdomen and chest upward to the lower lip, originating from 會陰 Huiyin (Ren 1), a point in the center of perineum, and terminating at 承漿 Chengjiang (Ren 24), a point at the depression in the middle of the mental labial groove, with 24 points (Fig.16). Indications are irregular menstruation, leukorrhea, hernia, enuresis, dysuresis, pain in the epigastrium and lower abdomen.

The most commonly used points of this channel and their indications are given below:

Points	Indications
中極 Zhongji (Ren 3)	pollution, impotence, irregular menstruation, leukorrhea, menorrhalgia, enuresis
關元 Guanyuan (Ren 4)	same as Zhongji, but also used for tonic purposes
氣海 Qihai (Ren 6)	menorrhalgia, irregular menstruation, pollution, abdominal pain, apoplexy (flaccid type)
神闕 Shenque (Ren 8)	diarrhea, abdominal pain, apoplexy (flaccid type)
中脘 Zhongwan (Ren 12)	gastralgia, vomiting, diarrhea, abdominal distension
膻中 Danzhong (Ren 17)	asthma, fullness of chest, chest pain, hiccup
天突 Tiantu (Ren 22)	asthma, cough, hiccup
廉泉 Lianquan (Ren 23)	aphasia, difficulty in swallowing, throat inflammation
承漿 Chengjiang (Ren 24)	facial paralysis, toothache, salivation

督脈 [dūmài]

the Du (Back Middle) Channel, or the Governing Meridian, running

286

from 長強 Changqiang (Du 1), a point at the back of the anus, along the midline of the back upward to the top of the head and then descending in the middle of the face down to 齦交 Yinjiao (Du 28), a point between the upper lip and the upper gum in the labial frenum, with 28 points (Fig.17). Indications are febrile diseases, stiffness and pain in the back, headache, mental disorder, epilepsy and hysteria.

The most commonly used points of this channel and their indications are given below:

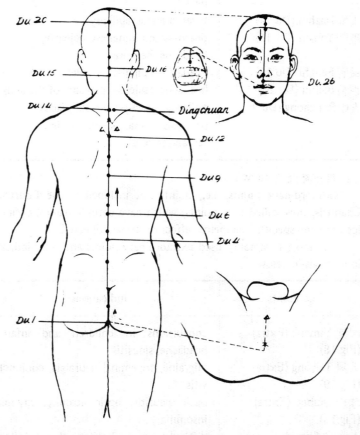

fig. 17

Points	Indications
長強 Changqiang (Du 1)	hematochezia, prolapse of the anus, hemorrhoid
命門 Mingmen (Du 4)	impotence, pollution, diarrhea, lumbago
脊中 Jizhong (Du 6)	epilepsy, diarrhea
至陽 Zhiyang (Du 9)	cough, jaundice, chest and back pain
身柱 Shenzhu (Du 12)	cough, epilepsy, stiffness and pain in the neck
大椎 Dazhui (Du 14)	fever, malaria, epilepsy
啞門 Yamen (Du 15)	deafness and muteness, epilepsy, headache, neurosis
風府 Fengfu (Du 16)	headache, epilepsy, apoplexy
百會 Baihui (Du 20)	headache, epilepsy, prolapse of the anus
人中 Renzhong (Du 26)	epilepsy, shock, sunstroke, facial paralysis, coma, convulsions in children and infants

經外奇穴 [jīngwàijīxué]

extraordinary points, i.e., points not included in the Fourteen Channels, now called new points, which have definite names, definite location and specific therapeutic effect on certain diseases.

The most commonly used extraordinary points and their indications are given below:

Points	Indications
印堂 Yintang (Extra) (Fig.18)	convulsions in children and infants, headache, sinusitis
太陽 Taiyang (Extra) (Fig.19)	migraine, trigeminal neuralgia, conjunctivitis
球後 Qiuhou (Extra) (Fig.18)	optic neuritis, optic atrophy, myopia, insomnia
上廉泉 Shanglianquan	difficulty in swallowing, throat inflam-

(Extra) (Fig.19)	mation
定喘 Dingchuan (Extra) (Fig.17)	cough, asthma
腰眼 Yaoyan (Extra) (Fig.10)	lumbago, irregular menstruation
子宮 Zigong (Extra) (Fig.16)	hysteroptosis, irregular menstruation
四縫 Sifeng (Extra) (Fig.20)	malnutrition syndrome in children, dyspepsia, whooping cough
十宣 Shixuan (Extra) (Fig.20)	coma, shock, apoplexy, sunstroke
膝眼 Xiyan (Extra) (Fig.6)	disorder of the knee joint
闌尾 Lanwei (Extra) (Fig.6)	appendicitis, paralysis of the lower limbs
膽囊 Dannang (Extra) (Fig.14)	diseases of the gallbladder
八風 Bafeng (Extra) (Fig.6)	redness and swelling, numbness and pain of the toes and dorsum of the foot

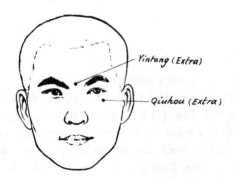

fig. 18

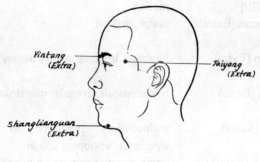

fig. 19

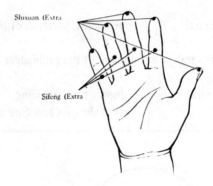

fig. 20

華佗夾脊穴 [huàtuó jiājǐxué]

Hua Tuo's Paravertebral Points (Extra), points said to have been originated by Hua Tuo: (1) from the 1st thoracic vertebra to the 5th lumbar vertebra, a point on either side of the vertebral process, 34 points in all; (2) on both sides of the spinal column, about 0.5 *cun* lateral to the midline, from the 1st cervical vertebra to the 4th sacral vertebra, altogether 28 points

Indications: mainly used for regulating the functioning of the internal organs and treating local disorders on the back along the spinal column

290

Points	Indications
Cervical 1—4	Diseases of the head region
Cervical 1—7	Diseases of the neck region
Cervical 4—Thoracic 1	Diseases of the upper extremities
Thoracic 1—7	Diseases of the chest region
Thoracic 8—12	Diseases of the abdominal region
Thoracic 11—Lumbar 5	Diseases of the lumbar region
Lumbar 2—Sacral 2	Diseases of the lower extremities
Lumbar 2—Sacral 4	Diseases of the urogenital system

特定穴 [tèdìngxué]

specific points: points on the Fourteen Channels with specific therapeutic effects, hence, specific names. They are 五輸穴 the Five Shu Points, 原穴 the Yuan Points, 絡穴 the Luo Points, 募穴 the Mu Points, 背俞穴 the Back Shu Points, 八會穴 the Eight Strategic Points, 郄穴 the Xi Points, 交會穴 the Crossing Points, 八脈交會穴 the Eight Confluent Points and 下合穴 the Xiahe Points

五輸穴 [wǔshūxué]

the Five Shu (Inductory) Points: five points on the Twelve Regular channels distributing distal to the elbow and knees, varying in their condition of the flow of vital energy and blood. They are: the Jing or the Well Points, the Xing or the Spring Points, the Shu or the Stream Points, the Jing or the River Points, the He or the Sea Points.

井穴 [jǐngxué]

the Jing or the Well Points, located at the end of the fingers or toes. Each of the Twelve Regular Channels has a Well Point, so there are twelve Well Points in all. They are:

少商 Shaoshang (Lu.11) 商陽 Shangyang (L.1.1.)
中冲 Zhongchong (P.9) 關冲 Guanchong (S.J.1)
少冲 Shaochong (H.9) 少澤 Shaoze (S.I.1)
隱白 Yinbai (Sp.1) 厲兌 Lidui (St.45)
大敦 Dadun (Liv.1) (足)竅陰 Foot-Qiaoyin (G.B.44)
湧泉 Yongquan (K.1) 至陰 Zhiyin (U.B.67)

Indications of these points are mental disorders and iritability.

滎穴 [xíngxué]

the Xing or Spring Points, located at the distal end of the limbs. Each of the Twelve Regular Channels has a Spring Point. They are used for treating febrile diseases.

魚際 Yuji (Lu.10)　　　二間 Erjian (L.I.2)
勞宮 Laogong (P.8)　　　液門 Yemen (S.J.2)
少府 Shaofu (H.8)　　　前谷 Qiangu (S.I.2)
大都 Dadu (Sp.2)　　　內庭 Neiting (St.44)
行間 Xingjian (Liv.2)　　俠溪 Xiaxi (G.B.43)
然谷 Rangu (K.2)　　　通谷 Tonggu (U.B.66)

俞穴 [shùxué]

(1) an acupuncture point in general; (2) the Shu or the Stream Points, located on the hands or feet. Each of the Twelve Regular Channels has a Stream Point. They are used for treating rheumatism.

太淵 Taiyuan (Lu.9)　　　三間 Sanjian (L.I.3)
大陵 Daling (P.7)　　　中渚 Zhongzhu (S.J.3)
神門 Shenmen (H.7)　　　後溪 Houxi (S.I.3)
太白 Taibai (Sp.3)　　　陷谷 Xiangu (St.43)
太冲 Taichong (Liv.3)　　足臨泣 Foot-Linqi (G.B.41)
太溪 Taixi (K.3)　　　束骨 Shugu (U.B.65)

經穴 [jīngxué]

(1) points on the Fourteen Channels; (2) the Jing or the River Points, of which each of the twelve Regular Channels has one. They are used for treating cough, asthma, disorders of the throat.

經渠 Jingqu (Lu.8)　　　陽溪 Yangxi (L.I.5)
間使 Jianshi (P.5)　　　支溝 Zhigou (S.J.6)
靈道 Lingdao (H.4)　　　陽谷 Yanggu (S.I.5)
商丘 Shangqiu (Sp.5)　　解溪 Jiexi (St. 41)
中封 Zhongfeng (Liv.4)　　陽輔 Yangfu (G.B.38)
復溜 Fuliu (K. 7)　　　昆侖 Kunlun (U.B.60)

合穴 [héxué]

the He or the Sea Points, located at the elbow or the knee. Each of the Twelve Regular Channels has a Sea Point, which is used for treating diseases of the Six Bowels, such as the stomach and the intestines.

尺澤 Chize (Lu.5)　　　曲池 Quchi (L.I.11)
曲澤 Quze (K.3)　　　天井 Tianjing (S.J.10)
少海 Shaohai (H.3)　　小海 Xiaohai (S.I.8)
陰陵泉 Yinlingquan (Sp.9)　足三里 Zusanli (Sf. 36)
曲泉 Ququan (Liv. 8)　　陽陵泉 Yanglingquan (G.B.34)
陰谷 Yingu (K.10)　　　委中 Weizhong (U.B. 40)

　　原穴 [yuánxué]

the **Yuan or Source Points**, where the condition of the vital energy is reflected and thus the pathological changes of internal organs are manifested. Each of the Twelve Regular Channels has a Source Point.

太淵 Taiyuan (Lu.9)　　京骨 Jinggu (U.B.64)
合谷 Hegu (L.I.4)　　　太溪 Taixi (K.3)
冲陽 Chongyang (St. 42)　大陵 Daling (P.7)
太白 Taibai (Sp.3)　　陽池 Yangchi (S.J.4)
神門 Shenmen (H.7)　　丘墟 Qiuxu (G.B.40)
腕骨 Hand-Wangu (S.I.4)　太冲 Taichong (Liv.3)

Indications: disorder of internal organs related to the respective channel.

　　絡穴 [luòxué]

the **Luo or the Connecting Points**. Each of the Fourteen Channels has a Luo Point to connect the respective Yang and·Yin Channel interior-exteriorly. The Spleen Channel has two Luo Points, hence fifteen in all, which are used to treat diseases of corresponding internal organs.

偏厲 Pianli (L.I.6)　　大鐘 Dazhong (K.4)
列缺 Lieque (Lu.7)　　飛揚 Feiyang (U.B.58)
公孫 Gongsun (Sp.4)　　外關 Waiguan (S.J.5)
豐隆 Fenglong (St.40)　　內關 Neiguan (P.6)
支正 Zhizheng (S.I.7)　　蠡溝 Ligou (Liv.5)
通裏 Tongli (H.5)　　　光明 Guangming (G.B.37)
大包 Dabao (Sp.21)　　長强 Changqiang (Du 1)
鳩尾 Jiuwei (Ren 15)

　　郄穴 [xìxué]

the **Xi or the Cleft Points**, where the energy of the channel accumulates deep. Each of the Twelve Regular Channels, together with the

Motility Channels of Yin and Yang, the Regulating Channels of Yin and Yang, has a Cleft Point, all together sixteen in number.

Indications of the Xi (Cleft) Points are acute cases and pains related to areas through which these channels run and internal organs related.

孔最 Kongzui (Lu.6)　　　　會宗 Huizong (S.J.7)
郄門 Ximen (P.4)　　　　　養老 Yanglao (S.I.6)
陰郄 Yinxi (H.6)　　　　　梁丘 Liangqiu (St.34)
溫溜 Wenliu (L.I.7)　　　　外丘 Waiqiu (G.B.36)
金門 Jinmen (U.B.63)　　　跗陽 Fuyang (U.B.59)
地機 Diji (Sp.8)　　　　　交信 Jiaoxin (K.8)
中都 Zhongdu (Liv.6)　　　陽交 Yangjiao (G.B.35)
水泉 Shuiquan (K.5)　　　　築賓 Zhubin (K.9)

募穴 [mùxué]

the Mu or the Front Points, located in the chest and abdomen, where the vital energy of respective internal organs of different channels expresses itself clearly and so if an internal organ is diseased, pathological reactions such as pain on pressure will be observed on corresponding point.

The Twelve Mu Points are used for diagnosing and treating diseases of corresponding internal organs.

中府 Zhonfu (Lu. 1)　　　中脘 Zhongwan (Ren 12)
膻中 Danzhong (Ren 17)　石門 Shimen (Ren 5)
巨闕 Juque (Ren 14)　　　京門 Jingmen (G.B.25)
期門 Qimen (Liv. 14)　　天樞 Tianshu (St. 25)
日月 Riyue (G.B.24)　　　關元 Guanyuan (Ren 4)
章門 Zhangmen (Liv. 13)　中極 Zhongji (Ren 3)

背俞穴 [bèishùxué]

the Back Shu Points, all located on the back, on the Urinary Bladder Channel (Fig. 10). If an internal organ is diseased, its corresponding Back Shu Point would show abnormal reactions such as pain on pressure.

294

Points	Indications
肺俞 Feishu (U.B.13) (lung)	cough, asthma, pneumonia, pulmonary tuberculosis
厥陰俞 Jueyinshu (U.B. 14)	cardiac diseases, neurasthenia, fullness of the chest
心俞 Xinshu (U.B. 15) (heart)	cardiac diseases, neurasthenia, epilepsy
肝俞 Ganshu (U.B. 18) (liver)	hepatitis, pain in the hypochondriac region, eye diseases
膽俞 Danshu (U.B.19) (gallbladder)	biliary cystitis, jaundice, low grade afternoon fever
脾俞 Pishu (U.B.20) (spleen)	chronic diarrhea, chronic hemorrhagic diseases, edema
胃俞 Weishu (U.B.21) (stomach)	gastric pain, gastric ulcer, nausea and vomiting
三焦俞 Sanjiaoshu (U.B. 22) (Triple Burners)	dyspepsia, edema, lumbago
腎俞 Shenshu (U.B.23) (kidney)	nephritis, impotence, irregular menstruation, chronic diarrhea, lumbago
大腸俞 Dachangshu (U.B. 25) (large intestine)	diarrhea, abdominal pain, dysentery, lumbago
小腸俞 Xiaochangshu (U.B.27) (small intestine)	diarrhea, abdominal pain, hematuresis
膀胱俞 Pangguangshu (U.B.28) (urinary bladder)	enuresis, retention of urine, pain in lumbosacral regions

八會穴 [bāhuìxué]
the **Eight Strategic or Influential Points**, with which eight kinds of bodily parts or elements are closely associated. So if anything has gone wrong with these parts or elements, the corresponding strategic point may be used in combination with other particular points for its treatment.
章門 Zhangmen (Liv.13)—associated with viscera

中脘 Zhongwan (Ren 12)—associated with bowels
膻中 Danzhong (Ren 17)—associated with vital energy
膈俞 Geshu (U.B.17)—associated with blood
陽陵泉 Yanglingquan (G.B.34)—associated with sinew
太淵 Taiyuan (Lu.9)—associated with vessels
大杼 Dashu (U.B.11)—associated with bones
懸鐘 Xuanzhon (G.B.39)—associated with marrow

交會穴 [jiāohuìxué]

the Crossing Points: Points where two or more channels cross each other, e.g., Sanyinjiao on the Spleen Channel is a point where the Spleen Channel, the Liver Channel and the Kidney Channel cross each other. So this point can be used to treat diseases of all these three channels. There are more than 90 such points on the body.

八脈交會穴 [bāmàijiāohuìxué]

the Eight Confluential Points: which are the points where the Eight Extraordinary Channels and the Twelve Regular Channels cross each other. Clinically they are used in pairs.

公孫 Gongsun (Sp. 4) and 内關 Neiguan (P.6) are used in combination to treat diseases of the heart, chest and epigastric region.

後溪 Houxi (S.I.3) and 申脈 Shenmai (U.B.62) are used in combination to treat disorders in the neck, shoulder, back, and inner canthus.

外關 Waiguan (S.J.5) and 足臨泣 Foot-Linqi (G.B.41) are used in combination to treat disorders of the mastoid region, cheek, and outer canthus.

列缺 Lieque (Lu.7) and 照海 Zhaohai (K.6) are used in combination to treat disorders of the throat, chest and lungs.

下合穴 [xiàhéxué]

the Xiahe or the Lower Corresponding Points—points on the three Yang Channels of the Foot corresponding to the six Bowels:

足三里 Zusanli (St.36), 上巨虚 Shangjuxu (St.37), 下巨虚 Xiajuxu (St.39), 陽陵泉 Yanglingquan (G.B.34), 委中 Weizhong (U.B.40) and 委陽 Weiyang (U.B.39) correspond to the *stomach*, the *large intestine*, the *small intestine*, the *gallbladder*, the *urinary bladder* and the Sanjiao (Triple Burners) respectively. These points are used to treat diseases of the Six bowels.

296

冲脉 [chōngmài]

the Chong or the Vital Channel, which originates from the uterus, comes into confluence with the Foot Shaoyin Channel and then runs upward along the two sides of the abdomen to the chest and then disperses. Its pathological manifestations are irregular menstruation, uterine bleeding and infertility.

带脉 [dàimài]

the Belt Channel, originating from the lower part of hypochondria and going round the waist. Its pathological manifestations are abdominal pain, weakness in the loins, irregular menstruation, leukorrhea.

陰維脈 [yīnwéimài]

the Regulating Channel of Yin, originating from the upper part of the inner ankle, running upward along the inner side of the lower limb, through the abdomen, the chest and the throat, terminating at the back of the neck. Its main pathological manifestation is angina pectoris.

陽維脈 [yángwéimài]

the Regulating Channel of Yang, originating from the lower part of the outer ankle running upward along the outer side of the lower limb, through the side of the trunk, the shoulder, the neck and terminating at the top of the head. Its pathological manifestation is fever with chills.

陰蹻脈 [yīnqiāomài]

the Motility Channel of Yin, originating from the inner side of the heel, running upward along the inner side of the lower limb, through the front private parts, the abdomen, the chest, the neck, either side of the nose and terminating in the eye. Its main pathological manifestation is sleepiness.

陽蹻脈 [yángqiāomài]

the Motility Channel of Yang, originating from the outer side of the heel, running upward along the outer ankle, the outer side of the lower limb, through the abdomen, the chest, the shoulder, the cheek, terminating at the back of the neck. Its pathological manifestations are mania and insomnia.

十二經筋 [shíèrjīngjīn]; 經筋 [jīngjīn]

muscles distributed along the Twelve Regular Channels. When a channel is diseased, it will be reflected in the impeded movement of the corresponding muscle group.

十二經別 [shíèrjīngbié]; 經別 [jīngbié]
collaterals or branches of the Twelve Regular Channels, which run in the deep part of the body to strengthen the communication between the interior and exterior channels of the Twelve Regular Channels in the trunk, and to serve as a supplementary passage for the flow of vital energy of the Regular Channels

十二皮部 [shíèr píbù]
the skin zones or cutaneous regions of the Twelve Regular Channels, which reflect the functioning condition of the latter. Pathologically, pathogenic factors may get into the body from the cutaneous regions to the interior channels. On the contrary, if an internal organ is diseased, it may be made known by changes on the skin zone through which the channel and collaterals run.

表經 [biǎojīng]
the exterior or outer channels, which are the Yang Channels, pertaining to the bowels and connecting with the viscera, and running on the exterior or outer side of the limbs. For example, the Large Intestine Channel of Hand Yangming is the exterior or outer channel of the Lung Channel of Hand Taiyin.

裏經 [lǐjīng]
the interior of inner channels, which are the Yin Channels, pertaining to the viscera and connecting with the bowels, and running on the interior or inner side of the limbs. For example, the Lung Channel of Hand Taiyin is the interior or inner channel of the Large Intestine Channel of Hand Yangming.

十五絡脈 [shíwǔ luòmài]
the fifteen main collaterals of the channels. Each of the Fourteen Channels has a collateral and together with the Great Collateral of the Spleen, there are fifteen collaterals in all, which communicate with the exterior and the interior of the body.

脾之大絡 [pí zhī dàluò]
the Great Collateral of the Spleen, which issues directly from this organ

孫絡 [sūnluò]

298

tertiary collaterals, subdivided small branches of the channel or capillaries

浮絡 [fúluò]

superficial collaterals, collaterals lying just beneath the skin

魚絡 [yúluò]

collateral on the palmar side of the root of the thumb. Its congestion is a sign of disorders of the Large Intestinal Channel.

胞絡 [bāoluò]; 胞脈 [bāomài]

collateral or channel of the womb, channels and collaterals connecting with the uterus, chiefly the Front Middle or the Conception Channel and Chong or the Vital Channel, governing menstruation, conception and pregnancy of women

陰絡 [yīnluò]

the Yin collaterals or branches: (1) collaterals or branches of the Three Yin Channels of Hand and Foot; (2) collaterals or branches going downward or deep

陽絡 [yángluò]

the Yang collaterals or branches: (1) collaterals or branches of the Three Yang Channels of Hand and Foot; (2) collaterals or branches running upward or superficially

灸法及其他由針刺演變之療法
Moxibustion and Other Techniques Derived from Acupuncture

艾 [ài]

moxa (Artemisia vulgaris)

艾絨 [àiróng]

moxa down, moxa wool, made of moxa leaves, fluffy and soft, the chief material for moxibustion

艾炷 [àizhù]

moxa cone, a cone-shaped mass made of moxa wool

艾條 [àitiáo]

moxa stick, a round long stick made of moxa wool

艾條灸 [àitiáojiǔ]
moxibustion with moxa stick, including mild moxibustion and pecking moxibustion

温和灸 [wēnhéjiǔ]
mild moxibustion with moxa stick: holding an ignited moxa stick about an inch from the patient's skin, keeping the spot warm and making it reddened, but not burned

雀啄灸 [quèzhuójiǔ]
pecking moxibustion with moxa stick: putting an ignited moxa stick near the skin surface of the patient, moving it up and down so as to give more heat to the applied spot

艾炷灸 [àizhùjiǔ]
moxibustion with ignited moxa cone, which may be applied directly or indirectly

直接灸 [zhíjiējiǔ]
direct moxibustion, application of ignited moxa cone directly on the skin surface

瘢痕灸 [bānhénjiǔ]
scar-producing moxibustion, one kind of direct moxibustion with ignited moxa cone till the skin is burned and then blisters, pustulates and leaves a scar

無瘢痕灸 [wúbānhénjiǔ]
non-scar-producing moxibustion, one kind of direct moxibustion with ignited moxa cone, which goes on only to such a degree as the skin is made red but not injured and so leaves no scar

間接灸 [jiànjiējiǔ]
indirect moxibustion, a kind of moxibustion with ignited moxa cone, performed by placing something (e. g., a piece of ginger, garlic, some salt, or a cake of beaten drug) between the moxa cone and the skin

隔薑灸 [géjiāngjiǔ]
indirect moxibustion with a slice of fresh ginger, performed by placing beneath the moxa cone a piece of ginger about 3 mm thick, with some pores made on it, till the treated area becomes red. It is used for treating vomiting, abdominal pain and diarrhea due to endogenous

cold.

隔蒜灸 [gésuànjiǔ]
indirect moxibustion with garlic slice, performed by placing a piece of fresh garlic about 3 mm thick with some pores made on it for treating sores and boils

隔鹽灸 [géyánjiǔ]
indirect moxibustion with salt, performed by placing salt into the umbilical depression to the brim and then putting a large ignited moxa cone on it, which is used for treating prostration, abdominal pain due to cold, acute vomiting and diarrhea

附子餅灸 [fùzǐbǐngjiǔ]
indirect moxibustion with a cake of aconitum variagatum mixed with some wine placed on the point beneath the moxa cone, used for treating impotence, chronic diarrhea

溫針灸 [wēnzhēnjiǔ]
moxibustion with warming needle, performed by placing a piece of ignited moxa stick on the handle of the needle after insertion, a practice used for treating rheumatic pains

一壯 [yī zhuàng]
one zhuang: the time taken and the therapeutic effect gained for burning a moxa cone as a unit in moxibustion

拔火罐 [báhuǒguàn]
cupping therapy: to suck by placing a vacuumized (usually by fire) cup or jar onto the affected or any part of the body surface for treating purposes

電針 [diànzhēn]
electro-acupuncture; galvano-acupuncture, acupuncture with electric stimulation after the needle has been inserted and normal sensation is felt

電測法 [diàncèfǎ]
electro-exploratory method, mostly used in auriculo-acupuncture, by which spots with best electric conductivity are located and used for needling points

穴位注射 [xuéwèi zhùshè]; 水針 [shuǐzhēn]
therapy of point injection (hydro-acupuncture), by which liquid

medicine is injected into the point so as to obtain therapeutic results through needling stimulation and pharmaceutical reaction. This method is mostly used in treating asthma, neurosis, gastralgia, facial paralysis, vomiting and sciatica.

穴位封閉 [xuéwèi fēngbì]
point block, block anaesthesia accomplished by injecting anaesthetic into acupuncture points, a method for treating pains of various kinds

針刺麻醉 [zhēncì mázuì]
acupuncture anaesthesia, anaesthetic effect obtained through needling so that surgical operation may be done while the patient remains conscious

電針麻醉 [diànzhēn mázuì]
electro-acupuncture anaesthesia, anaesthesia induced by electro-acupuncture

針麻誘導 [zhēnmá yòudǎo]
induction of acupuncture anaesthesia, procedure of manual or electric stimulation to raise the pain threshold of the patient before surgical operation

頭皮針療法 [tóupízhēn liáofǎ]; 頭針療法 [tóuzhēn liáofǎ]
scalp-acupuncture, also called head-acupuncture, by which the corresponding functional areas of the cerebral cortex on the scalp are needled to treat encephalopathy of various kinds, such as cerebral embolism

耳針療法 [ěrzhēn liáofǎ]
ear-acupuncture therapy or auriculo-acupuncture, by which specific points on the ear are needled to treat a large variety of diseases, such as asthma, gastric troubles, neurasthenia, skin diseases, hypertension, enuresis, etc. and also for acupuncture anaesthesia

鼻針療法 [bízhēn liáofǎ]
nose-acupuncture therapy, needling specific points on the nose for therapeutic purposes. Indications are the same as those for ear-acupuncture therapy.

埋綫療法 [máixiàn liáofǎ]
thread imbedding therapy: Catgut is imbeded in the point to bring

prolonged constant stimalation for treating purposes. Indications are gastric and duodenal ulcer, asthma, pain in the loins and the back, etc.

指壓療法 [zhǐyā liáofǎ]
finger-pressure therapy, performed by pressing and rubbing a given point with finger(s) for treating purposes. Indications are syncope, hysteria, epilepsy, toothache, etc.

指壓麻醉 [zhǐyā mázuì]
finger-pressure anaesthesia, a method to induce anaesthesia by pressing definite point(s) with the fingers, usually for extracting teeth

金針撥障法 [jīnzhēn bō zhàngfǎ]
loop couching, i. e., extracting cartaracts with acupncture technique. A special needle is inserted into the eye through an incision to remove the cataract from the pupil and then leave it in the lower part within the eye to restore eyesight.

XI Diseases and Symptoms of Various Branches of Medicine

時 病
Seasonal Diseases

時病〔shíbìng〕; 時令病〔shílìngbìng〕
seasonal diseases, including infectious diseases

時疫〔shíyì〕; 天行時疫〔tiānxíng shíyì〕
seasonal epidemic disease

病候〔bìnghòu〕
outward manifestation of disease; symptoms and signs

陰病〔yīnbìng〕
Yin diseases: (1) a general designation for diseases of insufficiency symptom-complex or of cold nature; (2) diseases of the Three Yin Channels

陽病〔yángbìng〕
Yang diseases: (1) a general designation for diseases of excessiveness symptom-complex or of heat nature; (2) diseases of the Three Yang Channels

卒病〔cùbìng〕; 暴病〔bàobìng〕
sudden attack of disease

新病〔xīnbìng〕
recent disease, usually referred to the onset of a new disease in addition to an old chronic illness

傷寒〔shānghán〕
(1) febrile diseases due to exogenous pathogenic factors; (2) affection by cold, manifested by chills and fever, hypohidrosis, headache, floating and tense pulse

熱病〔rèbìng〕
(1) febrile diseases due to exogenous factor; (2) disease due to summer heat

304

温病 [wēnbìng]
acute febrile diseases, mostly infectious

温(瘟)疫 [wēnyì]
epidemic infectious diseases

风温 [fēngwēn]
(1) an acute febrile disease caused by wind, prevailing in spring and winter, marked by fever, chills, headache, cough, etc., in the early stage; (2) symptom-complex of wind in acute febrile disease, usually occurring after diaphoresis, marked by high fever, spontaneous sweating, heaviness of the body, sleepiness, etc.

春温 [chūnwēn]
infectious febrile diseases in spring, such as epidemic meningitis

暑病 [shǔbìng]
acute disease due to summer heat, such as sunstroke

阳暑 [yángshǔ]
affection due to heat in summer, usually referred to sunstroke by direct exposure to sunshine

阴暑 [yīnshǔ]
affection due to cold in summer, e.g., due to exposure to cold draught or excessive cold drinks

伤暑 [shāngshǔ]; 感暑 [gǎnshǔ]
exposure to summer heat, a general term for cases of heat-stroke, especially for mild ones

中暑 [zhòngshǔ]
sunstroke; heatstroke

暑厥 [shǔjué]
heat syncope, a severe case of sunstroke marked by loss of consciousness and cold limbs

暑温 [shǔwēn]
infectious febrile diseases in summer, such as encephalitis B, malignant malaria, etc.

湿病 [shībìng]
diseases caused by dampness, usually with symptoms such as distending pain and swelling of joints, heaviness sensation of the body, watery diarrhea, edema, etc.

濕溫 [shīwēn]
infectious febrile disease caused by dampness, prevalent in summer and autumn, marked by prolonged fever, general aches and pains with heaviness, stuffiness in the chest and distension in the abdomen, greasy fur of the tongue, etc. as seen in typhoid and paratyphoid fever

秋燥 [qīuzào]
seasonal diseases in autumn caused by dryness, marked by fever with dry throat, dry cough, dry skin, etc.

冬溫 [dōngwēn]
infectious febrile diseases in winter

外感 [wàigǎn]
affection due to exogenous pathogenic factors

寒熱 [hánrè]
(1) cold and heat—two of the Eight Principal Symptom-complexes; (2) chills and fever

畏寒 [wèihán]
intolerance of cold

惡寒 [wùhán]
aversion to cold; chills

憎寒 [zēnghán]
shaking chills during fever

戰慄 [zhànlì]; 寒戰 [hánzhàn]
shiver, chills and trembling, as seen in cases of malaria

惡風 [wùfēng]
aversion to wind, suggesting that the superficial resistance is injured by exogenous pathogenic factors

發熱惡寒 [fārè wùhán]
fever with chills

寒熱往來 [hánrè wǎnglái]
alternate spells of fever and chills

身熱 [shēnrè]
feverishness

發熱 [fārè]
fever

外感發熱 [wàigǎn fārè]

fever caused by exogenous pathogenic factors

惡熱 [wùrè]

aversion to heat during fever

壯熱 [zhuàngrè]

strong heat, i.e., high fever caused by excessive pathogenic factors, as a manifestation of the syndrome of Qi (secondary defensive) system in febrile diseases

灼熱 [zhuórè]

burning heat—a description of high fever with the patient's skin hot to touch

煩熱 [fánrè]

fever with irritability and fidget, usually due to the presence of intense internal heat with impairment of the vital energy and essence

潮熱 [cháorè]

hectic fever; tidal fever, fever recurring daily, in most cases in the afternoon, like the regular rise and fall of the tide

陰虛潮熱 [yīnxū cháorè]

hectic fever due to consumption of vital essence, as seen in cases of tuberculosis

日晡潮熱 [rìbū cháorè]

tidal fever recurring daily in the afternoon, especially that caused by accumulation of evil heat in the intestine, known as tidal fever of Yangming or Splendid Yang

煩渴 [fánkě]

fidget and thirstiness, a symptom of impairment of body fluid caused by intense heat

上火 [shànghuǒ]

suffering from excessive internal heat with symptoms such as constipation, inflammation of the nasal and oral cavity, conjunctival congestion, etc.

神昏 [shénhūn]

loss of consciousness

譫語 [zhānyǔ]

delirium

躁狂 [zàokuáng]

mania

煩躁 [fánzào]

irritability and restlessness

躁煩 [zàofán]

restlessness due to deficiency of Yang, marked by involuntary movement of the limbs with cold body, no desire to drink, fine and feeble pulse

心中懊憹 [xīn zhōng àonóng]

distressing burning sensation in the epigastrium, seen in acute febrile disease or gastritis

心煩 [xīnfán]

fidgets, usually caused by endogenous heat

手足躁擾 [shǒu zú zàorǎo]

restless involuntary movement of the limbs

痙病 [jìngbìng]

spasmodic symptoms, especially those seen in febrile disease, such as opisthotonus, convulsions, trismus, etc.

項強 [xiàngjiáng]

rigid neck

角弓反張 [jiǎogōngfǎnzhāng]

opisthotonus

轉筋 [zhuànjīn]

spasm of the gastrocnemius muscles

拘攣 [jūluán]

contracture of the limbs, a sign of dysfunction of the *liver* usually caused by pathogenic factor of wind

拘急 [jūjí]

contracture or subjective sensation of contraction, e.g., of limbs (in cases of affection by exogenous factors or insufficient blood nourishment), flanks (in cases of stagnancy in the *liver*), and lower abdomen (in cases of insufficient vital function of the *kidney*)

抽筋 [chōujīn]

spasms of muscles

筋惕肉瞤 [jīn tì ròu shùn]

twitching of muscles

身瞤動 [shēn shùn dòng]
twitching of skeletal muscles due to deficiency of vital energy and
loss of body fluid

但欲寐 [dàn yù mèi]
sleepiness

結胸 [jiéxiōng]
accumulation of excessive harmful factor in the chest, manifested
by tenderness and fullness sensation in costal region with fever and
sweating, or by pain and tenderness from the epigastrium to lower
abdomen with constipation and thirst

胸悶 [xiōngmèn]
oppressed feeling in the chest, usually due to dampness and heat or
phlegm stagnated in the middle portion of the body involving the chest

痞滿 [pǐmǎn]
stuffiness and fullness sensation in the chest and abdomen due to
obstructed flow of vital energy

胸痞 [xiōngpǐ]
stuffiness in the chest

心下痞 [xīnxiàpǐ]
stuffiness in the gastric region, soft and painless on pressure

心下痞硬 [xīnxià pǐyìng]
stuffiness and rigidity of the gastric region

心下逆滿 [xīnxià nìmǎn]
distension in the gastric region with belching or nausea

少腹硬滿 [shàofù yìngmǎn]
resistance and distension of the lower abdomen due to blood
stasis or retention of urine

風寒感冒 [fēnghán gǎnmào]
affection due to wind and cold, manifested by chilliness and mild
fever, sweatlessness, headache, stuffed and running nose, sneezing,
general aching, floating and tense pulse, etc.

風熱感冒 [fēngrè gǎnmào]
affection due to wind and heat, manifested by fever with mild
chilliness, headache, sore throat, cough and expectoration of yellowish
sputum, thirst, rapid pulse, etc.

瘧 [nüè]; 瘧病 [nüèbìng]; 瘧疾 [nüèjī]
malaria

瘧母 [nüèmǔ]; 勞瘧 [láonüè]
chronic malaria with splenomegaly

白痢 [báilì]
"white dysentery", dysentery with whitish mucous purulent stool

濕熱痢 [shīrèlì]
"damp-heat dysentery", dysentery with frequent bloody mucoid stool, tenesmus, and burning sensation at the anus

疫毒痢 [yìdúlì]
epidemic toxic dysentery

噤口痢 [jìnkǒulì]
"food-denial dysentery", a severe case of dysentery, usually the patient loses appetite utterly and vomits whatever he eats or drinks

休息痢 [xiūxīlì]
intermittent chronic dysentery

遷延痢 [qiānyánlì]
persistent dysentery

久痢 [jiǔlì]
chronic dysentery

赤痢 [chìlì]
"red dysentery", dysentery with bloody stool

赤白痢 [chìbáilì]
"red-white dysentery", dysentery with frequent stool containing blood and mucus

裏急後重 [lǐjíhòuzhòng]
tenesmus

下迫 [xiàpò]
an urgent desire for defecation but ineffectual

下墜 [xiàzhuì]
straining at stool, tenesmus

注洩 [zhùxiè]
spouting diarrhea; watery diarrhea

熱瀉 [rèxiè]
"heat diarrhea", diarrhea due to accumulated heat in the large

intestine, with stinky, yellow stool accompained by abdominal pain, burning sensation at the anus, etc.

子午痧 [zǐwǔshā]

"meridian sickness", an acute disease accompanied by abdominal pain, vomiting, chills, perspiration and thirst, usually fatal within a few hours

絞腸痧 [jiǎochángshā]

acute intestinal colic, an acute illness marked by severe abdominal pain associated with an urgent desire for vomiting and defecation but ineffectual

霍亂 [huòluàn]

choleraic disease, any disease characterized by sudden and drastic vomiting and diarrhea, including acute gastro-enteritis, food poisoning and cholera

霍亂轉筋 [huòluàn zhuànjīn]

spasm of the gastrocnemius muscles following drastic vomiting and diarrhea

胃家實 [wèijiāshí]

"solid stomach and intestine", accumulation of evil heat in the stomach and intestine, which often results in the damage of fluid and brings on such symptoms as high fever, persistent thirst, profuse sweating, full and gigantic pulse, constipation or discharge of hard fecal masses, abdominal pain, etc.

發黃 [fāhuáng]

yellow discoloration of the skin and the sclera of the eye

黃疸 [huángdǎn]

jaundice

急黃 [jíhuáng]

fulminant jaundice, a critical case of jaundice with sudden onset, rapid deterioration and poor prognosis, accompanied by high fever, impairment of consciousness, abdominal distension, ascites, hematemesis, etc., as seen in fulminant hepatitis

大頭瘟 [dàtóuwēn]

infection with swollen head, an infectious febrile disease with flushed swollen face, including erysipelas of the face, epidemic parotitis, etc.

腮腫 [sāizhǒng]
cheek swelling, i.e., mumps

痄腮 [zhàsāi]
mumps, epidemic parotitis

發頤 [fāyí]
suppurative inflammation in the cheek, in most cases referred to purulent parotitis

百日咳 [bǎirìké]; 鷺鷥咳 [lùsīké]; 頓咳 [dùnké]
whooping cough

痘 [dòu]
pea-like skin sores, as seen on the skin of smallpox and chickenpox patients

痘瘡 [dòuchuāng]
smallpox

疹 [zhěn]
rash; skin eruption

癮疹 [yǐnzhěn]; 風疹塊 [fēngzhěnkuài]
urticaria; nettle rash; hives

風疹 [fēngzhěn]; 風痧 [fēngshā]
rubella

麻疹 [mázhěn]; 痧子 [shāzhǐ]
measles

麻毒入營 [mádú rù yíng]
measles with the Ying (nutrient) system involved, measles accompanied with high fever, delirium, convulsion, or loss of consciousness

麻毒陷肺 [mádú xiàn fèi]
measles with the lung involved, i.e., measles complicated by pneumonia

爛喉痧 [lànhóushā]; 喉痧 [hóushā]; 喉疹 [hóuzhěn]
scarlet fever

白喉 [báihóu]
diphtheria

疫喉 [yìhóu]
epidemic throat diseases, including diphtheria and scarlet fever

312

內科雜病
Miscellaneous Internal Diseases

雜病 [zábìng]
miscellaneous internal diseases, excluding those caused by exogenous pathogenic factors

宿疾 [sùjí]
old chronic disease

固(痼)疾 [gùjí]
obstinate chronic disease

隱疾 [yǐnjí]
occult disease, euphemism for venereal disease or impotence

廢疾 [fèijí]
crippling disease

主證 [zhǔzhèng]
main symptoms, which serve as the principal guidance for making diagnosis

風寒咳嗽 [fēnghán késòu]
cough due to wind and cold, accompanied by frothy sputum, stuffed nose, chilliness or aversion to cold, sweatlessness, general aching, etc.

風熱咳嗽 [fēngrè késòu]
cough due to wind and heat, accompanied with sticky sputum, fever, thirst, sore throat, etc.

痰咳 [tánké]; 痰濕咳嗽 [tánshī késòu]
productive (wet) cough, cough with copious expectoration, relieved when phlegm is discharged

乾咳 [gānké]
dry (unproductive) cough

喘 [chuǎn]; 喘促 [chuǎncù]; 上氣 [shàngqì]
asthma; dyspnea

短氣 [duǎnqì]
shortness of breath

少氣 [shǎoqì]
asthenic breathing, lack of strength to breathe, due to deficiency of vital energy, manifested by low voice in speaking, listlessness and lassitude

咳逆上氣 [kénì shàngqì]
cough with dyspnea

喘促 [chuǎncù]; 喘急 [chuǎnjí]
dyspnea and tachypnea

喘鳴 [chuǎnmíng]
dyspnea with wheezing

痰喘 [tánchuǎn]
asthma caused by excessive phlegm marked by tachypnea with phlegmatic sound, cough, stuffiness of the chest, etc.

寒痰 [hántán]
cold phlegm, thin and foamy sputum, usually due to cold

水飲 [shuǐyǐn]
fluid exudate from internal organs as a result of pathological changes

痰飲 [tányǐn]
retention of phlegm and fluid: (1) a general term for retention of phlegm and fluid in any part of the body; (2) a particular designation for retention of fluid in the gastro-intestinal tract, e.g., gastric retention in cases of pyloric stenosis

熱痰 [rètán]; 火痰 [huǒtán]
heat-phlegm, also called **fire-phlegm**: (1) a case of phlegm aggravated by taking pungent and hot food, being too thickly clothed or owing to abnormally hot weather; (2) phlegm lingering in the Heart Channel, joined and aggravated by heat, giving rise to mania, palpitation, etc.

頑痰 [wántán]
chronic case of phlegm retention, e.g., bronchial asthma with repeated attacks, mania, epilepsy, etc.

肺癰 [fèiyōng]
lung abscess

虛勞 [xūláo]
general debility; consumption

314

癆瘵 [láozhài]
phthisis, chronic infectious consumptive diseases such as pulmonary tuberculosis

骨蒸 [gǔzhēng]
"bone steaming", a term for hectic fever and night sweating, symptoms of consumptive disease

勞倦 [láojuàn]; 勞傷 [láoshāng]
illness caused by overexertion, with the vital energy of the *spleen* damaged, manifested by fatigue, lassitude, fidget, shortness of breath on exertion, spontaneous sweating, etc.

五勞 [wǔláo]
(1) five factors causing fatigue or overstrain: looking, lying, sitting, standing or walking for too long a time; (2) five kinds of consumptive diseases: consumption of *lung, liver, heart, spleen,* and *kidney*

虛損 [xūsǔn]
deficiency and impairment of Yin, Yang, vital energy or blood in viscera and bowels

虛煩 [xūfán]
fidget due to deficiency of vital essence which brings on endogenous heat

虛熱 [xūrè]
fever due to deficiency of Yin, Yang, vital energy or blood

五心煩熱 [wǔxīn fánrè]
sensation of heat felt in the chest, palms and soles, a common symptom in consumptive disease or deficiency of Yin, manifesting asthenic fire or endogenous heat produced as a result of consumption of vital essence

內傷發熱 [nèishāng fārè]
fever due to internal injury, i.e., due to disorder of internal organs caused by emotional strains, improper diet, overwork, sexual intemperance, etc.

陰虛發熱 [yīnxū fārè]
fever due to deficiency of Yin (vital essence), marked by tidal fever, sensation of heat felt in the chest, palms and soles, accompanied by night sweating, dryness in the mouth, reddened tongue, fine and

315

rapid pulse

陽虛發熱 [yángxū fārè]

fever due to deficiency of Yang (vital function), marked by fever often appearing in the morning, accompanied by spontaneous sweating, intolerance of wind, lassitude, anorexia, feeble pulse, etc.

血虛發熱 [xuèxū fārè]

fever due to deficiency of blood

乾血癆 [gānxuèláo]

consumption with blood stasis and blood deficiency, seen mostly in women, often accompanied with menopenia or amenia

健忘 [jiànwàng]

amnesia, forgetfulness

多夢 [duōmèng]

dreamfulness

怔忡 [zhēngchōng]

continuous violent palpitation

心悸 [xīnjì]

palpitation

心動悸 [xīndòngjì]

palpitation with visible throbbing of the heart

心痛徹背 [xīntòng chè bèi]

pectoral pains radiated to the back

胸痹 [xiōngbì]

pectoral pain with stuffiness

真心痛 [zhēnxīntòng]

true heartache, corresponding to angina pectoris, so named to distinguish it from gastralgia which was also called heartache or cardialgia in ancient times

厥心痛 [juéxīntòng]

pectoral pains or gastralgia with cold limbs

自汗 [zìhàn]

spontaneous perspiration, sweating in the daytime spontaneously (not caused by physical exertion, thick clothing, fever, etc.) usually due to insufficiency of vital evergy, especially of defensive energy

盜汗 [dàohàn]

night sweat, sweat during sleep, usually due to the action of endogenous heat brought on by consumption of vital essence

氣虛自汗 [qìxū zìhàn]
spontaneous sweating due to deficiency of vital energy, i.e., due to lowered superficial resistance (defensive energy), usually accompanied by fatigue, weakness and aversion to wind

陽虛自汗 [yángxū zìhàn]
spontaneous sweating due to deficiency of Yang

陰虛盜汗 [yīnxū dàohàn]
night sweat due to deficiency of Yin

大汗 [dàhàn]
profuse sweating which may result in excessive loss of fluid and collapse

冷汗 [lěnghàn]
cold sweat

戰汗 [zhànhàn]
general perspiration following shivering, seen in the course of febrile disease, which may lead to subsidence of fever and then recovery, or to collapse

眩暈 [xuànyūn]
vertigo; dizziness

瞑眩 [míngxuàn]
dizziness and nausea, usually referred to those caused by the side-effect of drugs

冒眩 [màoxuàn]; 眩冒 [xuànmào]
dizziness and fainting

掉眩 [diàoxuàn]
vertigo with tremor, usually due to dysfuntion of the *liver* (a symptom of endogenous wind in the *liver*)

頭重 [tóuzhòng]
heaviness of the head, usually due to exogenous or endogenous dampness

頭風 [tóufēng]
severe intermittent headache

偏頭痛 [piāntóutòng]; 偏頭風 [piāntóufēng]

hemicrania; migraine

風热頭痛 [fēngrè tóutòng]
headache due to wind and heat, usually associated with fever, thirst, constipation, floating and rapid pulse, etc.

内傷頭痛 [nèishāng tóutòng]
headache due to internal damage of vital energy, blood, etc., marked by its slow and intermittent onset

肝陽頭痛 [gānyáng tóutòng]
headache due to exuberance of Yang (Vital function) of the liver, accompanied with dizziness, irritability, peevishness, bad sleep and taut pulse

氣虚頭痛 [qìxū tóutòng]
headache due to deficiency of vital energy, i.e., due to lowered functional activities of the *spleen* to send up adequate vital essence and energy to the head, marked by its aggravation during exertion, associated with anorexia and lassitude

百合病 [bǎihébìng]
"lily disease", an ancient term for neurosis with mental strain, listlessness, sleeplessness, anorexia, sham heat and sham cold, bitterness in the mouth, yellow urine, rapid pulse, etc. It is so called because it can be effectively treated by administering *Bulbus Lilii.*

癫狂 [diānkuáng]
depressive-maniac insanity

癫 [diān]
insanity with emotional depression

狂 [kuáng]
mania with emotional excitement

癇證 [xiánzhèng]; 羊癇風 [yángxiánfēng]
epilepsy

驚癇 [jīngxián]
(1) epilepsy induced by fright; (2) infantile convulsion

臟躁 [zàngzào]
hysteria

梅核氣 [méihéqì]
globus hystericus

318

奔豚 [bēntún]
"running piggy", a feeling of masses of gas ascending within the abdomen like running piggies, usually seen in cases of gastro-intestinal neurosis

不得眠 [bùdémián]; 不寐 [bùmèi]; 失眠 [shīmián]
insomnia

卒中 [cùzhòng]
stroke, a sudden and severe attack, as of apoplexy

中風 [zhòngfēng]
apoplexy

眞中風 [zhēnzhòngfēng]
true apoplexy: (1) apoplexy with chills and fever (2) apoplexy with hemiplegia as its sequela

口噤 [kǒujìn]
trismus

失語 [shīyǔ]
aphasia

偏枯 [piānkū]; 半身不遂 [bànshēnbùsuí]
hemiplegia; paralysis of one side of the body

喎僻不遂 [wāipìbùsuí]
mouth and eyes awry and hemiplegia, usually seen after cerebral apoplexy

麻木 [mámù]
numbness

厥 [jué]; 厥證 [juézhèng]
(1) syncope, a temporary loss of consciousness; (2) cold limbs

昏厥 [hūnjué]
a fainting spell

手足厥冷 [shǒuzú juélěng]; 手足逆冷 [shǒuzú nìlěng]; 四逆 [sìnì]
cold limbs up to above the knees and elbows with sudden loss of consciousness, occurring in syncope or shock

蛔厥 [huíjué]
acute abdominal pain with cold limbs due to ascariasis, as seen in biliary ascariasis

热厥 [rèjué]
collapse due to excessive evil heat in the interior of the body

热深厥深 [rèshēn juéshēn]
The deeper does evil heat penetrate, the colder are the limbs—a symptom of syncope or shock in acute febrile diseases.

痿證 [wěizhèng]
flaccid paralysis of limbs

痹 [bì]
(1) **obstruction** of vital energy and blood flow, usually bringing on pains; (2) **diseases of obstruction** due to pathogenic factors blocking in various parts of the body including internal organs; (3) **rheumatic or rheumatoid arthritis** due to wind, cold and dampness blocking in the channels of limbs

歷節風 [lìjiéfēng]
arthritis, swollen and painful joints with limitation in motion, including acute rheumatic arthritis, rheumatoid arthritis and gout

三痹 [sānbì]
three kinds of rheumatic or rheumatoid arthritis: 行痹 [xíngbì] or arthritis with migratory pain, 着痹 [zhuóbì]or arthritis with fixed pain and heaviness, and 痛痹 [tòngbì] or arthritis with severe pain

热痹 [rèbì]
arthralgia due to heat, marked by pain, heat, redness and swelling of the joints, usually seen in acute rheumatic arthritis

風痹 [fēngbì]; 行痹 [xíngbì]
arthralgia due to wind, marked by migratory pains

寒痹 [hánbì]; 痛痹 [tòngbì]
arthralgia due to cold, marked by severe pain exaggerated by cold

濕痹 [shībì]; 着痹 [zhuóbì]
arthralgia due to dampness, marked by swelling with heaviness sensation in joints with fixed or localized pain

口淡 [kǒudàn]
tastelessness in the mouth, mostly due to insufficient functioning of the *spleen* and *stomach*

口甜 [kǒutián]
sweetness in the mouth, usually seen in cases with dampness and

heat in the *spleen* and *stomach*

口苦 [kǒukǔ]

bitterness in the mouth, seen in cases with excessive heat, especially of the *liver* and *gallbladder*

口酸 [kǒusuān]

sourness in the mouth, usually seen in cases of indigestion

口鹹 [kǒuxián]

saltiness in the mouth, usually due to deficiency of the *kidney*

口糜 [kǒumí]

oral erosion

口臭 [kǒuchòu]

halitosis, foul breath

胃痛 [wèitòng]; 胃脘痛 [wèiwǎntòng]; 心下痛 [xīnxiàtòng]

stomachache; gastralgia; cardialgia, pain in the stomach

肝胃氣痛 [gānwèi qìtòng]

gastralgia due to perverted flow of vital energy of the liver, usually caused by emotional disturbance

泛惡 [fàn è]; 惡心 [ěxīn]

nausea

乾嘔 [gān ǒu]

retching; dysemesis; vomiturition

熱嘔 [rèǒu]

vomiting due to heat, spouting vomiting immediately after food-taking due to accumulated heat in the *stomach* or this organ being attacked by evil heat, as seen in cases of acute gastritis, cholecystitis, etc.

反胃 [fǎnwèi]

regurgitation

朝食暮吐 [zhāoshí mùtù]

vomit in the evening what was eaten in the morning

暮食朝吐 [mùshí zhāotù]

vomit in the morning what was eaten in the previous evening

噎嗝 [yēgé]

difficulty in swallowing, often caused by cancer of the esophogus

上膈 ［shànggé］

obstruction in the upper, vomiting instantly after intake of food

下膈 ［xiàgé］

obstruction in the lower, vomiting in the evening of undigested food taken during the day

呃逆 ［ènì］

hiccup; hiccough

嘈雜 ［cáozá］

distress in the stomach, with a feeling of emptiness and uneasiness

燒心 ［shāoxīn］

heartburn

吞酸 ［tūnsuān］; 反酸 ［fǎnsuān］

acid regurgitation

噯氣 ［àiqì］; 噫氣 ［yīqì］

belching; eructation

噯腐 ［àifǔ］

belching with fetid odour

傷食 ［shāngshí］

indigestion caused by improper diet or overeating

宿食 ［sùshí］; 食滯 ［shízhì］; 食積 ［shíjī］

retention or stagnancy of undigested food in the stomach and intestine

停食 ［tíngshí］

food stagnancy in the stomach and intestine; dyspepsia

納呆 ［nàdāi］

want of appetite; anorexia

關格 ［guāngé］

obstruction and rejection: (1) vomiting and retention of urine and stool occurring simultaneously; (2) retention of urine and stool; (3) a kind of very strong pulse indicating divorce of Yin and Yang

吐矢 ［tǔshǐ］

vomiting fecal matter, seen in cases with enteric obstruction

脾約 ［píyuē］

lack of intestinal fluid causing difficulty in defecation

瀉泄 ［xièxiè］

322

diarrhea

便溏 [biàntáng]

loose bowel

溏便 [tángbiàn]

sticky loose stool

五更瀉 [wǔgēngxiè]

"fifth-watch diarrhea": diarrhea occurring before dawn daily, due to deficiency of fire in the Vital Gate to warm the *stomach* and *spleen*

下利清谷 [xiàlì qīnggǔ]

diarrhea with fluid stool containing undigested food

滑洩 [huáxiè]

incessant diarrhea, usually due to dysfunction of the *spleen*

飧洩 [sūnxiè]

diarrhea with undigested food discharged, usually accompanied by borborygmi and pains in the abdomen, due to hypofunction of the *spleen* induced by stagnancy of vital energy of the *liver*

腸鳴 [chángmíng]; 腹鳴 [fùmíng]

borborygmi

中滿 [zhōngmǎn]

fullness sensation in the abdomen, usually due to dysfunction of the *spleen* and *stomach*

腫脹 [zhǒngzhàng]

general edema with abdominal distension

單腹脹 [dānfùzhàng]

simple abdominal distension without edema of the limbs, as seen in cases of liver cirrhosis with ascites

臌脹 [gǔzhàng]

distension of abdomen with gas or fluid

氣臌 [qìgǔ]

tympanites, abdominal distension with gas

水臌 [shuǐgǔ]

ascites; dropsy of the abdomen, abdominal distension with fluid

蟲積 [chóngjī]

intestinal parasitic disease

痞塊 [pǐkuài]

mass or lump in the abdomen

癥瘕積聚 [zhēng jiā jī jù]

mass in the abdomen: 癥 and 積 which are caused by stasis of blood have fixed shape and are immovable, with a fixed pain (localized in the same place), if ever present; 瘕 and 聚 which are caused by stagnation of vital energy usually have no fixed shape and are easily movable, or appear and disappear from time to time, with a migratory pain, if ever present, 癥 and 瘕 are usually referred to lumps or masses in the lower abdomen of woman.

水氣 [shuǐqì]

(1) **disease due to water retention,** characterized by edema; (2) **edema**

水腫 [shuǐzhǒng]

edema, pathogenesis of which is associated with dysfunction of the *lung, spleen* and *kidney*

虛腫 [xūzhǒng]

edema due to deficiency of Yang (vital function) of the *kidney* or the *spleen*

目巢上微腫 [mùcháo shàng wēi zhǒng]

edematous eyelids

跗腫 [fūzhǒng]

edema of instep

陽水 [yángshuǐ]

edema of Yang nature, i.e., edema due to dysfunction of the *lung* which appears on the eyelids or face first; usually with symptoms of heat and excessiveness

風水 [fēngshuǐ]

edema due to affection by wind such as that seen in cases of acute nephritis

陰水 [yīnshuǐ]

edema of Yin nature, i.e., edema due to dysfunction of the *spleen* and the *kidney*, which appears on the lower limbs first, usually with symptoms of cold and deficiency

血證 [xuèzhèng]

(1) **bleeding disease** such as hemoptysis, epistaxis, hematuria, etc.;

324

(2) **blood troubles including bleeding, blood stasis and evil heat in blood**

失血 ［shīxuè］

hemorrhage, a general term for various kinds of bleeding

夺血 ［duóxuè］

(1) loss of blood; (2) dehydration of blood, e.g., resulting from massive sweating

鼻衄 ［bínǜ］

epistaxis; bleeding from the nose

衄血 ［nǜxuè］

(1) epistaxis; (2) non-traumatic external bleeding

咯血 ［kǎxuè］

hemoptysis

咳血 ［kéxuè］; 痰血 ［tánxuè］

coughing blood; bloody sputum brought up when coughing

吐血 ［tùxuè］

spitting blood

呕血 ［ǒuxuè］

vomiting blood; hematemesis

溲血 ［sōuxuè］; 血尿 ［xuèniào］

hematuria

便血 ［biànxuè］

bleeding per rectum, including bloody stool and passage of pure blood

近血 ［jìnxuè］

near-by bleeding, i.e., bleeding into the alimentary tract near the anus, referred to bleeding in the rectum or anus, the discharged blood being fresh red

远血 ［yuǎnxuè］

distant bleeding, i.e., bleeding into the alimentary tract distant from the anus, usually the blood discharged being dark or black

蓄血 ［xùxuè］

stagnated blood accumulated in a channel or an organ, e.g., in the uterus (manifested by distension and pain in the lower abdomen, chills and fever, delirium or other mental disorders at night), in the

325

middle portion of the body cavity with pain, tenderness and resistance over the epigastrium as symptoms

血枯 [xuèkū]
blood exhaustion, disease caused by massive loss of blood

血脱 [xuètuō]
blood prostration: (1) collapse resulting from massive hemorrhage; (2) general debility caused by chronic hemorrhage

肌膚甲錯 [jīfū jiǎcuò]
scaly dry skin, a symptom of blood stasis, also seen in pellagra

消渴病 [xiāokěbìng]
diabetes, a general term for diseases with symptoms of excessive thirst, polyuria and wasting, including diabetes mellitus and insipidus, etc.

三消 [sānxiāo]
three types of diabetes according to pathogenesis, symptomatology and course of development marked by three polys: polydypsia, polyphagia and polyuria

上消 [shàngxiāo]; 肺消 [fèixiāo]
upper (or lung) diabetes, characterized by polydypsia

中消 [zhōngxiāo]; 胃消 [wèixiāo]; 脾消 [píxiāo]
middle (or stomach, or spleen) diabetes, characterized by polyphagia, emaciation, constipation, etc.

下消 [xiàxiāo]; 腎消 [shènxiāo]
lower (or kidney) diabetes, characterized by polyuria with thick suspension in the urine, impotence, etc.

消穀善飢 [xiāogǔ shànjī]
eating much yet ever feeling hungry, one of the main symptoms of hyperfunction of the *stomach*, as seen in diabetes mellitus

淋證 [lìnzhèng]
urination disturbance including pains during urination, pollakiuria, dysuria, and dripping of urine

淋濁 [lìnzhuó]
urination disturbance with turbid discharge, in most cases referred to gonorrhea

五淋 [wǔlìn]

five kinds of urination troubles: urinary disturbances due to urolithiasis, due to dysfunction of the urinary bladder, with chyluria, caused by over-strain, and with hematuria

石淋 [shílìn]
urolithiasis, urinary disturbance associated with the presence of urinary calculi

氣淋 [qìlìn]
urination disturbance due to dysfunction of the urinary bladder or hypofunction of the kidney, marked by fullness in the lower abdomen with dysuria and pain in the urethra after urination

勞淋 [láolìn]
urination disturbance caused by overstrain, marked by dripping of urine with dull pains, usually seen in chronic cases

熱淋 [rèlìn]
urination disturbance due to dampness and heat, marked by frequent and painful urination with scanty red and hot urine, accompanied by fever and chills, lumbago, fullness and pains in the lower abdomen, corresponding to acute urinary infection in most cases

血淋 [xuèlìn]
urination disturbance with hematuria

溺赤 [nìchì]; 尿赤 [niàochì]
red, brown urine

小便不利 [xiǎobiàn bùlì]
difficulty in urination; deficient secretion of the urine

小便頻數 [xiǎobiàn pínshuò]
frequent urination

小便失禁 [xiǎobiàn shījìn]
incontinence of urine

小便淋漓 [xiǎobiàn lìnlí]
continuous dripping of urine, usually associated with frequent and scanty urination

遺溺 [yínì]; 遺尿 [yíniào]
enuresis

失溲 [shīsōu]
incontinence of urine

癃閉 [lóngbì]

difficulty in urination (癃) **or anuria** (閉), seen in diseases of urinary bladder and urethra with retention of urine, or in renal failure with extreme suppression of urine secretion

二便不通 [èr biàn bùtōng]

constipation and ischuria

腰酸 [yāosuān]

distress in loins, weekness, heaviness and distension felt in the lower back and hypochondriac regions

腰痛 [yāotòng]

lumbago

夢遺 [mèngyí]

nocturnal emission

滑精 [huájīng]

spermatorrhea, involuntary seminal discharge

陽痿 [yángwěi]

impotence

早洩 [zǎoxiè]

prospermia

莖中痛 [jīngzhōngtòng]

pains in the penis

奪精 [duójīng]

great loss of semen, manifested by listlessness, impairment of hearing and eye-sight, etc.

不育 [bùyù]

sterility

疝 [shàn]; 疝氣 [shànqì]; 小腸氣 [xiǎochángqì]; 小腸氣痛 [xiǎocháng qìtòng]

(1) **hernia**; (2) **diseases of the genitalia,** e.g., painful swelling of testicle or scrotum; (3) **severe pain in the lower abdomen with constipation and ischuria**

328

婦產科病症
Gynecological and Obstetrical Diseases

經帶胎產 [jīng dài tāi chǎn]
illnesses with abnormal menstruation, leukorrhagia, or occurring
during pregnancy or parturition, four general categories of obstetrical
and gynecological diseases
月經 [yuèjīng]; 月事 [yuèshì]; 月信 [yuèxìn]; 經水 [jīngshuǐ]
menstruation; menses
天癸 [tiānguǐ]
(1) sex-stimulating essence of the kidney in both sexes; (2) menstruation
天癸竭 [tiānguǐ jié]
(1) exhaustion of the sex-stimulating essence; (2) cease of menstruation; menopause
月經病 [yuèjīngbìng]
menopathy
月經不調 [yuèjīng bùtiáo]
menstrual disorders, abnormal menstruation, irregular menstruation and other menstrual complaints
月經提前 [yuèjīng tíqián]
advanced menstruation, menstruation coming one week or more
ahead of due time
月經錯後 [yuèjīng cuòhòu]
retarded menstruation, menstruation coming one week or more
after due time
經亂 [jīngluàn]
menoxenia; irregular menstruation
月經過多 [yuèjīng guòduō]
menorrhagia, abnormally profuse menstruation
月經過少 [yuèjīng guòshǎo]
menopenia, abnormally scanty menstruation
停經 [tíngjīng]
ceasing of menstruation during pregnancy, lactation or some

chronic diseases

經閉 [jīngbì]

amenia; amenorrhea; menostasis, absence or suppression of the menstruation

經斷 [jīngduàn]; 經絕 [jīngjué]

menopause

痛經 [tòngjīng]; 行經腹痛 [xíngjīngfùtòng]

dysmenorrhea; menorrhalgia

倒經 [dàojīng]; 逆經 [nìjīng]

vicarious menstruation, menstrual flow from some part other than vagina, especially from nose

崩漏 [bēnglòu]

uterine bleeding, excessive uterine bleeding occurring not in the regular menstruation period or incessant dripping of blood

漏下 [lòuxià]

mild persistent vaginal bloody discharge

崩證 [bēngzhèng]

sudden profuse uterine bleeding

帶下 [dàixià]

(1) morbid leukorrhea; (2) (in a broad sense) gynecological diseases

白帶 [báidài]

leukorrhea

赤帶 [chìdài]

pinkish leukorrhea

赤白帶 [chìbáidài]

pinkish leukorrhea mixed with white matter

陰挺 [yīntǐng]

prolapse of uterus

妊娠 [rènshēn]; 重身 [chóngshēn]

pregnancy; gestation

不孕 [bùyùn]

infertility

胎元 [tāiyuán]

(1) embryo within mother's womb; (2) essence that feeds the fetus; (3) placenta

330

臍帶 [qídài]
umbilical cord by which the fetus is attached to the placenta
惡阻 [èzǔ]
morning sickness, nausea and vomiting during early pregnancy
子煩 [zǐfán]
irritability during pregnancy
子嗽 [zǐsòu]
cough during pregnancy
子瘖 [zǐyīn]
hoarseness or aphonia during pregnancy
子腫 [zǐzhǒng]
edema during pregnancy
子滿 [zǐmǎn]
general edema during pregnancy, accompanied by abdominal distension and asthma
子癇 [zǐxián]; 子冒 [zǐmào]
(1) eclampsia of pregnancy; (2) puerperal eclampsia
胎動不安 [tāidòng bùān]
continuous moving of the fetus causing pain in lower abdomen—a sign of threatened abortion
胎漏 [tāilòu]; 胞漏 [bāolòu]
placenta leakage, bloody discharge from the uterus of a pregnant woman but without abdominal pain
胎元不固 [tāiyuán bùgù]
fetus unconsolidated, liable to abort
滑胎 [huátāi]
habitual abortion
小產 [xiǎochǎn]
miscarriage, abortion after three months' pregnancy
息胞 [xībāo]; 胞衣不下 [bāoyībùxià]
detention of the afterbirth
惡露 [èlù]
lochia
惡露不下 [èlù bùxià]
retaining of lochia

惡露不止 [èlù bùzhǐ]
incessant dripping of lochia over a period of 2-3 weeks after childbirth

產後發熱 [chǎnhòu fārè]
postnatal fever, fever after childbirth due to various causes such as infection, blood deficiency, blood stasis, etc.

產後血暈 [chǎnhòu xuèyūn]
faint after childbirth due to excessive loss of blood

蓐勞 [rùláo]
general weakness after childbirth due to loss of blood and exhaustion of vital energy

產後腹痛 [chǎnhòu fùtòng]
postpartum abdominal pain

缺乳 [quērǔ]
lack of milk secretion after childbirth

兒科病症
Children's Diseases

純陽之體 [chúnyáng zhī tǐ]
major Yang constitution, referred to a child's body, characterized by fullness of vitality while healthy and exuberance of Yang (e.g., liability to high fever and impairment of fluid) while ill

驚風 [jīngfēng]
infantile convulsion

急驚風 [jí jīngfēng]
acute infantile convulsion

慢驚風 [màn jīngfēng]
chronic infantile convulsion

驚厥 [jīngjué]
(1)faint from fright; (2)convulsion

天釣 [tiāndiào]
infantile convulsion with eyes turned upward, salivation and cyanosis, due to accumulation of heat in the *heart* and *lung*.

瘈瘲 [qìzòng]

clonic convulsion, a convulsion marked by alternating contraction and relaxing of the muscles

撮口 [cuōkǒu]

trismus neonatorum

臍風 [qífēng]

tetanus neonatorum due to infection of the umbilicus

胎毒 [tāidú]

fetus-toxicosis, boils, blisters, eczema, etc. of newborns which were considered in ancient times to be due to endogenous toxicity of the pregnant mother in the fetus stage

胎热 [tāirè]

fetus-fever, a febrile disease of the newborn alleged to the mother's improper diet and medication during pregnancy

胎黄 [tāihuáng]; 胎疸 [tāidǎn]

infantile jaundice

流涎 [liúxián]

salivation; ptyalism, excessive flow of saliva

口糜 [kǒumí]

oral ulceration, usually due to accumulation of heat in the Spleen Channel

口疳 [kǒugān]

oral sores (of malnourished children), aphthous ulcer

疳 [gān]; 疳积 [gānjī]

infantile malnutrition due to digestive disturbance or intestinal parasites with symptoms of wasting, pallor or sallowness, potbelly, chronic diarrhea, etc..

蛔疳 [huígān]

malnutrion due to ascariasis

蟲积 [chóngjī]

intestinal parasitosis, mostly seen in children marked by sallowness, emaciation, potbelly, fits of umbilic pain

乳积 [rǔjī]

indigestion due to improper milking

遺尿 [yíniào]

(1) nocturnal enuresis; bed-wetting; (2) incontinence of urine

夜啼 [yètí]

morbid night crying of babies, in most cases due to cold in the *spleen* (marked by pallor, hands and abdomen cold to touch, coiled posture of the baby suggesting abdominal pain) or heat in the *heart* (marked by flushed face, fever, irritability)

不乳 [bùrǔ]

inability (of a new-born baby) to suck milk due to oral trouble

傷乳 [shāngrǔ]

infantile dyspepsia, caused by improper breast feeding

溢乳 [yìrǔ]; 傷乳吐 [shāngrǔtù]

regurgitation of milk due to over-feeding, usually accompanied with fever, abdominal distension, etc.

五遲 [wǔchí]

Five Retardations: retarded in standing, walking, hair-growing, tooth eruption and speaking—striking features of retarded growth

五軟 [wǔruǎn]

Five Softs: soft head, soft neck, soft limbs, soft muscles and soft mouth (weakness in chewing)—striking features of delayed growth and mental retardation

鷄胸 [jīxiōng]

chicken breast, deformity of chest in which the sternum is prominent, usually due to rickets

龜背 [guībèi]

humpback like a tortoise-shell, a kind of deformity in children due to underdevelopment and malnutrition, as seen in rickets

臍突 [qítū]; 臍疝 [qíshān]

protruded umbilicus; umbilical hernia

苦夏 [kǔxià]

summer affliction of children marked by anorexia and loss of weight

疰夏 [zhùxià]

summer consumption, a children's disease usually occuring in summer, with symptoms of dyspepsia, lassitude and wasting, or with persistent fever

334

外 證
Superficial Surgical Lesions

外證 [wàizhèng]
superficial surgical lesions such as boils, erysipelas, scabies, scrofula, etc.

瘡瘍 [chuāngyáng]
suppurative infection on body surface

癤 [jiē]
furuncle; boil

髮際瘡 [fàjìchuāng]
small boils near the hairline, usually at the back of one's neck

臁瘡 [liánchuāng]
chronic ulcer on the shank

癰 [yōng]
carbuncle

發背 [fābèi]
subcutaneous inflammation on the back

瘩背 [dábèi]
carbuncle around the shoulder blades

腸癰 [chángyōng]
intestinal abscess, appendicitis, usually including its complcations

臍癰 [qíyōng]
infection of the umbilicus

疔 [dīng]
deep-rooted boil

紅絲疔 [hóngsīdīng]
"red-thread boil", a boil complicated by acute inflammation of the adjacent lymphatic vessel which looks like a piece of red thread under the skin

疔瘡走黃 [dīngchuāng zǒuhuáng]
septicemia induced by boils and carbuncles

疔疽 [dīngjū]

deep-rooted boil on the face, especially under the nose or on either side of the mandible, often causing sharp local pain, and liable to cause severe complications if treated improperly

疽 [jū]
deep-rooted ulcer

瘭疽 [biāojū]
panaris, especially referred to pyogenic infection of the tissues on the palmar side of the finger tip

脱疽 [tuōjū]
gangrene of the extremities, especially referred to thromboangiitis

丹毒 [dāndú]; 火丹 [huǒdān]
erysipelas

流火 [liúhuǒ]
erysipelas on leg

缠腰火丹 [chányāo huǒdān]; 缠腰蛇丹 [chányāo shédān]; 蛇串疮 [shéchuànchuāng]; 火带疮 [huǒdài chuāng]
herpes zoster; acute posterior ganglionitis

無名腫毒 [wúmíng zhǒngdú]
nameless poisoning swelling, a kind of local inflammation on the body surface, often hard, red and painful

燒傷 [shāoshāng]
burns

金瘡 [jīnchuāng]
incised wound

金瘡痙 [jīnchūangjìng]; 破傷風 [pòshāngfēng]
tetanus

褥瘡 [rùchuāng]
bedsore

凍瘡 [dòngchuāng]; 凍風 [dòngfēng]
chilblain; frostbite

閃挫 [shǎncuò]
sudden strain or contusion of the muscle

挫傷 [cuòshāng]
contusion

閃傷 [shǎnshāng]

wrench, soft tissue injury due to a sudden wrench of the body

闪腰 [shǎnyāo]

sudden strain of lumbar muscles

伤筋 [shāngjīng]

injury of muscles and-tendons

扭伤 [niǔshāng]

sprain

瘀伤 [yūshāng]

contusion wound with ecchymosis

落枕 [làozhěn]

stiff neck caused by improper posture in sleeping

岩 [yán]

cancer; carcinoma

失荣 [shīróng]

cancer on the neck or near the ear

瘰疬 [luǒlì]

scrofula, mainly referred to tuberculosis of the cervical lymph-nodes

瘿 [yǐng]

goiter

气瘿 [qìyǐng]

soft goiter, mainly referred to simple goiter

肉瘿 [ròuyǐng]

"fleshy" goiter, mostly referred to nodular goiter and endemic goiter

石瘿 [shíyǐng]

hard goiter, as seen in cases of thyroid adenoma and carcinoma

乳漏 [rǔlòu]

lacteal fistula

乳癖 [rǔpǐ]

nodules in breast, as seen in cases of chronic cystic mastitis

乳中结核 [rǔ zhōng jiéhé]; 乳核 [rǔhé]

hard mass in breast, seen in tuberculosis or carcinoma of breast

乳癰 [rǔyōng]

acute mastitis; abscess of the breast

337

乳疽 [rǔjū]
intramammary abscess
内痔 [nèizhì]
internal hemorrhoids
外痔 [wàizhì]
external hemorrhoids
内外痔 [nèiwàizhì]
mixed hemorrhoids
脱肛 [tuōgāng]
prolapse of the rectum
肛漏 [gānglòu]
anal fistula
肛裂 [gāngliè]
anal fissure
肛瘘 [gānglòu]
anal fistula
流痰 [líután]; 骨痨 [gǔláo]; 疮痨 [chuāngláo]
tuberculosis of the bone and joints
流注 [liúzhù]
wandering abscess, an abscess that burrows in the deep tissues and finally appears at a considerable distance from the place where it started
痱 [fèi]
miliaria; prickly heat
粉刺 [fěncì]; 酒刺 [jiǔcì]
acne
疣 [yóu]
wart
白癜风 [báidiànfēng]; 白驳风 [báibófēng]
vitiligo
白屑风 [báixièfēng]
seborrhea sicca
牛皮癣 [niúpíxuǎn]
"cattle-hide tinea", including neurodermatitis and chronic eczema
白疕 [báibì]; 蛇虱 [shéshī]

psoriasis (ancient names for psoriasis)

秃瘡 [tūchuāng]

scabby scalp, usually referred to white ringworm

癬疥 [xuǎnjiè]

skin diseases

疥瘡 [jièchuāng]

scabies

濕疹 [shīzhěn]

eczema

浸淫瘡 [jìnyínchuāng]

acute eczema

脚濕氣 [jiǎo shīqì]

tinea of the foot

黃水瘡 [huángshuǐchuāng]

impetigo

手癬 [shǒu xuǎn]

ringworm on the hand

鵝掌風 [ézhǎngfēng]

"goose-foot tinea"; tinea manuum, fungus infection of the hand

腋臭 [yèxiù]

armpit odour

麻風 [máfēng]; 癘風 [lìfēng]

leprosy

五官病症
Diseases of Eye, Ear, Nose, Mouth and Throat

火眼 [huǒyǎn]

inflammed eye, i.e., conjunctivitis

風火眼痛 [fēnghuǒ yǎntòng]; 風熱眼 [fēngrèyǎn]

acute conjunctivitis

天行赤目 [tiānxíng chìmù]

prevalent redness of the eyes, i.e., acute infectious conjunctivitis

眼緣赤爛 [yǎnyuán chìlàn]

redness and ulceration of the margin of eyelid, i.e., tarsitis

沙眼 [shāyǎn]

trachoma

胬肉攀睛 [núròu pān jīng]

pterygium of the eye extending over a part of the cornea

星翳 [xīngyì]

dotted nebula, small opaque dots on the cornea

翳 [yì]

nebula, slight corneal opacity

鼻塞 [bísāi]

stuffed nose

鼻淵 [bíyuān]

sinusitis

酒渣鼻 [jiǔzhābí]

rosacea

暴聾 [bàolóng]

sudden loss of hearing, mostly due to trauma, infection, or flaming up of the internal fire, e.g. excessive five of the *liver*

重聽 [zhòngtīng]

hard of hearing

耳鳴 [ěrmíng]

tinnitus

鵝口瘡 [ékǒuchuāng]

thrush, a disease usually of infants, with a milky-white adhesion in mouth and throat and pus formation

牙風 [yáfēng]

tooth decay, toothache

牙宣 [yáxuān]

exposure of the root of the tooth as the result of atrophy of the gum

走馬牙疳 [zǒumǎ yágān]

noma

舌岩 [shéyán]; 舌菌 [shéjūn]

tongue cancer

舌癰 [shéyōng]

tongue ulcer

喉癰 [hóuyōng]

throat abscesses, including retropharyngeal abscess, peritonsillar abscess, etc.

乳蛾 [rǔé]

acute tonsillitis

暴喑 [bàoyīn]

sudden loss of voice

XII Distinguished Physicians and Well-known Medical Works in History

名 醫
Distinguished Physicians

岐伯 [qíbó]

Qi Bo. Legend has it that Qi Bo was a famous physician in the reign of Huangdi, the Yellow Emperor (an ancient emperor during 2698—2589 B.C.). He was asked by the Emperor to taste various kinds of herbs and to study medicine and pharmacy. The first and greatest medical work in China Huangdi Nei Jing (黃帝內經)"Huangdi's Internal Classic", or "Canon of Medicine", mainly consists of questions and answers between the Yellow Emperor and Qi Bo on problems of medicine and pharmacy.

雷公 [léigōng]

Lei Gong: (1) said to be a famous physician in the reign of the Yellow Emperor. Discussions between the Emperor and Lei Gong on medicine and pharmacy as well as on acupuncture and moxibustion are recorded in "Canon of Medicine"; (2) 雷斅 [léi xiào], a pharmacist in the North and South Dynasties (317—617A.D.) who wrote Lei Gong Pao Zhi Lun (雷公炮炙論)"Lei's Method of Preparing Drugs"

醫和 [yī hé]

Yi He (about 600 B.C.), a famous physician in the Period of Spring and Autumn (722—221 B.C.), who put forward the theory that abnormality in the six climatic conditions in nature, namely, cloudy (陰),sunny(陽), windy (風), rainy (雨), gloomy (晦), and bright (明), would lead to various kinds of diseases

扁鵲 [biǎnquè]

Bian Que (about 500 B.C.), also known as Qin Yue-ren (秦越人), a native of Mozhou (鄚州), now Renqiu County (任邱縣),Hebei Province (河北省), the earliest noted physician who was good at various subjects in medicine, versed in diagnosis and treatment, especially in pulse-taking and acupuncture. He was ascribed the authorship of some medical works such as Bian Que Nei Jing (扁鵲內經) "The Internal Classic of Bian Que" and Bian Que Wai Jing (扁鵲外經) "The External Classic of Bian Que", all of which have been lost.

淳于意 [chúnyú yì]

Chunyu Yi (about 205—? B.C.), also called Cang Gong (倉公), "the Reverend Master of Granary", for having been put in charge of the public granary of Qi Kingdom (齊國), who was a native of Linzi (臨菑) Shandong Province (山東省) and a well-known physician with rich experience in treating diseases. He paid much attention to pulse-taking and was credited to have devised the method of keeping complete clinical records and case histories to estimate the percentage of successes and failures and thus to find a guide to further predictions.

張機 [zhāng jī]

Zhang Ji (150?—219?A.D.), also called Zhang Zhong-jing (張仲景), a native of Nanyang (南陽), Henan Province (河南省). One of the most influential physicians in the history of Chinese medicine, Zhang Ji was the first to advocate the methods of analysing and differentiating pathological conditions in accordance with the Six Channels and the Eight Principal Syndromes and has been considered the founder of the principle of treating diseases according to the method of differentiating symptoms and signs. He was ascribed the authorship of several medical books on various topics, the most important of which now extant are Shang Han Za Bing Lun (傷寒雜病論) "Treatise on Febrile and Miscellaneous Diseases" and Jin Kui Yao Lue Fang Lun (金匱要略方論) "Synopsis of Prescriptions of the Golden Chamber".

華陀 [huà tuó]

Hua Tuo (?—208 A.D.), also known as Hua Fu (華勇) or Hua Yuan-hua (華元化), a native of Bo County (亳縣), Anhui Province (安徽省), the most famous surgeon and at the same time master of about all branches of medicine, who was said to have performed many major operations including abdominal section with herbal anesthesia and to be the first to recommend therapeutic gymnastics called the Frolics of Five Animals. We also owe the practice of hydrotherapy and acupuncture to him. The book Zhong Zang Jing (中藏經) was ascribed to hlm but it was in fact compiled by an unknown author during the Six Dynasties.

王熙〔wáng xī〕

Wang Xi (about 210–285 A.D.), also called Wang Shu-he (王叔和), a native of Gaoping (高平), Shanxi Province (山西省), versed in pulse-taking, commissioner of the Imperial Academy of Medicine, and author of Mai Jing (脈經) "The Pulse Classic", the first comprehensive book on sphymology now extant in China. He perfected and systemized the art of pulse-taking, yet emphasized the use of all the four methods of diagnosis, viz. inspection, audio-olfactive investigation, interrogation, and palpation and sphygmology. He rearranged Zhang Zhong-jing's "Treatise on Febrile and Miscellaneous Diseases" and hence contributed much for preserving that important classic on medicine.

皇甫謐〔huángfǔ mì〕

Huangfu Mi (214–282 A.D.), also called Huangfu Shi-an (皇甫士安), a native of Andingchaona (安定朝那), now Pingliang (平涼), Gansu Province (甘肅省), a literary man who, suffering from rheumatism, began to study medicine. He became a famous acupuncturist and com-piled the book Zhen Jiu Jia Yi Jing (針灸甲乙經) "A Classic of Acu-puncture and Moxibustion" or "Systematic Classic of Acu-moxither-apy", the first monograph exclusively on the subject, in which the art of acupuncture is explained minutely.

葛洪〔gě hóng〕

Ge Hong (281–341 A.D.), born in Jurong (句容), Jiangsu Province (江蘇省), more popularly known as Ge Zhi-chuan (葛椎川), and Bao Pu Zi (抱朴子), a famous physician and world known alchemist, author of Bao Pu Zi (抱朴子), a treatise on alchemy, dietetics and some magical practices, and Zhou Hou Bei Ji Fang (肘後備急方) "A Hand-book of Prescriptions for Emergencies". In this medical work there are many valuable descriptions and records about diseases as well as their treatments.

龔慶宣〔gōng qìngxuān〕

Gong Qing-xuan, an expert in the North and South Dynasties (317–617 A.D.). He compiled the book Liu Juan-zi Gui Yi Fang

(劉涓子鬼遺方) "Remedies Left Over by Ghosts", the earliest extant medical book on surgery.

陶弘景 [táo hóngjǐng]

Tao Hong-jing (452–536 A.D.), also called Tao Tong-ming (陶通明), a native of Danyang (丹陽), now Nanjing (南京) of Jiangsu Province (江蘇省), a Taoist specialized in the study of herbs. He compiled Ben Cao Jing Ji Zhu (本草經集注) "Commentary on Sheng Nong's Herbal", one of the most valuable materia medica in China, describing 730 varities of medical substances including vegetable, animal or mineral drugs.

雷斆 [léi xiào]

Lei Xiao (about 500 A.D.), great pharmacist and author of Lei Gong Pao Zhi Lun (雷公炮炙論) "Lei's Treatise on Preparing Drugs", a standard work dealing with the processes of the preparation of drugs which appeared in the 10th century and had been in use for centuries before Ming Dynasty

甄權 [zhēn quán]

Zhen Quan (about 540–643A.D.), a physician in the Tang Dynasty, born in Fugou (扶溝), Henan Province (河南省). He was a great expert in acupuncture and was the author of Zhen Fang (針方) "Needling Prescriptions" and Ming Tang Ren Xing Tu (明堂人形圖) "Figures of the Human Body."

巢元方 [cháo yuánfāng]

Chao Yuan-fang (550–630 A.D.), imperial physician of Emperor Yangdi (楊帝) of the Sui Dynasty. He took charge of the compilation of the well-known book Zhu Bing Yuan Hou Zong Lun (諸病源候總論) "General Treatise on the Etiology and Symptomatology of Diseases", which was the first Chinese work in this category and remained a book of reference for a long time and is still valued much.

楊上善 [yáng shàngshàn]

Yang Shang-shan, a physician on the turn of the Sui and Tang Dynasties, who was appointed imperial physician in 605–616A.D. and was an expert in the art of healing. He was one of the earliest physicians who made notes and commentaries on "Internal Classic" or "Canon of Medicine" and was the author of Huangdi Nei Jing Tai Su (黃帝內經太

素) "Fundamentals of Huangdi's Internal Classic", which is an important reference book for studying "Internal Classic".

孫思邈 [sūn sīmiǎo]

Sun Si-miao (581–682 A.D.), a native of Huayuan (華原), now Yao County (耀縣), Shanxi Province (陝西省), who was a prominent physician of Tang Dynasty and the author of Qian Jin Yao Fang (千金要方)"Prescriptions Worth A Thousand Gold"(652A.D.) and Qian Jin Yi Fang (千金翼方) "Supplement to Prescriptions Worth A Thousand Gold" (682 A.D.). His works have been considered as an agglomeration of the medical achievements before the 7th century.

蘇敬 [sū jìng]

Su Jing (7th century), also known as Su Gong (蘇恭), a court official in Tang Dynasty. Seeing the necessity of the systematization of the herbals, he submitted a written statement to the Emperor and was ordered by the Emperor Gao Zong (高宗) to review traditional herbals with Changsun Wu-ji (長 孫 無 忌), Li Ji (李勣), Xu Xiao-chong (許孝崇) and others, a staff of 22 scholars and physicians. As a result of their hard work, in 659 A.D., Xin Xiu Ben Cao (新修本草) "Newly-Compiled Materia Medica" or Tang Ben Cao (唐本草)"The Tang Materia Medica" was published as the first official pharmacopoeia in China.

鑒真 [jiànzhēn]

Jian Zhen (688–763A.D.),a native of Jiangyang County (江陽縣), now Yangzhou (揚州), Jiangsu Province (江蘇省), an outstanding Buddhist monk as well as a physician. Invited by Japanese monks he set off for Japan. Having overcome a lot of unthinkable difficulties and suffered great losses, including the loss of his eyesight, he got to Japan at last and spent the later part of his life there. He enjoyed great popularity among the Japanese people not only for his preaching Buddhism among them but also for having introduced into that country traditional Chinese medicine and other arts and techniques.

王燾 [wáng tāo]

Wang Tao (about 702–772A.D.), a native of Mei County (郿縣), Shanxi Province (陝西省) and a distinguished physician of Tang Dynasty. Trying to cure his sick mother, he made up his mind to go in for

346

medicine. Having worked in the imperial library for twenty years and read a lot of medical books, he compiled a book of his own, entitled Wai Tai Mi Yao (外台秘要) "Medical Secrets of an Official" (752 A.D.), an exhaustive study of every branch of medicine.

王冰 [wáng bīng]

Wang Bing, a physician in the Tang Dynasty, who was good at the art of healing and health preservation. He spent altogether twelve years in rearranging and revising Su Wen (素問) "Plain Questions", one of the two component parts of "Internal Classic", into 24 volumes, on which he made notes, commentaries and supplements.

咎殷 [zǎn yīn]

Zan Yin, a native of Chengdu(成都), Sichuan Province (四川省), who was a specialist in women's diseases in the 9th century, and the author of Jing Xiao Chan Bao (經效產寶) "Tested Treasures in Obstetrics", which was written during 852–856A.D. and was one of the earliest books on obstetrics existing to-day

王維一 [wáng wéiyī]

Wang Wei-yi (about 987–1067A.D.), a distinguished acupuncturist in North Song Dynasty who sponsored the casting of two life-size, hollow bronze figures, on the surface of which were marked the distribution and courses of the Channels and the exact location of the points; and took charge of the compilation of a very important book entitled Tong Ren Shu Xue Zhen Jin Tu Jing (銅人俞穴針灸圖經)"Illustrated Manual on the Points for Acupuncture and Moxibustion as Found on the Bronze Figure" (published in 1207A.D.). This facilitated the locating of acupuncture points and the teaching of acupuncture.

蘇頌 [sū sòng]

Su Song (1209–1101A.D.), not a physician but an official, who compiled Tu Jing Ben Cao (圖經本草) "Illustrated Herbal" (1062) in 21 volumes, the appended pictures in which were collected from different provinces by the order of the Emperor. This was the first complete herbal with detailed pictorial illustrations of each medicament.

沈括 [shěn kuò]

Shen Kuo (1030–1095A.D.),also called Shen Cun-zhong (沈存中), a native of Qiantang (錢塘), now Hangzhou (杭州), Zhejiang Province

(浙江省). Though more famous as a scientist, he was renowned in medical circle for his treatise of therapeutics and medicine, entitled Su Shen Liang Fang (蘇沈良方) "Best Formulas Collected by Su Shi and Shen Kuo".

錢乙 [qián yǐ]

Qian Yi (about 1032–1113 A.D.), also called Qian Zhong-yang (錢仲陽), born in Yunzhou (鄆州), now Dongping (東平) Shandong Province (山東省), a distinguished pediatrist who was appointed court physician in 1090 A.D., whose experience as a pediatrician for more than 40 years was collected and edited by his student Yan Xiao-zhong (閻孝忠) in the book Xiao Er Yao Zheng Zhi Jue (小兒藥證直訣) "Key to Therapeutics of Children's Diseases" in 3 volumes in 1119 A.D. It was one of the earliest pediatric books in ancient China and had profound influence upon the development of this subject. He was the first to give valuable differentiation of measles, scarlet fever, chickenpox and smallpox. He pointed out the peculiar features of pediatrics and put forward some new methods of diagnosis and therapies.

龐安時 [páng ānshí]

Pang An-shi (11th century), a native of Qishui (蘄水), now Qichun (蘄春), Hubei Province (湖北省), a celebrated physician known for having written several medical works, among which the most widely read was a detailed and comprehensive treatise on various kinds of fevers under the title of Shang Han Zong Bing Lun (傷寒總病論) "General Discourse on Febrile Diseases" (1100 A.D.)

唐慎微 [táng shènwēi]

Tang Shen-wei, also called Tang Shen-yuan (唐審元), a native of Chong Qing (崇慶), Sichuan Province (四川省) and a physician especially proficient in therapeutics, who declined the offer of being appointed an official and devoted his life to medical practice and collecting folk recipes. He wrote Jing Shi Zheng Lei Bei Ji Ben Cao (經史證類備急本草) "Classic Classified Materia Medica for Emergencies" in 1108 A.D., a work in 31 volumes, which comprehensively summed up the knowledge about herbals at that time, and submitted it to the Emperor who changed the title to Da Guan Ben Cao (大觀本草).

成無己 [chéng wújǐ]

Cheng Wu-ji (1062–1155A.D.) a native of Liaoshe (聊攝), now Liaocheng (聊城), Shandong Province (山東省), known for his assiduous study of Zhang Zhong-jing's classical work "Treatise on Febrile and Miscellaneous Diseases". He wrote several books on its comment, his Zhu Jie Shang Han Lun (注解傷寒論) "Commentary on the Treatise on Febrile Diseases" (1144 A.D.) being considered the earliest of its kind in Chinese medical literature.

許叔微 [xǔ shūwéi]

Xu Shu-wei (1079–1154? A.D.), a native of Zhenzhou (眞州), now Yizheng (儀徵), Jiangsu Province (江蘇省), a famous physician in the 12th century and a close follower of Zhang Zhong-jing. He prepared graphic illustrations of 36 varieties of the pulse based on Zhang Zhong-jing's work, and propounded the theory of using drugs in relation to the intensity of the disease. He was the author of several medical works, among which Lei Zheng Pu Ji Ben Shi Fang (類證普濟本事方) "Classified Effective Prescriptions for Universal Relief" (1132?) in 10 volumes has been one of his most widely read.

陳言 [chén yán]

Chen Yan, also called Chen Wu-ze (陳無擇), the author of San Yin Ji Yi Bing Zheng Fang Lun (三因極一病證方論) "A Treatise on the Three Categories of Pathogenic Factors of Diseases", a work of 18 volumes published in 1174 A.D., in which causes of diseases were grouped under three headings after Zhang Zhong-jing's theory

張元素 [zhāng yuánsù]

Zhang Yuan-su, also called Zhang Jie-gu (張潔古), a native of Yizhou (易州), now Yi Shui (易水), Hebei Province (河北省), who lived in the 13th century and made the bold announcement that in view of the different conditions between the ancient and modern times it was impossible to treat new diseases with old methods. He therefore discarded obsolete traditional formulas and devised a system of his own. Most of the doctors of the Jin Yuan period (1115–1368A.D.) were influenced by his teachings. He was the author of Zhen Zhu Nang (珍珠囊) "The Pearl Bag" and some other medical works. Among his disciples were such eminent doctors as Li Gao (李杲) and Wang Hao-gu (王好古).

劉完素 [liú wánsù]

Liu Wan-su (about 1120–1200 A.D.), also called Liu Shou-zhen (劉守眞), a native of Hejian (河間), Hebei Province (河北省), who propounded the theory that diseases were caused by excessive heat in the body and advocated the use of medicines of cold nature and thus started the Cold School of Medicine. He was the author of Su Wen Xuan Ji Yuan Bing Shi (素問玄機原病式) "Etiology Based on Su Wen" and some other medical works and had much influence on the School of Epidemic Febrile Diseases in the Ming and Qing Dynasties.

張從正 [zhāng cóngzhèng]

Zhang Cong-zheng (about 1156–1228 A.D.), also called Zhang Zi-he (張子和), a native of Kaocheng(考城), Henan Province (河南省), once a court physician, with rich experience in various branches of medicine, who compared a disease to a foreign substance in the organism which should be attacked and driven out by drastic drugs, such as diaphoretics, emetics and purgatives and thus started the Attack or Purgation School. He was the author of Ru Men Shi Qin(儒門事親) "The Literati's Care of Their Parents", which was completed by his disciple Ma Zhi-ji (麻知己).

李杲 [lǐ gǎo]

Li Gao (1180–1252A.D.), also called Li Ming-zhi (李明之) or Li Dong-yuan (李東垣), a native of Zhengding (正定), Hebei Province (河北省). Being a disciple of Zhang Yuan-su, he held that diseases, apart from external changes, were mainly caused by "internal injury" of the *spleen* and *stomach* (i.e., intemperance in drinking and eating or overwork) and advocated cure by regulating the *spleen* and the *stomach* and nourishing the original Qi (vital energy). He was considered the founder of the School for Strengthening Spleen and Stomach. His master piece was Pi Wei Lun (脾胃論) "Treatise on Spleen and Stomach".

宋慈 [sòng cí]

Son Ci (1186–1249A.D.), also called Song Hui-fu (宋惠父), a native of Jianyang (建陽), Fujian Province (福建省), author of Xi Yuan Ji Lu (洗冤集錄) "Instructions to Coroners", published in 1247A.D., a treatise on forensic medicine written on the basis of his personal experience as a judge and his profound knowledge of previous works on the subject, which exerted a great influence on Chinese jurisprudence. The book has been translated into several foreign languages.

陳自明 [chén zìmíng]

Chen Zi-ming (about 1190–1272 A.D.), also called Chen Liang-fu (陳良甫), a native of Linchuau (臨川), now Fuzhou (撫州), Jiangxi Province (江西省), a distinguished gynecologist who belonged to a family of medical practitioners for many generations and was the author of two important books: Fu Ren Da Quan Liang Fang (婦人大全良方) "The Complete Effective Prescriptions for Diseases of women" and Wai Ke Jing Yao (外科精要) "Essence of Surgery".

陳文中 [chén wénzhōng]

Chen Wen-zhong, the most noted pediatrist in the 13th century, and author of Xiao Er Dou Zhen Fang Lun (小兒痘疹方論) "Treatise on Smallpox and Measles in Children" published in 1241 A.D., and Xiao Er Bing Yuan Fang Lun (小兒病源方論) "Treatise on Etiology of Children's Diseases", which appeared in 1253 A.D.

危亦林 [wēi yìlín]

Wei Yi-lin (1277–1347A.D.), also called Wei Da-zhai (危達齋), a native of Nanfeng (南豐), Jiangxi Province (江西省), claimed to be a born physician and famous in bone-setting. From the experience of his own and the findings of his ancestors, not a few of whom were noted physicians, he compiled a large number of prescriptions in book form entitled Shi Yi De Xiao Fang (世醫得效方) "Effective Formulas Tested by Physicians for Generations".

羅天益 [luó tiānyì]

Luo Tian-yi, also called Luo Qian-fu (羅謙甫), a physician in the Yuan Dynasty (1279–1368A.D.), who was a native of Zhending (正定), Hebei Province (河北省). He had learned medicine from Li Gao (李杲) for more then ten years and was once an imperial doctor in the army. Combining his tutor Li Gao's theories with those of other schools and adding his own experience as well, he wrote Wei Sheng Bao Jian (衞生寶鑒) "The Precious Mirror of Hygiene".

滑壽 [huá shòu]

Hua Shou (1304–1386A.D.), also called Hua Bai-ren (滑伯仁), originally a native of Xuchang (許昌), Henan Province (河南省), later moved to Yizhen (儀眞), Jiangsu Province (江蘇省) and Yuyao (余姚) of Zhejiang Province (浙江省); author of a very useful treatise on acupuncture Shi Si Jing Fa Hui (十四經發揮) "The Expounding of the Fourteen Channels", published in 1341 A.D. He recomposed the "Difficult Classic" or "Classic on Medical Problems" or Nan Jing Ben Yi (難經本義) "The Genuine Meaning of the Difficult Classic", which appeared in 1361 A.D. He was good at differential diagnosis and use of drugs and was particularly skilful in acupuncture. His study of channels and points contributed much for the development of this branch of medicine.

葛乾孫 [gě qiánsūn]

Ge Qian-sun (1305–1353A.D.), also called Ge Ke-jiu (葛可久), a native of Changzhou (長州), now Wu County (吳縣), Jiangsu Province (江蘇省). As his father was a noted physician, he naturally carried on his father's profession, treating diseases effectively with herbal medicines, needling and massage. He was the author of Shi Yao Shen Shu (十藥神書) "A Miraculous Book of Ten Recipes", which was a wonderful record of diagnosis and treatment of pulmonary tuberculosis.

王好古 [wáng hàogǔ]

Wang Hao-gu, also called Wan Jin-zhi (王進之), or Wang Hai-zang (王海藏), a native of Zhaozhou (趙州), now Zhao County (趙縣), Hebei Province (河北省); a distinguished physician in the 13th century, whose chief contribution was that he strongly advocated the use of tonics and stimulants for infectious diseases in the later stage when the metabolic function is weakened, and avoidance of purgatives. Five of his publications are still in existence, including Tang Ye Ben Cao (湯液本草) "Materia Medica of Decoction" (1298 A.D.)

曾世榮 [zēng shìróng]

Zeng Shi-rong (1252–1330A.D.), a most skilful children's physician with over fifty years of experience, author of Huo You Kou Yi (活幼口議) "Discussions on Life-saving of Infants and Children"(1283 A.D.) and Huo You Xin Shu (活幼新書) "A New Book for Saving the Life of Infants and Children", published in 1294 A.D., whose special contribution to pediatrics lay in the skill in grouping the different natures and forms of what was in fact a single disease, thus aiding the

352

practitioners in diagnosis

朱震亨 [zhū zhènhēng]

Zhu Zhen-heng (1280–1358A.D.), a native of Danxi (丹溪), Jinhua (金華), in Zhejiang Province (浙江省), also known as Master of Danxi (丹溪先生), who thought indulgence was the root of all troubles and exhorted the value of tonics for the purpose of making up the deficit in Yin. He advocated the theory that Yang was always in excess while Yin was often deficient, and thus belonged to the School for Nourishing the Yin. He was the author of Ge Zhi Yu Lun (格致余論) "On Inquiring the Properties of Things" (1347A.D.), and Ju Fang Fa Hui (局方發揮) "An Expounding of the Formularies of the Bureau of the People's Welfare Pharmacies".

忽思慧 [hū sīhuì]

Hu Si-hui, a great dietitian of Mogolian nationality in the 14th century, who had been chef of the imperial household of Yuan Dynasty for more than ten years before he compiled on the basis of his own experience and his knowledge of herbal medicines the famous book Yin Shan Zheng Yao (飲膳正要) "Principles of Correct Diet", published and presented to the emperor in 1330 A.D.

倪維德 [ní wéidé]

Ni Wei-de, an eye specialist in the 14th century and author of the valuable book on the causes and mechanism of eye diseases Yuan Ji Qi Wei (元機啓微) "Revealing the Mystery of the Origin", which was published in 1370 A.D.

樓英 [lóu yīng]

Lou Ying (1320–1389A.D.), also called Lou Gong-shuang(樓公爽) or Lou Quan-shan (樓全善), a native of Xiaoshan (蕭山), Zhejiang Province (浙江省), author of Yi Xue Gang Mu (醫學綱目) "Compendium of Medicine", which appeared in 1565 A.D. In this book diseases were classified into various types and categories according to Yin-Yang and viscera and this practical system of classification was found to be very helpful in differential diagnosis and treatment.

寇平 [kòu píng]

Kou Ping, an outstanding pediatrician in the 15th century, the author of Quan You Xin Jian (全幼心鑒) "Directions in Pediatrics"

(1451 A.D.), in which indigestion or unsuitable food was held to be mainly responsible for children's illnesses

虞摶 [yú tuán]

Yu Tuan (1438-1517 A.D.), also called Yu Tian-min (虞天民), a native of Yiwu (義烏), Zhejiang Province (浙江省), who adapted over thirty precious medical works and edited his own Yi Xue Zheng Zhuan (醫學正傳) "Orthodox Medical Record" (1515 A.D.)

薛鎧 [xuē kǎi]

Xue Kai, also called Xue Liang-wu (薛良武), a native of Suzhou (蘇州), Jiangsu Province (江蘇省), a distinguished imperial physician, especially well-known in pediatrics, author of Bao Ying Cuo Yao (保嬰撮要) "Essentials for the Care of Infants" (1556 A.D.), in which the importance of giving the right dosage of drugs to infants and children according to age was stressed and the severing of the umbilical cord by cautery was recommended

汪機 [wāng jī]

Wang Ji (1463-1539 A.D.), also called Wang Sheng-zhi (汪省之) or Wang Shi-shan (汪石山), a native of Qimen (祁門), Anhui Province (安徽省); son of a noted physician and author of several medical books such as Zhen Jiu Wen Da (針灸問答) "Catechism on Acupuncture and Moxibustion" (1530 A.D.), which is clear, simple and kept to essentials, and is very useful for beginners, Wai Ke Li Li (外科理例) "Surgery with Illustrations" (1531 A.D.), Yi Xue Li Li (醫學理例) "Principles of Medicine". etc.

薛己 [xuē jǐ]

Xue Ji (about 1488-1558 A.D.), also called Xue Xin-fu (薛新甫), son of Xue Kai (薛鎧), a famous physician versed in various subjects of medicine. He compiled many medical works such as Nu Ke Cuo Yao (女科撮要) "Essentials of Obstetrics and Gynecology" (1548 A.D.).His and his father's works were edited by Wu Guan (吳琯) and entitled Xue Shi Yi An (薛氏醫案) "Xues' Medical Records", which consists of 24 books such as Wai Ke Shu Yao (外科樞要) "Essentials of Surgery" (1571 A.D.), etc.

王鑾 [wáng luán]

Wang Luan, a pediatrician in the 16th century; author of You Ke

Lei Cui (幼科類萃) "Collection of Pediatric Cases" (1534 A.D.), a comprehensive work summarizing the current knowledge on the subject in which each ailment was dealt with according to pulse diagnosis, method of treatment, acupuncture and prescriptions.

盧和 [lú hé]

Lu He, a distinguished herbalist in the 16th century, author of Shi Wu Ben Cao (食物本草) "Dietary Materia Medica", in which Lu gave explanations on the laxative value of vegetables and their good effect on the health of man. He advocated vegetable diet and advised that meat should be eaten sparingly.

孫一奎 [sūn yīkuí]

Sun Yi-kui (1520-1600 A.D.), also called Sun Wen-yuan (孫文垣) or Sun Dong-su (孫東宿), a native of Xinan (新安), Anhui Province (安徽省); author of Chi Shui Xuan Zhu (赤水玄珠) "Black Pearl of the Red River", Yi Zhi Xu Yu (醫旨緒余) "Supplement to Principles of Medicine" and Yi An (醫案) "Medical Records", collected by his sons Tai-lai (泰來) and Ming-lai (明來), in which he advocated the combination of various schools and maintained that a doctor should be conversant with all the theories in order to master the whole art of healing, and one's chief aim should be the conquest of diseases

徐春甫 [xú chūnfǔ]

Xu Chun-fu, also called Xu Ru-yuan (徐汝元), a native of Qimen (祁門), Anhui Province (安徽省), who lived in the 16th century and was the author of Gu Jin Yi Tong Da Quan (古今醫統大全) "A Complete Work of Ancient and Modern Medicine" (1556 A.D.), in which rich and valuable materials in various fields of medicine were accumulated. He recommended that healthy people should avoid company of anyone with consumptive diseases, mainly pulmonary tuberculosis.

李梴 [lǐ yán]

Li Yan, also called Li Zhai-jian (李齋健), a native of Nanfeng (南豐), Jiangxi Province (江西省); a physician who lived in the 16th century and who summarized the prescriptions used at that period in medical practice and divided them into 18 different kinds. He was the author of Yi Xue Ru Men (醫學入門) "Elementary Medicine"

(1575 A.D.) and Xi Yi Gui Ge (習醫規格) "Rules for Medical Study" (1575 A.D.)

萬全 [wàn quán]

Wan Quan, also called Wan Mi-zhai (萬密齋), a native of Luotian (羅田), Hubei Province (湖北省); a distinguished pediatrist of the Ming Dynasty. Born in a family of physicians for three generations, he inherited their rich clinical experiences, especially in pediatrics and surgery. He advocated that a child should be frequently exposed to sunlight and fresh air, trained to resist cold, protected from being frightened and should not be overfed or given too much drug treatment. He was the author of Dou Zhen Shi Yi Xin Fa (痘疹世醫新法) "Experiences in the Treatment of Smallpox and Rash Handed Down through Generations", You Ke Fa Hui (幼科發揮) "Expounding of Pediatrics" (1579 A.D.) and Yu Ying Jia Mi (育嬰家秘) "Family Secrets in Child Care", etc.

李時珍 [lǐ shízhēn]

Li Shi-zhen (1518-1593 A.D.), also called Li Dong-bi (李東壁) or Li Bin-hu (李瀕湖), a great physician and naturalist. He was a native of Qizhou (蘄州), now Qichun (蘄春), Hubei Province (湖北省) and born in a physician's family. His father Li Yan-wen (李言聞) was an accomplished medical practitioner. After three unsuccessful attempts of higher official examinations, Li Shi-zhen decided to carry on his father's profession. He concentrated his mind on medical studies and his medical skill gained a wide recognition by his contemporaries. He wrote a dozen of medical works among which Ben Cao Gang Mu (本草綱目) "Compendium of Materia Medica" is the greatest. The other works written by Li include Bin Hu Mai Xue (瀕湖脈學) "The Pulse Studies of Bin-hu" and Qi Jing Ba Mai Kao (奇經八脈考) "A Study on the Eight Extra Channels", etc.

楊繼洲 [yáng jìzhōu]

Yang Ji-zhou (1522-1620 A.D.), also called Yang Ji-shi (楊濟時), a native of Sanqu (三衢), now Qu County (衢縣), Zhejiang Province (浙江省). His grandfather had been an imperial physician. He succeeded his grandfather's profession, and was especially skilful in acupuncture. He compiled a very comprehensive and at the same time practical

356

book Zhen Jiu Da Cheng (針灸大成) "Compendium of Acupuncture and Moxibustion" (1601 A.D.), based on Gad Wu's (高武) and others' works on the subject. Hence, his work served as a link between the past and the future.

王肯堂 [wáng kěntáng]

Wang Ken-tang (1549–1613 A.D.), also called Wang Yu-tai (王宇泰) or Wang Sun-an (王損庵). After being a court official for some years, he returned to his native place and became a physician, devoting most of his time to reading and collecting facts until he became a famous physician of his time. He was the author of Liu Ke Zheng Zhi Zhun Sheng (六科證治准繩) "Standards of Diagnosis and Treatment of Six Branches of Medicine" (1602 A.D.), which had the largest circulation of medical books in the 17th century.

李中立 [lǐ zhōnglì]

Li Zhong-li, also called Li Zheng-yu (李正宇), a native of Yongqiu (雍邱), now Qi County (杞縣), Henan Province (河南省); author of Ben Cao Yuan Shi (本草原始) "Origin of Materia Medica" (1612 A.D.), a most practical book for pharmacists. Li had drawn the illustrations for the medical substances himself, with their properties and methods of preparation described in detail. His book may be considered as one of the earliest works in the field of pharmacognosy.

李濂 [lǐ lián]

Li Lian, also called Li Chuan-fu (李川父), a literary man in the Ming Dynasty. He had been an official in Shanxi Province (山西省) and was famous for his command of old Chinese language and literature. He wrote Yi Shi (醫史) "History of Medicine", which deals with the lives of distinguished physicians and is the earliest extant biography of ancient medical professionals.

高武 [gāo wǔ]

Gao Wu, also called Gao Mei-gu (高梅孤), born in Yin County (鄞縣), Zhejiang Province (浙江省), a specialist in needling in the Ming Dynasty (1368-1644 A.D.). He compiled Zhen Jiu Jie Yao (針灸節要) "Extracts of the Principles of Acupuncture and Moxibustion" on the basis of "Internal Classic" and "Classic of Medical Problems". He also compiled Zhen Jiu Ju Yin (針灸聚英) "Essentials of Acupuncture and Moxibustion". To help locate the needling points, he made three bronze figures as models, a man, a woman and a child.

趙獻可 [zhào xiànkě]

Zhao Xian-ke, also called Zhao Yang-kui (趙養葵), born in Yin County (鄞縣), Zhejiang Province (浙江省), a physician in the Ming Dynasty. He was the author of Yi Guan (醫貫) "Key Link of Medicine". He advocated Xue Ji's (薛己) theory and particularly developed the theory of the "Vital Gate", attaching special importance to the function of this organ and maintained that reinforcement of the fire of the "Vital Gate" should be stressed in the treatment of diseases.

陳實功 [chén shígōng]

Chen Shi-gong (1555-1636 A.D.), also called Chen Yu-ren (陳毓仁)or Chen Ru-xu (陳若虛), a native of Nantong (南通), Jiangsu Province (江蘇省), who was a distinguished surgeon with his 40 years' practical experience summarized in his book Wai Ke Zheng Zong (外科正宗) "Orthodox Manual of Surgery", which appeared in 1617 A.D.

繆希雍 [miào xīyōng]

Miao Xi-yong (1556-1627? A.D.), also called Miao Zhong-chun (·繆仲淳), born in Changshu (常熟), Jiangsu Province (江蘇省), a physician in the Ming Dynasty, who often treated the poor free of charge. He was an expert on meteria medica and was the author of Sheng Nong Ben Cao Jing Shu (神農本草經疏) "Annotation on Sheng Nong's Herbal" and Xian Xing Zhai Yi Xue Guang Bi Ji (先醒齋醫學廣筆記)"Extensive Notes on Medicine", which impress the readers of his knowledge and clinical experience in medicine, surgery, gynecology and pediatrics.

張介賓 [zhāng jièbīn]

Zhang Jie-bin (about 1563-1640 A.D.), also called Zhang Jing-yue (張景岳), a native of Shanyin (山陰), now Shaoxing (紹興), Zhejiang Province (浙江省), author of several books on specified subjects, such as pulse, gynecology, pediatrics and surgery. Being especially versed in Nei Jing "Internal Classic", Zhang was the author of Lei Jing (類經) "Systematic Compilation of the Internal Classic". His complete works Jing Yue Quan Shu (景岳全書)"Jing Yue's Complete Works" appeared in 1624 A.D.

吳有性 [wú yǒuxìng]

Wu You-xing (1582-1652 A.D.), also called Wu You-ke (吳又可), a native of Gusu (姑蘇), now Wu County (吳縣), Jiangsu Province (江蘇省), a forerunner epidemiologist, author of Wen Yi Lun (溫疫論) "Treatise on Acute Epidemic Febrile Diseases" (1642 A.D.), a book devoted to the special study of several kinds of epidemic diseases being prevalent then in many parts of China. He put forward the theory of Li-qi (戾氣), pestilential factors, and made much contribution to the understanding of the role of certain infectious factors in the etiology of communicable diseases.

喻昌 [yù chāng]

Yu Chang (about 1585-1664 A.D.), also called Yu Jia-yan (喻嘉言), a native of Xinjian (新建), Jiangxi Province (江西省) who practised medicine in Changshou (常熟), Jiangsu Province (江蘇省), a well-known skilful practitioner and the author of Shang Lun Zhang Zhong-jing Shang Han Lun (尚論張仲景傷寒論) "A Critical Study of Zhang Zhong-jing's Treatise on Febrile Diseases" or simply Shang Lun Pian (尚論篇) "Critical Study" (1948 A.D.) and Yi Men Fa Lu (醫門法律) "Principles and Prohibitions of Medical Profession", in which Yu showed the rare courage to express his views freely to correct the errors or criticize the teachings of the old masters, throwing considerable light on the two classics "Treatise on Febrile Diseases" and "Synopsis of Prescriptions of the Golden Chamber."

武之望 [wǔ zhīwàng]

Wu Zhi-wang, also called Wu Shu-qing (武叔卿), a physician in the Ming Dynasty, born in Shanxi Province (陝西省). He compiled Ji Yin Gang Mu (濟陰綱目)"Outline of Therapeutics for Diseases of Women" on the basis of Wang Ken-tang's Nü Ke Zheng Zhi Zhun Sheng(女科證治準繩) "Standards for Diagnosis and Treatment of Women's Diseases". which has been circulated far and wide. Another book entitled Ji Yang Gang Mu (濟陽綱目) "Outline of Therapy for Diseases of Men" was also written by him.

陳司成 [chén sīchéng]

Chen Si-cheng,also called Chen Jiu-shao (陳九韶), born in Haining

(海寧), Zhejiang Province (浙江省), a physician in the Ming Dynasty, specialized in treating syphilis, who wrote Mei Chuang Mi Lu (霉瘡秘錄) "Secret Records of Syphilis", which not only sums up the experiences of his physician ancestors but also provides new records of diagnosis and treatment of the disease and is the first monograph on syphilology in China.

李中梓 [lǐ zhōngzǐ]

Li Zhong-zi, also called Li Shi-cai (李士材), born in Songjiang (松江), Jiangsu Province (江蘇省), a physician in the Ming Dynasty. On the basis of "Internal Classic" and "Treatise on Febrile Diseases" and with reference to those works written by other distinguished physicians and without neglecting his own experience in clinical practice, he wrote and compiled many books such as Nei Jing Zhi Yao (內經知要) "Essentials of Internal Classic", Yi Zong Bi Du (醫宗必讀) "Required Readings for Medical Professionals". etc.

傅仁宇 [fù rényǔ]

Fu Ren-yu, also called Fu Yun-ke (傅允科), a famous oculist in the Ming Dynasty, who had clinical experience for more than 30 years and wrote Shen Shi Yao Han (審視瑤函) "A Precious Book of Ophthamology", also entitled Yan Ke Da Quan (眼科大全) "A Complete Work of Ophthalmology" (1644 A.D.), which consists of detailed descriptions of the symptoms, diagnosis and treatment of eye diseases and is hence regarded as a comprehensive summing-up of eye troubles at that time.

汪昂 [wāng áng]

Wang Ang (1615-? A.D.), also called Wang Ren-an (汪訒安), born in Xiuning (休寧), Anhui Province (安徽省), a physician in the Qing Dynasty who wrote a number of medical books such as Yi Fang Ji Jie (醫方集解) "Collection of Prescriptions with Exposition", Tang Tou Ge Jue (湯頭歌訣) "Recipes in Rhymes". He held a correct and broad-minded attitude toward the introduction of Western medicine to China at the end of Ming Dynasty and wrote that it was the brain, not the heart that was the seat of mental activities from whence intelligence and memory sprang.

張璐 [zhāng lù]

Zhang Lu (1617-167? A.D.), also called Zhang Lu-yu (張路玉), or Zhang Shi-wan (張石頑), a native of Changzhou (長洲), now Wu County (吳縣), Jiangsu Province (江蘇省). He devoted most of his time to reading and writing and was the author of many medical works. The most famous work Yi Tong (醫通) "On Medicine" in 16 volumes took him fifty years to complete, in which various methods of vaccination or variolation and the spread of this practice in China at that time were given in detail. He emphasized the good points of the Warm Tonic School (溫補派) and was one of its chief protagonists.

李用粹 [lǐ yòngcuì]

Li Yong-cui, also called Li Xing-an (李惺安) or Li Xiu-zhi (李修之), a native of Shanghai, a physician in Qing Dynasty, who compiled Zheng Zhi Hui Bu (證治滙補) "A Supplement to Diagnosis and Treatment", a book of limpid style and of practical value.

柯琴 [kē qín]

Ke Qin (1662-1735 A.D.), also called Ke Yun-bo (柯韻伯), or Ke Si-feng (柯似峰), a physician at the beginning of Qing Dynasty, born in Cixi (慈溪), Zhejiang Province (浙江省), who wrote Shang Han Lun Zhu (傷寒論注) "Annotation of Treatise on Febrile Diseases", Shang Han Lun Yi (傷寒論翼) "Supplementary Treatise on Febrile Diseases", Shang Han Fu Yi (傷寒附翼) "Extra Additions to Treatise on Febrile Diseases". The three books combined were called Shang Han Lai Su Ji (傷寒來蘇集) "Recovery from Febrile Diseases".

葉桂 [yè guì]

Ye Gui (1667-1746 A.D.), also called Ye Tain-shi (葉天士) or Ye Xiang-yan (葉香岩), a native of Suzhou (蘇州), Jiangsu Province (江蘇省) and a renowned physician for his remarkable diagnosis and methods of treatment, a recognized leader of the School of Epidemic Febrile Diseases (溫病學). Ye introduced the use of aromatic stimulants in the treatment of epidemic fevers with great success. His lectures and teachings were edited by his disciple and was entitled Wen Re Lun (溫熱論) "On Epidemic Fevers" (1746 A.D.).

尤怡 [yóu yí]

You Yi (?-1749 A.D.), who was also called You Zai-jing (尤在涇), born in Changzhou (長州), Jiangsu Province (江蘇省), a physician in the Qing Dynasty. When he was young, he was poor but studied very hard, and used to earn a living by selling the characters he had written. He was clever at writing poems and prose but he went in for medicine later. He made a good study on "Treatise on Febrile Diseases" and "Synopsis of Prescriptions of the Golden Chamber" and wrote Shang Han Guan Zhu Ji (傷寒貫珠集), "A String of Beads from Treatise on Febrile Diseases", Jin Kui Yi (金匱翼) "Supplementary Prescriptions of the Golden Chamber", etc. The medical records of his patients were arranged in order by his descendants in book form entitled Jing Xiang Lou Yi An (靜香樓醫案)"Medical Case Records by the Master of Quiet Fragrant Chamber".

陳復正 ［chén fùzhèng］

Chen Fu-zheng, also called Chen Fei-xia(陳飛霞), born in Luofu (羅浮), Guangdong Province (廣東省), a physician in the Qing Dynasty. When he was a child, he used to be in poor health. Later he studied Taoism and the art of medicine and alchemy. He excelled as a pediatrist and was particularly good at treating contagious eruptive fevers and infantile convulsions. He was the author of You You Ji Cheng (幼幼集成) "A Complete Work on Pediatrics" with a comprehensive description of children's diseases and a collection of simple and useful prescriptions.

薛雪 ［xuē xuě］

Xue Xue (1681-1700 A.D.), also called Xue Sheng-bai (薛生白) or Xue Yi-piao (薛一瓢), a native of Suzhou (蘇州), Jiangsu Province (江蘇省).He was as famous a physician as his contemporary Ye Tian-shi (葉天士) and specially skilful in treating epidemic febrile diseases. He was the author or Shi Re Tiao Bian (濕熱條辨), "Detailed Analysis of Dampness and Heat", which conveys his original views in this field and has proved to be an aid to the study of epidemic febrile diseases.

徐大椿 ［xú dàchūn］

Xu Da-chun (1693-1771 A.D.), also called Xu Ling-tai (徐靈胎),or Xu Da-ye (徐大業), a native of Wu County (吳縣), Jiangsu Province (江蘇省). He was a versatile genius, his knowledge embracing astronomy and water conservancy, furthermore, he was good at writing poems and essays. After having practised medicine for fifty years, he

362

retired and lived seclusively on Huixi (洄溪), the Winding Stream, hence the name the Old Man on the Winding Stream (洄溪老人). He was the author of numerous books, such as Nan Jing Jing Shi (難經經釋) "Explanation of Difficult Classic", Yi Guan Bian (醫貫砭) "A Critique on Key Link of Medicine" and Yi Xue Yuan Liu Lun (醫學源流論) "on the Origin and Source of Medicine". He did not cling to conventional methods, but advocated that physicians had to learn the properties of drugs, and was opposed to abusing drastic drugs hot in nature and pungent in flavour as tonics.

何夢瑤 [hé mèngyáo]

He Meng-yao (1694-? A.D.), an official as well as a literary man and physician, a native of Nanhai (南海), Guangdong Province (廣東省). He was clever at writing poems and essays and was the author of a good number of books, such as Yi Bian (醫偏) "Fundamentals of Medicine", Ben Cao Yun Yu (本草韻語) "Herbal in Rhymes", Sheng Xiao Jiao Qi Mi Fang (神效脚氣秘方) "Wonderful Recipes for Beriberi", Fu Ke Liang Fang (婦科良方) "Prescriptions or Gynecology". You Ke Liang Fang (幼科良方) "Prescriptions for Pediatrics", Dou Zhen Liang Fang (痘疹良方) "Prescriptions for Poxes and Measles", etc.

傅山 [fù shān]

Fu Shan (1607-1684 A.D.), also called Fu Qing-zhu (傅青主) or Fu Gong-chi (傅公池). a native of Yangqu (陽曲) , now Taiyuan (太原), Shanxi Province (山西省). He made himself master of such a versatility of subjects that he was a well-known poet, painter, calligrapher and distinguished physician. After the fall of the Ming Dynasty, he resigned from work and took part in fighting against the rule of the Qing government. In the field of medicine, he left us such books as Bian Zheng Lu (辨證錄) "Notes on Diagnosis", Shi Shi Mi Lu (石室秘錄) "Secret Records in Stone House", Dong Tian Ao Zhi (洞天奧旨) "Mysterious Teachings in Cave", etc. Since the author was against the government, his real name was not made known. The above-mentioned books had been rearranged and republished by Chen Shi-duo (陳士鐸) under the name of Xian Shou (仙授) "God's Teaching". Certain parts of the book were extracted and published again in the middle of the 19th century, entitled Fu Qing-zhu Nü Ke (傅青主女科) "Fu Qing-

363

zhu's Works on Women's Diseases" or "Fu Qing-zhu's Obstetrics and Gynecology" and Fu Qing-zhu Nan Ke（傅青主男科）"Fu Qing-zhu's works on Men's Diseases".

沈金鰲［shěn jīn áo］

Shen Jin-ao (1717-1776 A.D.), also called Shen Qian-lu (沈芊綠), born in Wuxi（無錫）, Jiangsu Province (江蘇省). He was the author of Shen Shi Zun Sheng Shu （沈氏尊生書）"On the Importance of Life Preservation" which deals with medical substances, pulse-feeling, febrile and miscellaneous diseases as well as gynecology and pediatries. The book is rich in content and has been very popular.

趙學敏［zhào xuémǐn］

Zhao Xue-min (about 1719-1805 A.D.), also called Zhao Shu-xuan （趙恕軒）or Zhao Yi-ji（趙依吉）, a native of Qiantang（錢塘）, now Hangzhou（杭州）, Zhejiang Province (浙江省); a physician and famous pharmacist in the Qing Dynasty, author of Ben Cao Gang Mu Shi Yi （本草綱目拾遺）"A Supplement to the Compendium of Materia Medica", (printed in 1765 A.D.), in which all the new drugs that had come into use since the Ming Dynasty were listed. He collected and systemized the folk healer Zhao Bai-yun's（趙伯雲）experiences in treating diseases in two books entitled Chuan Ya Nei Pian(串雅內編)"Internal Treatise on Folk Medicine" and Chuan Ya Wai Pian (串雅外編)"Extra Treatise on Folk Medicine".

程國彭［chéng guópéng］

Cheng Guo-peng, also called Cheng Zhong-ling（程鍾齡）, a native of Tiandu（天都）, now She County（歙縣）, Anhui Province (安徽省); a celebrated physician in the Qing Dynasty who had practised medicine for thiry years and was the author of Yi Xue Xin Wu（醫學心悟）"Medicine Comprehended", which is both concise and practical and consequently is often referred to by medical practitioners. He was also the author of Wai Ke Shi Fa（外科十法）"Ten Methods in Surgery".

鄭梅間［zhèng méijiān］

Zheng Mei-jian, also called Zheng Shu-fu（鄭樞扶）, born in She County（歙縣）, Anhui Province（安徽省）, a laryngologist in the Qing Dynasty. As it had been the profession of his family for generations, he was not wanting in practical experience. His widely read book Chong

Lou Yu Yao (重樓玉鑰) "Jade Key to the Secluded Chamber" deals exclusively with laryngology. It involves the anatomy and physiology of larynx and pharynx, as well as the diagnosis, treatment and prognosis of their diseases. A special volume on the needle treatment of laryngeal diseases in included.

吳瑭 ［wú táng］

Wu Tang(about 1758-1836 A.D.), also called Wu Ju-tong (吳鞠通), a native of Huaiyin (淮陰), Jiangsu Province (江蘇省), an authority on acute epidemic febrile diseases; author of Wen Bing Tiao Bian (溫病條辨) "Detailed Analysis of Epidemic Febrile Diseases" (1798 A.D.), in which he summarized his own experiences in the treatment of epidemic febrile diseases for years and made distinctions between different fevers and devised new methods of treatment with success.

陳念祖 ［chén niànzǔ］

Chen Nian-zu (about 1753-1823 A.D.), also called Chen Xiu-yuan (陳修圓) or Chen Shen-xiu (陳慎修), a native of Changle (長樂), Fujian Province (福建省), born in a poor family, who had to make a living by practising medicine. His talent and industry soon made him a skilful physician and prolific writer who compiled many popular works which have been widely read both by professionals and laymen, such as Shang Han Lun Qian Zhu (傷寒論淺注) "Simplified Commentary on Treatise on Febrile Diseases", Yi Xue San Zi Jing (醫學三字經) "The A.B.C. of Medicine", Jin Kui Yao Lue Qian Zhu (金匱要略淺注) "Simplified Commentary on the Synopsis of the Golden Chamber", Changsha Fang Ge Kuo (長沙方歌括) "Formulas of Zhang Zhong-jing in Verse", Shi Fang Ge Kuo (時方歌括) "Popular Remedies in Verse", etc.

王清任 ［wáng qīngrèn］

Wang Qing-ren (1768-1831 A.D.), also called Wang Xun-chen (王勳臣), a native of Yutian (玉田), Hebei Province (河北省), Who practised medicine in Beijing for scores of years. He stressed the importance of studying new facts and of innovation, and was famous for being the author of Yi Lin Gai Cuo(醫林改錯)"Errors of Medicine Corrected" in which the author drew the sketches of the internal organs and corrected a number of mistakes in the previous conceptions on the basis of personal observation of many exposed bodies in public cemeteries.

There are also quite a few new conceptions and ideas about medicine in this book.

林佩琴 [lín pèiqín]

Lin Pei-qin, also called Lin Yun-he (林雲和) or Lin Xi-tong (林羲桐), born in Danyang (丹陽), Jiangsu Province (江蘇省), a physician in Qing Dynasty, who made researches into medical books for dozens of years. Integrating the strong points of various medical schools with his own clinical experience, he compiled Lei Zheng Zhi Cai (類證治裁) "Treatment of Different Kinds of Diseases", emphasizing that diagnosis and treatment must be based on an overall analysis and differentiation of symptoms and signs. It quotes the theories of different medical schools which are well selected and are of practical value.

吳其浚 [wú qíjùn]

Wu Qi-jun (1789-1846 A.D.), also called Wu Yue-zhai (吳瀹齋), born in Gushi (固始), Henan Province (河南省), an official as well as a botanist. Having devoted his whole life to the study of plants, he compiled Zhi Wu Ming Shi Tu Kao Chang Bian (植物名實圖考長編) "A Lengthy Compilation of Plants with Illustrations", and Zhi Wu Ming Shi Tu Kao (植物名實圖考) "An Illustrated Book on Plants". The Former includes the arrangement and classification of medicinal plants recorded in ancient books while the latter contains those the author had seen with his own eyes and with illustrations and descriptions. Both serve as a supplement to Li Shi-chen's "Compendium of Materia Medica" and exert some influence on the study of medicinal botany, and general botany, in China and abroad.

陸懋修 [lù màoxiū]

Lu Mao-xiu, also called Lu Jiu-zhi (陸九芝), born in Yuanhe (元和), Jiangsu Province (江蘇省), in a doctor's family, a wellknown physician who wrote Shi Bu Zhai Yi Shu (世補齋醫書) "A Book on Medicine". He clung to the old tradition so closely that he was opposed to Wang Qing-ren's proposal of making anatomical observation of the viscera of the human body.

王泰林 [wáng tàilín]

Wang Tai-lin (1798-1862 A.D.), also called Wang Xu-gao (王旭高), born in Wuxi (無錫), Jiangsu Province (江蘇省), who learned medic-

366

ine from his uncle, and at first was good at surgery, later specialized in internal medicine. He made a detailed study of the diagnosis and treatment of liver complaints. He was the author of Yi Fang Zheng Zhi Hui Bian (醫方證治滙編) "A Collection of Classified Prescriptions with Diagnosis and Treatment" and Yi Xue Chu Yan (醫學芻言) "Preliminary Remarks on Medicine", etc. His case records were collected by Fang Geng-xia (方耕霞) in book form entitled Wang Xu-gao Yi An (王旭高 醫案) "Medical Case Records by Wang Xu-gao".

吳尚先 [wú shàngxiān]

Wu Shang-xian (about 1806-1886 A.D.), also called Wu Shi-ji (吳師機) or Wu An-ye (吳安業) or Wu Zun (吳樽). He was born in a well-to-do family and had passed the government official examination, yet he went in for medicine and initiated economical methods of treatment for those who could not afford high charges for medical care and advocated external therapies, such as ointment and plasters, hydrotherapy, breathing therapy, cautery and moxibustion. He was the author of Li Yue Pian Wen (理瀹骈文) "A Rhymed Discourse on New Therapeutics" (1864 A.D.).

王世雄 [wáng shìxióng]

Wang Shi-xiong (1808-1866? A.D.), also called Wang Meng-ying (王孟英), born in Qiantang (錢塘), Zhejiang Province (浙江省). Owing to his original views on the diagnosis and treatment of febrile diseases, he became a well-known specialist in this field. He compiled Wen Re Jing Wei (溫熱經緯) "An Outline of Epidemic Febrile Diseases", Huo Luan Lun (霍亂論) "On Acute Diseases with Vomiting and Diarrhea", etc., and put all the case records of his patients in the book Wang Shi Yi An (王氏醫案) "Wang's Medical Case Records".

雷豐 [léi fēng]

Lei Feng, also called Lei Shaoyi (雷少逸), born in Qu County (衢縣), Zhejiang Province (浙江省), a physician at the end of Qing Dynasty, specialized in treating epidemic febrile diseases, who wrote Shi Bing Lun (時病論) "On Seasonal Diseases", which was widely read because the methods of treatments and prescriptions recommended proved highly effective.

唐宗海 [táng zōnghǎi]

Tang Zong-hai (1851-1918 A.D.), also called Tang Rong-chuan (唐容川), a physician at the end of Qing Dynasty, born in Peng County (彭縣), Sichuan Province (四川省). He was one of those who first tried to unite traditional Chinese medicine and Western medicine. He was the author of Zhong Xi Hui Tong Yi Jing Jing Yi (中西滙通醫經精義) "Essentials of Confluent Traditional Chinese and Western Medicine". He had tried his best to prove that traditional Chinese medicine was not unscientific and pointed out that both Chinese and Western medicines were worthy of note. He was also the author of Xue Zheng Lun (血證論) "Treatise on Blood Troubles" in which some special methods of treating bleeding diseases are given.

何炳元 [hé bǐngyuán]

He Bing-yuan (1861-1929A.D.), also called He Lian-chen (何廉臣), or He Yin-yan (何印岩), born in Shaoxing (紹興), Zhejiang Province (浙江省), who had studied both traditional Chinese and Western medicine. Comparing the two with each other, he came to the conclusion that Western medicine was not perfect and traditional Chinese medicine should not in any case be neglected. He had been chairman of the Medical Association in Shaoxing and editor of "Shaoxing Medical Journal". He was the author of a number of books, such as Zhong Feng Xin Quan (中風新詮) "A New Exposition of Apoplexy", Xin Yi Zong Bi Du (新醫宗必讀) "A New Selection of Required Readings for Medical Professionals, Nei KeZheng Zhi Quan Shu (內科證治全書) "A Complete Book on Internal Medicine", Quan Guo Ming Yi Yan An Lei Bian (全國名醫驗案類編) "A Classified Collection of Successful Medical Case Records of Noted Chinese Physicians", etc.

丁甘仁 [dīng gānrén]

Ding Gan-ren (1866-1926A,D.), also called Ding Ze-zhou (丁澤周), born in Chang-zhou (常州), Jiangsu Province (江蘇省) and later lived in Shanghai. In 1916 he set up the Shanghai Institute of Traditional Chinese Medicine, the Women's Institute of Traditional Chinese Medicine, and the Guangyi Hospital of Traditional Chinese Medicine. He was the author of Hou Sha Zheng Zhi Gai Yao (喉痧證治概要) "An Outline of Diagnosis and Treatment of Scarlet Fever". He made great contribution to the training of physicians of the traditional school. The book Ding Gan-ren Yi An (丁甘仁醫案) "Ding Gan-ren's Medical Case Records" was compiled by his students.

張錫純 [zhāng xīchún]

Zhang Xi-chun (1860-1933 A.D.), also called Zhang Shou-fu (張壽甫), born in Yanshan (鹽山), Hebei Province (河北省), who made researches into ancient medical books and advocated the combination of traditional Chinese and Western Medicine. Having practised medicine for scores of years, he succeeded in making numerous effective prescriptions. He was the author of Yi Xue Zhong Zhong Can Xi Lu (醫學衷中參西錄) "Records of Traditional Chinese Medicine in Combination with Western Medicine", which is widely read.

惲鐵樵 [yùn tiěqiáo]

Yun Tie-qiao (1878-1935 A.D.), also called Yun Shu-jue (惲樹珏), born in Wujin (武進), Jiangsu Province (江蘇省), a modern physician. When he was young, he studied literature, later because of his poor health and the death of his children, he went in for Chinese and Western medicine. He had run medical schools and taken part in the campaign of opposing defamation and extermination of traditional Chinese medicine. He advocated supplementing Chinese medicine with Western medical theories. He wrote more than 20 books, such as Qun Jing Jian Zhi Lu (羣經見智錄) "Wisdom Exposed in Medical Classics", Shang Han Lun Yan Jiu (傷寒論研究) "Research into Treatise on Febrile Diseases", Mai Xue Fa Wei (脈學發微) "Detailed Study of Pulse Lore", etc.

名 著
Well-Known Medical Works

黃帝內經 [huángdì nèi jīng]

Huangdi Nei Jing, "Huangdi's Internal Classic", or "Canon of Medicine", the oldest and greatest medical classic extant in China, with its authorship ascribed to the Ancient Emperor Huangdi (2698-2589 B.C.). Actually the work was a product of various unknown authors in the Warring States Period (475-221 B.C.). The book consists of two parts: Su Wen (素問) or "Plain Questions", and Ling Shu (靈樞) or "Miraculous Pivot", also known as "Canon of Acupuncture".

素問 [sù wèn]

Su Wen, "Plain Questions", also called Huangdi Nei Jing Su Wen (黃帝內經素問) "Plain Questions of Huangdi's Internal Classic", originally consisting of 9 volumes, with 81 articles. After Wei Jin Dynasties there were left only 8 volumes. In the Tang Dynasty when Wang Bing (王冰) made notes and commentaries on the book, he divided it into 24 volumes and supplemented some of the lost articles. In Northern Song Dynasty Lin Yi (林億) et al, read proofs and made notes on it again, and all later extant editions were based on this one. The book includes a variety of subjects, such as human anatomy and physiology, causes of diseases, pathology, diagnosis, differentiation of symptoms and signs, treatment, disease prevention, health preservation, man and nature, the application of the theories of Yin and Yang and of the Five Elements in medicine, the theory of the promotion of the flow of vital energy, etc. The books is prized by physicians of all generations.

靈樞 [líng shū]

Ling Shu, "Miraculous Pivot", one of the two parts of "Internal Classic", also called Huangdi Nei Jing Ling Shu Jing (黃帝內經靈樞經) "Miraculous Pivot of Huangdi's Internal Classic". The subjects of "Miraculous Pivot" are similar to those of "Plain Questions", but the former has a more detailed description of channels and needling and is less detailed in theories concerning the circular movement of the Five Elements. In introducing basic theories and clinical practice, the two books supplement each other. This books as well as "Plain Questions" is prized by physicians of all generations.

類經 [lèi jīng]

Lei Jing, "Systematic Compilation of the Internal Classic", compiled by Zhang Jie-bin (張介賓) and published in 1624 A.D. which is a rearrangement of Nei Jing "Internal Classic". The books consists of 12 categories, including hygiene, Yin Yang, organ pictures, pulse, channels, sapors, theories of treatment, acupuncture, etc. It has been considered by students of Nei Jing "Internal Classic" as one of the most important reference books in the study of this classic.

内經知要 [nèi jīng zhī yào]

Nei Jing Zhi Yao, "Essentials of Internal Classic", compiled by Li Nian-e (李念莪) in the Ming Dynasty. The books is divided into 8 parts, including Yin Yang, pulse, channels, principles of treatment, etc. Combining basic with clinical theories, the author made extracts and ex-positions of "Internal Classic". The books is clearly written and well organized.

難經 [nán jīng]

Nan Jing, "Difficult Classic" or "Classic on Medical Problems", a book appeared in the 1st or 2nd century B.C. Its authorship is unknown, though tradition ascribes it to Qin Yue-ren (秦越人). It deals with fundamental medical theories and expounds the main points of Nei Jing "Internal Classic" in the form of questions and answers. The points of acupuncture and moxibustion, the method of needling, the physiological and pathological conditions of the Channels and Collaterals, and the method of feeling the pulse are all discussed.

難經本義 [nánjīng běnyì]

Nan Jing Ben Yi, "The Genuine Meaning of the Difficult Classic" compiled by Hua Shou (滑壽) and published in 1366 A.D., a most influential book among complementary works of "Difficult Classic" or "Classic on Medical Problems"

傷寒雜病論 [shānghán zábìng lùn]

Shang Han Za Bing Lun, "Treatise on Febrile and Miscellaneous Diseases", written by Zhang Zhong-jing (張仲景) at about the beginning of the 3rd century, in which diagnosis and treatment of fevers and other miscellaneous diseases were dealt with. The book was rearranged by Wang Shu-he (王叔和) in the Jin Dynasty, and later in the Song Dynasty it was divided into two books by Jiao Zheng Yi Shu Ju (校正醫書局) "Bureau for Censoring and Publishing Medical Books", namely, Shan Han Lun (傷寒論) "Treatise on Febrile Diseases" and Jin Kui Yao Lue Fang Lun (金匱要略方論) "Synopsis of Prescriptions of the Golden Chamber"

傷寒論 [shānghán lùn]

Shang Han Lun, "Treatise on Febrile Diseases", a new edition of

Zhang Zhong-jing's（張仲景）book "Treatise on Febrile and Miscellaneous Diseases",rearranged by Wang Shu-he（王叔和）in 10 volumes, in which acute febrile diseases are analysed and differentiated in accordance with the theory of the Six Channels. The book has long been one of the most influential works in the history of Chinese medicine.

金匱要略方論 ［jīnkuì yàolüè fāng lùn］

Jin Kui Yao Lue Fang Lun, "Synopsis of Prescriptions of the Golden Chamber", or simply Jin Kui Yao Lue（金匱要略）written by Zhang Zhong-Jing（ 張仲景 ）at the beginning of the 3rd century and was rearranged by Wang Shu-he（王叔和）in three volumes. It deals mainly with miscellaneous diseases of internal medicine, and a part of surgical and women's diseases in addition. There are 25 chapters, including 262 prescriptions.

金匱要略心典 ［jīnkuì yàolüè xīndiǎn］

Jin Kui Yao Lue Xin Dian, "Commentaries on Synopsis of Prescriptions of the Golden Chamber" which was written by You Yi（尤怡）in the Qing Dynasty and published in 1732. This book comments on "Synopsis of Prescriptions of the Golden Chamber" briefly and to the point, with all the theories and major problems clearly explained and some mistakes corrected. The unintelligible places in the original book are left untouched rather than wrongly interpreted.

金匱翼 ［jīnkuì yì］

Jin Kui Yi, "Supplements to Commentaries on Synopsis of Prescriptions of the Golden Chamber" written by You Yi（ 尤怡 ）and published in 1768. This is to supplement the book Jin Kui Yao Lue Xin Dian (金匱要略心典) "Commentaries on Synopsis of Prescriptions of the Golden Chamber". The book deals exclusively with miscellaneous diseases of internal medicine which are divided into 48 families (groups). It is succinct in wording and the prescriptions chosen are of practical value.

脈經 ［mài jīng］

Mai Jing, "The Pulse Classic", written by Wang Shu-he (王叔和) in the 3rd century, generally acknowledged as the standard work on the subject and the earliest comprehensive work dealing with sphygmology now extant

瀕湖脈學 [bīnhú mài xué]

Bin Hu Mai Xue, "The Pulse Studies of Bin-hu" written by Li Shizhen（李時珍）in 1564 A.D., in which 27 kinds of pulses and their diagnostic value are given in detail in lucid verses. The book has been very popular for centuries.

諸病源候總論 [zhū bìng yuán hòu zhǒnglùn]

Zhu Bing Yuan Hou Zhong Lun, "General Treatise on the Etiology and Symptomology of Diseases", compiled by Chao Yuan-fang (巢元方) et al., in 610 A.D. in 50 volumes with etiology and symptoms of various diseases given in detail. It consists of 67 categories with 1.720 entries.

三因極一病證方論 [sān yīn jí yī bìng zhèng fāng lùn]

San Yin Ji Yi Bing Zheng Fang Lun, "A Treatise on the Three Categories of Pathogenic Factors of Diseases" written by Chen Yan（陳言）in 1174 A.D., who classified the causes of diseases into external,internal and miscellaneous ones which are regarded as neither external nor internal

神農本草經 [shénnóng běncǎo jīng]

Shen Nong Ben Cao Jing, "Shen Nong's Herbal" or "The Herbal", the earliest materia medica, believed to be a product of the 1st century B.C. with its authorship attributed to the ancient emperor and "the Divine Peasant" Shen Nong, in which 365 kinds of drugs were listed and divided into three classes: superior, common and inferior

名醫別錄 [míngyī biélù]

Ming Yi Bie Lu, "Transactions of Famous Physicians",a book on pharmacology, compiled by Tao Hong-jing（陶弘景）on the basis of "Shen Nong's Herbal". He expounded "Shen Nong's Herbal" on the one hand, and supplemented it with 365 kinds of medicinal substances on the other.

本草拾遺 [běncǎo shíyí]

Ben Cao Shi Yi, "A Supplement to the Herbal". It was written in 10 volumes by Chen Cang-qi（陳藏器）in the Tang Dynasty (8th century). The book mainly added in those medicinal substances not included in Xin Xiu Ben Cao（新修本草）"Newly-Revised Materia Medica of Tang".

唐本草 [táng běncǎo]；新修本草 [xīnxiū běncǎo]

Tang Ben Cao, "The Tang Materia Medica", or Xin Xiu Ben Cao, "Newly-Compiled Materia Medica of Tang", which was compiled by Su Jing (蘇敬) and 22. other scholars. It listed 844 medical substances. Since it was sponsored by the Tang Dynasty government, it is considered to be the earliest pharmacopoeia published officially in the world.

經史證類備急本草 [jīng shǐ zhèng lèi bèijí běncǎo]
Jing Shi Zheng Lei Bei Ji Ben Cao, "Classic Classified Materia Medica for Emergencies", or Zheng Lei Ben Cao (證類本草) "Classified Materia Medica" for short, compiled by Tang Shen-wei (唐愼微) at the end of the 11th century. It listed 1,746 kinds of medicine with directions for use and preparation, and many new prescriptions were added. The book laid a solid foundation for the development of the knowledge of Ben Cao.

湯液本草 [tāngyè běncǎo]
Tang Ye Ben Cao, "Materia Medica of Decoction", which was written by Wang Hao-gu (王好古) and published in 1289 A.D., with a list of 238 kinds of drugs. The flavour, taste, therapeutic properties as well as the mutual influence of medicines when used in combination are given in detail.

救荒本草 [jiùhuāng běncǎo]
Jiu Huang Ben Cao, "Herbal for Relief of Famines", compiled by Zhu Su (朱橚) in 1404 A.D., listing 414 plants which might be used for food against famine

本草綱目 [běncǎo gāngmù]
Ben Cao Gang Mu, "Compendium of Materia Medica", compiled by Li Shi-Zhen (李時珍), a gigantic and most comprehensive work published in 1590 A.D., in 52 volumes which took the author 30 years for its completion. It listed 1,892 medical substances, more than 1,000 illustrations and over 10,000 prescriptions with detailed description of the appearance, properties, method of collection, preparation and use of each substance. This book is far more than a pharmaceutical compendium, it is also a comprehensive work on various branches of natural history including botany, zoology, mineralogy and metallurgy.

本草備要 [běncǎo bèiyào]
Ben Cao Bei Yao, "Essentials of Materia Medica", written by Wang

Ang (汪昂) and published in 1694. It was a simple but important book on pharmacology, dealing first with the "nature of drugs" and then describing the properties and tastes, uses and indications, etc. of 470 kinds of commonly used drugs with over 400 illustrations.

本草綱目拾遺 [běncǎo gāngmù shíyí]

Ben Cao Gang Mu Shi Yi, "A Supplement to the Compendium of Materia Medica", written by Zhao Xue-min (趙學敏) in 1765 A.D. It listed 716 medical substances which had not been included in Li Shi-zhen's "Compendium of Materia Medica", with some imported ones from abroad.

珍珠囊藥性賦 [zhēnzhūnáng yàoxìng fù]

Zhen Zhu Nang Yao Xing Fu, "Nature of the Drugs of the Pearl Bag in Songs", also known as Lei Gong Yao Xing Fu (雷公藥性賦) "Lei Gong's Nature of Drugs in Songs", written by Yuan Shan Dao Ren (元山道人) at the beginning of Ming Dynasty, which describes in detail the indications and cautions for the use of 90 kinds of common drugs and introduces 1,406 medical substances in the form of songs and notes

用藥法象 [yòng yào fǎ xiàng]

Yong Yao Fa Xiang. "Rules in the Use of Drugs", written by Li Gao (李杲), in which drugs are classified according to their therapeutic properties into 4 kinds: to ascend, to descend, to float and to sink

雷公炮炙論 [léigōng pàozhì lùn]

Lei Gong Pao Zhi Lun, "Lei's Method of Preparing Drugs", written by Lei Xiao (雷斅) in the 5th century, in which the fundamental processes of preparing drugs were dealt with. It is one of the earliest extant books on this subject.

炮炙大全 [pàozhì dàquán]

Pao Zhi Da Quan, "A Complete Handbook on the Preparation of Drugs", compiled by Miao Xi-yong (繆希雍) and Zhuang Ji-guang (莊繼光) on the basis of Lei's work on the subject with some additions made of the new methods then popular among the people

飲膳正要 [yǐnshàn zhèng yào]

Yin Shan Zheng Yao, "Principles of Correct Diet" written by Hu Si-hei (忽思慧). It lists the food and drink of the royal family and the nobility, and describes with illustrations the nature, taste and indications of about 200 different kinds of medicinal herbs which can be used as food.

植物名實圖考 [zhíwù míng shí tú kǎo]

Zhi Wu Ming Shi Tu Kao, "An Illustrated Book of Plants", written by Wu Qi-jun (吳其濬) in 38 volumes and published in 1848, a book on botany which includes no less than 1,714 plant species. The author made a comparatively detailed description of the shape, color, nature, taste, usage and growing area of the plants. His drawings of them were vivid and true of life.

植物名實圖考長編 [zhíwù míng shí tú kǎo chángbiān]

Zhi Wu Ming Shi Tu Kao Chang Bian, "A Lengthy Compilation of Plants with Illustrations". It was written by Wu Qi-jun (吳其濬) in 22 volumes and was published in 1848. Based on data from ancient literature, it was compiled to form a pair to "An Illustrated Book of Plants" (植物名實圖考).788 plant substances are listed in the book.

全國中草藥滙編 [quánguó zhōngcǎoyào huìbiān]

Quan Guo Zhong Cao Yao Hui Bian, "A Compilation of Chinese Medicinal Herbs", in two volumes with a list of about 2,200 herbal medicines. The names, sources, morphology, environment, cultivation, collection and preparation, chemistry, pharmacology, nature, taste, uses, indications and administration of the medicine are given in detail, with pictures of the living plants. The first volume was published in 1975 by the People's Health Publishing House.

肘後備急方 [zhǒuhòu bèijí fāng]

Zhou Hou Bei Ji Fang, "A Handbook of Prescriptions for Emergencies", written by Ge Hong (葛洪 281-341 A.D.). The prescriptions recorded are simple and the drugs used are common and effective. Many valuable descriptions of diseases and treatments are recorded.

備急千金要方 [bèijí qiānjīn yàofāng]

Bei Ji Qian Jin Yao Fang, "Prescriptions Worth a Thousand Gold for Emergencies" or (千金要方) Qian Jin Yao Fang, "Prescriptions Worth a Thousand Gold", compiled by Sun Si-miao (孫思邈) at the end of the 7th century in 30 volumes, with general introduction, prescriptions of various clinical branches, diet, pulse-taking, acupuncture, etc.

千金翼方 [qiānjīn yì fāng]

Qian Jin Yi Fang, "A Supplement to the Prescriptions Worth a Thousand Gold", compiled by Sun Si-miao (孫思邈) at the end of the 7th century in 30 volumes, including various medical branches such as herbals, febrile diseases, obstetrics and gynecology, pediatrics, miscellaneous diseases of internal medicine, pulse-taking, acupuncture, diet, etc. This work together with (千金要方) Qian Jin Yao Fang "Prescriptions Worth a Thousand Gold" have been considered as an agglomeration of the medical achievements before the Tang Dynasty.

外台秘要 [wàitái mìyào]

Wai Tai Mi Yao, "Medical Secrets of an Official", compiled by Wang Tao (王燾) in 752 A.D. in 40 volumes in which a comprehensive and exhaustive study of medicine is made with 1,104 categories of medical problems discussed and over 6,000 prescriptions recorded

太平聖惠方 [tàipíng shènghuí fāng]

Tai Ping Sheng Hui Fang, "The Peaceful Holy Benevolent Prescriptions" or simply Sheng Hui Fang (聖惠方) "Holy Benevolent Prescriptions", compiled by Wang Huai-yin (王懷隱) in 992 A.D. in ten volumes, recording 16,834 prescriptions of various medical branches with discussions on diagnosis and pathology of various diseases

太平惠民和劑局方 [tàipíng huímín héjìjú fāng]

Tai Ping Hui Min He Ji Ju Fang, "Formularies of the Bureau of People's Welfare Pharmacies" or simply He Ji Ju Fang (和劑局方) "Formularies of the Bureau of Pharmacy", compiled by Chen Shi-wen (陳師文) et al., in 1151 A.D., in 10 volumes, consisting of 14 categories and 788 prescriptions which were popular and effective. Most of the medicines were in pill or powder form, ready for use and storage.

普濟本事方 [pǔjì běnshì fāng]

Pu Ji Ben Shi Fang, "Effective Prescriptions for Universal Relief", also called Lei Zheng Pu Ji Ben Shi Fang (類證普濟本事方) "Classified Effective Prescriptions for Universal Relief" or Ben Shi Fang (本事方) "Effective Prescriptions", a book in 10 volumes, which was written by Xu Shu-wei (許叔微) in Southern Song Dynasty and published in the middle of the 12th century. It mainly deals with common diseases related to internal medicine, listing 23 kinds of treatment with more than 300 prescriptions. To the end of each precription are appended the author's proved case records.

济生方 [jìshēng fāng]

Ji Sheng Fang, "Recipes for Saving Lives", also called Yan Shi Ji Sheng Fang (嚴氏濟生方) "Yan's Recipes for Saving Lives", a book in 10 volumes, which was written by Yan Yong-he (嚴用和) in 1253 A.D. It consists of 79 articles dealing with diseases of internal medicine, surgery and gynecology. It includes over 450 recipes, all of which were proved effective by the author.

世醫得效方 [shìyī déxiào fāng]

Shi Yi De Xiao Fang, "Effective Formulas Tested by Physicians for Generations", compiled by Wei Yi-lin (危亦林) in 1345 A.D., on the basis of the author's family experiences as physicians for five successive generations, in which are listed prescriptions for children's diseases, internal medicine, ophthalmology, oral diseases, dentistry, bone-setting, war wounds, ulcers and carbuncles

局方發揮 [júfāng fāhuī]

Ju Fang Fa Hui, "An Expounding of the Formularies of the Bureau of the People's Welfare Pharmacies", written by Zhu Zhen-heng (朱震亨) in the 14th century, who pointed out and criticized the mechanical and indiscriminate use of the formularies of the People's Welfare Pharmacies which were popular then.

普濟方 [pǔjì fāng]

Pu Ji Fang, "Prescriptions for Universal Relief", a most complete collection of prescriptions (with 61, 739 prescriptions and 239 illustrations) in 168 volumes, which was written by Teng Hong (滕弘) et al. under the patronage of Zhu Su (朱橚) and issued in 1406 A.D.

奇效良方 [qíxiào liángfāng]

Qi Xiao Liang Fang, "Wonderful Well-tried Recipes", a book in 69 volumes with its authorship ascribed to Dong Su (董宿) and Fang Xian (方賢). It was published in 1470. According to the principles of treatment of different diseases, it divides recipes into 64 families, such as wind, cold, heat, etc., which are subdivided into still smaller groups. It lists more than 7,000 recipes, most of which are passed down from the

Song and Ming Dynasties, and at the same time states the methods of needling and bone-setting.

醫方集解 [yīfāng jíjiě]

Yi Fang Ji Jie, "Collection of Prescriptions with Exposition" which was written by Wang Ang (汪昂) in the Qing Dynasty and published in 1682. The book lists about 700 prescriptions, divided into 21 classes, such as tonifying, sudorifying, vomiting inducing, etc. It describes in detail the combination of ingredients, properties, and indications of each recipe with reference to the theories of various schools.

湯頭歌訣 [tāngtóu gējué]

Tang Tou Ge Jue, "Recipes in Rhymes", written by Wang Ang (汪昂) in the Qing Dynasty and published in 1694. Over 300 recipes are selected and written in more than 200 songs. To each song are appended simple notes so that it may be made easier for beginners to learn by heart. The book is very popular.

串雅內、外編 [chuànyǎ nèi wài biān]

Chuan Ya Nei Wai Bian, "Bound Volume of Treatises on Folk Medicine", a joint edition of the two books "Treatise on Folk Medicine" and "The Extra Treatise on Folk Medicine" written by Zhao Xue-min (趙學敏) in 1759 A.D. on the basis of the recipes employed by folk healers and reference materials in medical works concerned. Each consisted of 4 volumes including simple, handy, cheap yet effective recipes, as well as methods of making drugs and of treating diseases of animals and plants.

理瀹駢文 [lǐyuè piánwén]

Li Yue Pian Wen, "A Rhymed Discourse on New Therapeutics", written by Wu Shang-xian (吳尚先), who was famous for practising folk medicine and advocating external therapies such as ointment and plasters, hydrotherapy, breathing therapy, cautery and moxibustion

溫疫論 [wēnyì lùn]

Wen Yi Lun, "Treatise on Acute Epidemic Febrile Diseases", written by Wu You-ke (吳又可) in 1642 A.D., a study of etiology and pathology of epidemic febrile diseases. The author pointed out it was Li Qi (戾氣), epidemic noxious air, that got into the human body through mouth and nose and caused epidemic febrile diseases.

溫熱論 ［wēnrè lùn］

Wen Re Lun, "Treatise on Epidemic Fevers", lectured by Ye Tian-shi (葉天士) and edited by his disciple in 1746 A.D., a book on the diagnosis and treatment of acute febrile diseases in which the theory of the development or transmission of the disease among the 4 systems: Wei (superficial resistance), Qi (energy), Ying (nutrition) and Xue (blood) was introduced

溫病條辨 ［wēnbìng tiáobiàn］

Wen Bing Tiao Bian, "Detailed Analysis of Epidemic Febrile Diseases", written by Wu Tang (吳瑭) in 1798 A.D., a development of Ye Tian-shi's "Treatise on Epidemic Fevers", in which differential diagnosis of diseases according to pathological changes of the Triple Burners was given in detail

溫熱經緯 ［wēnrè jīngwěi］

Wen Re Jing Wei, "An Outline of Epidemic Febrile Diseases", written by Wang Meng-ying (王孟英) in 1852 A.D. in 5 volumes. The author threw light on the cause of epidemic fevers, their signs and symptoms, and methods of treatment on the basis of the theories stated in "Internal Classic" and "Treatise on Febrile and Miscellaneous Diseases" and with reference to the view points of distinguished physicians in Qing Dynasty such as Ye Gui (葉桂), Xue Xue (薛雪), Chen Ping-bo (陳平伯), Yu Shi-yu (余師愚), etc.

時病論 ［shíbìng lùn］

Shi Bing Lun, "On Seasonal Diseases", written by Lei Feng (雷豐) in 1882, a book of practical value, mainly dealing with febrile diseases of the four seasons. It states the cause, symptoms and treatment of the diseases and introduces the author's own prescriptions and the recipes commonly employed.

脾胃論 ［píwèi lùn］

Pi Wei Lun, "Treatise on the Spleen and Stomach", written by Li Gao (李杲) and published in the 13th century. On the authority of the view point "Man lives on water and grain" expressed in "Internal Classic", the author emphasized and explained the importance of nourishing the *spleen* and the *stomach*. For curing *spleen* and *stomach* troubles caused by improper diet or fatigue, he recommended Bu Zhong Yi Qi

Tang (補中益氣湯) "Decoction for Reinforcing the Middle Barner and Replenishing Vital Energy" and Sheng Yang Yi Wei Tang (升陽益胃湯) "Decoction for Activating Vital Function and Replenishing the *stomach*", which produce good effect.

十藥神書 [shíyào shénshū]

Shi Yao Shen Shu, "A Miraculous Book of Ten Recipes", written by Ge Qian-sun (葛乾孫) in 1348 A.D., containing 10 recipes, namely, three remedies for hemoptysis, three for cough, one hypnotic and three nutrients, all of which were sound remedies for treating consumptions, specially pulmonary tuberculosis.

證治滙補 [zhèngzhì huìbǔ]

Zheng Zhi Hui Bu, "Supplement to Diagnosis and Treatment", a book in 8 volumes, which was written by Li Yong-cui (李用粹) and published in 1687 A.D. The book mainly deals with miscellaneous diseases of internal medicine, recording more than 80 kinds of diseases with their diagnoses, methods of treatment and prescriptions.

類證治裁 [lèizhèng zhìcái]

Lei Zheng Zhi Cai. "Treatment of Different Kinds of Diseases" written by Lin Pei-qin (林佩琴) in 1839. The author differentiated and analyzed various diseases of internal medicine, gynecology and surgery according to their cause and clinical manifestation; and introduced concrete therapy and prescriptions. To many diseases were appended case records for reference. This book integrates the good points of various schools and is quite influential in medical circles.

血證論 [xuèzhènglùn]

Xue Zheng Lun, "Treatise on Blood Troubles", written by Tang Rong-chuan (唐容川) and published in 1884 A.D. It deals with the diagnosis and treatment of various blood troubles, including a general introduction and over 170 diseases. The author broke fresh ground in this field.

經效產寶 [jīngxiào chǎnbǎo]; 產寶 [chǎnbǎo]

Jing Xiao Chan Bao or simply **Chan Bao, "Tested Treasures in Obstetrics"**, written by Zan Yin (昝殷) in 852-856 A.D., the earliest book exclusively on obstetrics in which diseases during pregnancy, at the time of parturition and after delivery are diagnosed and treated.

衛生家寶產科備要 [wèishēng jiābǎo chǎnkē bèiyào]
Wei Sheng Jia Bao Chan Ke Bei Yao, "A Precious Medical Book on Obstetrics for Home Use", a valuable book on obstetrics compiled by Zhu Duan-zhang (朱端章) and published in 1184 A.D. The author pooled together the knowledge of obstetrics and of nursing infants from all previous medical works.

婦人大全良方 [fùrén dàquán liángfāng]; 婦人良方大全 [fù rén liángfāng dàquán]
Fu Ren Da Quan Liang Fang or **Fu Ren Liang Fang Da Quan "The Complete Effective Prescriptions for Diseases of Women"** or simply Fu Ren Liang Fang (婦人良方) "Effective Prescriptions for Diseases of Women", written by Chen Zi-ming (陳自明), which is the first and most important treatise on gynecology and obstetrics. It was first published in 1237 A.D.

濟陰綱目 [jìyīn gāngmù]
Ji Yin Gang Mu, "Compendium of Therapy for Women's Diseases", a book on obstetrics and gynecology in 5 volumes, written by Wu Zhi-wang (武之望) and published in 1620. In 1665 Wang Qi (汪琪) made commentaries on the book and reedited it into 14 volumes without changing its content. It was written on the basis of Wang Ken-tang's (王肯堂) Fu Ke Zheng Zhi Zhun Sheng (婦科證治準繩) "Standards of Diagnosis and Treatment in Gynecology". Troubles with menstruation, leucorrhea, pregnancy and parturition are divided into different topics with discussions and prescriptions of practical value.

傅青主女科 [fùqīngzhǔ nǚkē]
Fu Qing Zhu Nü Ke, "Fu Qing-zhu's Obstetrics and Gynecology", also known as Nü Ke (女科) "Obstetrics and Gynecology", a book in 2 volumes written by Fu Shan (傅山). It was completed in the 17th century and first published in 1827. The book consists of 77 articles dealing with the diagnosis and treatment of diseases concerned with obstetrics and gynecology. Its language is simple and its prescriptions are practical. In addition to this book, the author wrote Chan Hou Bian (產後編) "Postpartum Care", dealing with the diagnosis and treatment of 43 kinds of diseases in the scope of obstetrics.

The combined edition of the two books is called Fu Shi Nü Ke Da Quan (傅氏女科大全) "Complete Works of Fu's Obstetrics and Gynecology".

小兒藥證直訣 [xiǎoér yàozhèng zhíjué]
Xiao Er Yao Zheng Zhi Jue, "Key to Therapeutics of Children's Diseases", written by Qian Yi (錢乙) generally aknowledged as the greatest pediatrist in Chinese medicine, and edited and published by his pupil Yan Ji-zhong 閻季忠) in 1119 A.D. in three volumes: one for diagnosis, one for case recording and one for prescriptions. The author emphasized the peculiarities of pediatrics and the characteristics of children's physiology and pathology.

幼幼新書 [yòuyòu xīnshū]
You You Xin Shu, "New Book for the Nursing of Children" or "New Pediatrics", a most comprehensive treatise on children's diseases in 40 volumes compiled by Liu Fang (劉昉), Wang Li (王歷) and Wang Shi (王湜) in 1132 A.D. dealing with etiology, diagnosis, therapies of various kinds of children's diseases, child care, etc.

小兒痘疹方論 [xiǎoér dòuzhén fānglùn]
Xiao Er Dou Zhen Fang Lun, "Treatise on Smallpox and Measles in Children", which was written by Chen Wen-zhong (陳文中), a noted pediatrist in the 13th century, and published in 1241 A.D.

幼幼集成 [yòuyòu jíchéng]
You You Ji Cheng, "A Complete Work on Pediatrics", written by Cheng Fu-zheng (陳復正) and published in 1750. He converged and reorganized the main contents of pediatrics in ancient books, adding in his own views as to some theoretical problems concerning the therapeutic methods of certain diseases, e.g. infantile convulsions.

劉涓子鬼遺方 [liújuānzǐ guǐyí fāng]
Liu Juan-zhi Gui Yi Fang, "Remedies Left Over by Ghosts", the earliest medical work on surgery, written by Gong Qing-xuan (龔慶宣) in 496—499 A.D., dealing mainly with the treatment of traumatic wounds, carbuncles, mastitis, burns, eczema, and scabies, with excellent remarks on surgical nursing, drainage and sterilization

理傷續斷秘方 [lǐshāng xùduàn mìfāng]
Li Shang Xu Duan Mi Fang, "Secrets of Treating Wounds and

Bone-Setting", also called (仙授理傷續斷秘方) Xian Shou Li Shang Xu Duan Mi Fang "Secrets of Treating Wounds and Bone-Setting Handed Down by the Fairy", the earliest book on bone-setting, written by Lin Dao Ren (藺道人) in about 846 A.D., with good remarks on traction, reunion, and fixation of fractured and dislocated bones

外科精要 [wàikē jīngyào]

Wai Ke Jing Yao, "Essence of Surgery", written by Chen Zi-ming (陳自明) and published in 1263 A.D., one of the earliest books under the title of surgery with differential diagnosis and treatment of furuncles, carbuncles, gangrene, ulcers and wounds

秘傳外科方 [mìchuán wàikē fāng]

Mi Chuan Wai Ke Fang, "Secret Methods of Surgery" by Zhao Yi-zhen (趙宜眞), which appeared in 1395 A.D. with 24 surgical illustrations

解圍元藪 [jiěwéi yuánsǒu]

Jie Wei Yuan Sou, "Source of Relief", a book specially devoted to leprosy, which was written by Shen Zhi-wen (沈之問) in the year 1550. It deals with the cause of leprosy, its various manifestations and relations to channels and lists no less than 249 prescriptions.

瘡瘍經驗全書 [chuāngyáng jīngyàn quánshū]

Chuang Yang Jing Yan Quan Shu, "A Complete Manual of Experiences in the Treatment of Sores", usually attributed to Dou Han-qing (竇漢卿) but was actually written by Dou's grandson. The book appeared in 1569 A.D., which deals with all diseases requiring surgical treatment, classified according to the various parts of the body.

外科啓玄 [wàikē qǐxuán]

Wai Ke Qi Xuan, "Revealing the Mystery of Surgery", written by Shen Gong-chen (申拱宸), published in 1604 A.D. The book begins with a general exposition of the various forms of therapy and then deals with different types of cases requiring surgical treatment. To each section is appended an illustration.

外科正宗 [wàikē zhèngzōng]

Wai Ke Zheng Zong, "Orthodox Manual of Surgery", written by Chen Shi-gong (陳實功) on the basis of forty years of personal experience, in which each disease is dealt separately with diagnosis, therapeutic methods and operations, case records and prescriptions. It was published in 1617 and has since been one of the most influential surgery books.

外科大成 [wàikē dàchéng]

Wai Ke Da Cheng, "A Complete Book on Surgery", written by Qi Kun (祁坤) in 1665. It gives an exhaustive description of diagnosis and treatment of surgical diseases and is the book upon which Yi Zong Jin Jian Wai Ke Xin Fa Yao Jue (醫宗金鑒外科心法要訣) "Golden Mirror of Medicine: Essentials of Surgical Treatment" is based.

銀海精微 [yínhǎi jīngwēi]

Yin Hai Jing Wei, "An Exhaustive and Comprehensive Survey of the Silvery Sea", or "Essentials of Ophthalmology", a book in 2 volumes, which appeared in the 13th century with its authorship attributed to Sun Si-miao (孫思邈)

秘傳眼科龍木論 [mìchuán yǎnkē lóngmù lùn]

Mi Chuan Yan Ke Long Mu Lun, "Long Mu's Secret Treatise on Eye Diseases", an anonymous book in ten volumes which appeared in the 13th century. It includes 72 kinds of eye diseases, glaucoma and cataract regarded as two chief ailments.

原 (元) 機啓微 [yuánjī qǐwēi]

Yuan Ji Qi Wei, "Revealing the Mystery of the Origin", written by Ni Wei-de (倪維德), published in 1370 A.D., which gives a systematic exposition of eye diseases not only as a local affliction but as part of defective functioning of the whole body, and often due to unhygienic conditions

審視瑤函 [shěnshì yáohán]

Shen Shi Yao Han, "A Precious Book of Ophthalmology", also entitled (眼科大全) Yan Ke Da Quan, "A Complete Work on Ophthalmology", a comprehensive and exhaustive treatise on eye diseases by Fu Yun-ke (傅允科), which appeared in 1644 in seven volumes, listing 108 kinds of eye troubles and their treatment.

洗冤集錄 [xǐyuān jílù]

Xi Yuan Ji Lu, "Instruction to Coroners", a book on forensic medicine, written by Song Ci (宋慈) and published in 1247 A.D.

The original book had 10 volumes, but after the Ming Dynasty, there were left only 4. It systematically summed up the achievements made before the Song Dynasty in this field, and introduced tests and identifications of toxicity and measures for emergency treatment. It also dealt with anatomy, pathology, bone-setting, surgical operations, etc. The book is of great value and has been translated into many foreign languages.

針灸甲乙經 [zhēnjiǔ jiǎyǐ jīng]

Zhen Jiu Jia Yi Jing, "A Classic of Acupuncture and Moxibustion", the earliest exclusive and systemized book on acupuncture and moxibustion, written by Huangfu Mi (皇甫謐) in about 259 A.D., in which the names and number of points of each channel and their exact locations were defined. It also dealt with the properties and indications of each point and the methods of manipulation.

銅人俞穴針灸圖經 [tóngrén shùxuè zhēnjiǔ tújīng]

Tong Ren Shu Xue Zhen Jiu Tu Jing, "Illustrated Manual on the Points for Acupuncture and Moxibustion as Found on the Bronze Figure", written by Wang Wei-yi (王惟一), published in 1027 A.D. in 3 volumes. The author made detailed studies and investigation of the acupuncture points and marked out a total of 657 points on the human body.

十四經發揮 [shísìjīng fāhuī]

Shi Si Jing Fa Hui, "Exposition of the Fourteen Channels", written by Hua Shou (滑壽), which appeared in 1341 A.D. and made a marked development of the channel theory

針灸聚英 [zhēnjiǔ jùyīng]

Zhen Jiu Ju Ying, "Essentials of Acupuncture and Moxibustion" written by Gao Wu (高武) in the Ming Dynasty, published in 1529 A.D. In the book the author brought together the theories of various schools concerning acu-moxibustion.

針灸問答 [zhēnjiǔ wèndá]; 針灸問對 [zhēnjiǔ wènduì]

Zhen Jiu Wen Da or Zhen Jiu Wen Dui, "Catechism on Acupuncture and Moxibustion", written by Wang Ji (汪機) in 1530 A.D. in which the theories and principles of acupuncture and moxibustion are expounded

386

針灸大成 [zhēnjiǔ dàchéng]
Zhen Jiu Da Cheng, "Compendium of Acupuncture and Moxibustion", written by Yang Ji-zhou (楊繼洲) in 1601 A.D., who clarified the confusions in points and channels and unified the divergent views concerning them

針刺麻醉 [zhēncì mázuì]
Zhen Ci Ma Zui, "Acupuncture Anaesthesia", published in 1972. In the book the history, characteristics, theories, methods of acupuncture anaesthesia and the points most commonly used for this purpose as well as the application of this art in various operations and the galvano-acupuncture anaesthesia-devices in common use are given in detail. It is a preliminary summing-up of the results of scientific research in this field.

中藏經 [zhōng zàng jīng]
Zhong Zang Jing, "Treasured Classic", a comprehensive book on medicine, with its authorship ascribed to Hua Tuo (華佗), hence also called "Hua's Zhong Zang Jing". But most probably it was written by an unknown author during the Six Dynasties (317-618 A.D.). The book includes 49 articles on diagnosis and treatment, pulse, internal organs, deficiency and excessiveness symptom-complexes, cold and heat symptom-complexes, etc, as well as a list of prescriptions.

儒門事親 [rúmén shìqīn]
Ru Men Shi Qin, "The Literati's Care of Their Parents", written by Zhang Zi-he (張子和), whose classification of diseases was based on Liu Wan-su's (劉完素) theory of six exogenous pathogenic factors and whose three methods of treatment were diaphoretics, emetics and purgatives

蘭室秘藏 [lánshì mìcáng]
Lan Shi Mi Cang, "A Secret Book Kept in Chamber", a comprehensive book on medicine, written by Li Gao (李杲) and published in 1276 A.D. The book deals with various kinds of diseases, which are classed into 21 groups. In the book the author's treatise on diseases of the *spleen* and *stomach* was especially prized by the later generations; the prescriptions listed were mostly created by himself.

丹溪心法 [dānxī xīnfǎ]

Dan Xi Xin Fa, "A Medical Book by Master of Danxi". It was written by Zhu Zhen-heng (朱震亨) in the Yuan Dynasty, but re-arranged and edited by his disciples. In 1481 A.D., the book was reedited with supplements and corrections by Cheng Chong (程充). At the beginning of the book, there are 6 treatises on medical theories and then 100 articles dealing with various diseases, most of which are concerned with internal medicine. The author's theory that "Yang was ever excessive and Yin ever deficient" is reflected in the whole book.

醫門法律 [yīmén fǎlǜ]
Yi Men Fa Lu, "Principles and Prohibitions of Medical Profession" written by Yu Chang (喩昌) in 1658 A.D. It explains the principles of diagnosis and treatment based on an overall differentiation of symptoms and signs; points out the errors usually made; and suggests prohibitions in this respect. Hence the title.

醫林改錯 [yīlín gǎicuò]
Yi Lin Gai Cuo, "Errors in Medicine Corrected", a book written by Wang Qing-ren (王清任) in 1830 A.D., who insisted on making anatomical observations and had made studies for dozens of years of internal organs of the human body. In the book not only did he correct certain mistakes made by the past generations concerning the internal organs but suggested new methods of treating blood stasis and hemiplegia. His method of activating blood circulation and removing blood stasis is still of practical value.

醫學衷中參西錄 [yīxué zhōngzhōng cānxī lù]
Yi Xue Zhong Zhong Can Xi Lu, "Records of Traditional Chinese and Western Medicine in Combination", written by Zhang Xi-chun(張錫純) and published in the years from 1918 to 1934. There were altogether 30 volumes in 7 issues. The revised edition consists of 5 parts, viz, prescriptions, medical substances, medical theories, notes and case records. The author tried his best to integrate traditional Chinese medicine with Western medicine.

名醫類案 [míngyī lèiàn]
Ming Yi Lei An, "Classified Medical Records of Distinguished Physicians" compiled by Jiang Guan (江瓘) and his son and comp-

leted in 1552 A.D. Afterwards Wei Zhi-xiu (魏之琇) revised the book, since then the new edition has been in circulation. The book deals with acute and chronic infectious diseases, other miscellaneous diseases concerned with internal medicine, surgery, gynecology, pediatrics, etc. The medical case records are written in detail; the methods of treatment and prescriptions are well chosen. Occasionally notes and commentaries are made by the authors.

醫貫 [yī guàn]

Yi Guan, "Key Link of Medicine", a book on medical theories, which was written by Zhao Xian-ke (趙獻可) in 1687 A.D. He supported Xue Ji's (薛已) views, advocating that "the fire of the Vital Gate" was the basis of the body, and emphasizing the importance of "genuine fire" and "genuine water". Throughout the book he suggested maintaining "the fire of the Vital Gate". This is an important reference book for studying the Vital Gate.

續名醫類案 [xù míngyī lèiàn]

Xu Ming Yi Lei An, "Classified Medical Records of Distinguished Physicians Continued" compiled by Wei Zhi-xiu (魏之琇), published in 1770 A.D. This is a continuation of the book Ming Yi Lei An 《名醫類案》 "Classified Medical Records of Distinguished Physicians" by Jiang Guan (江瓘).

臨證指南醫案 [línzhèng zhǐnán yīàn]

Lin Zheng Zhi Nang Yi An, "Medical Records as a Guide to Diagnosis" written by Ye Gui (葉桂) in 10 volumes. Later the book was rearranged by Hua Xiu-yun (華岫雲) et al. and published in 1766 A.D. Of the 10 volumes, 8 were devoted to miscellaneous diseases of internal medicine, one to gynecology and one to pediatrics.

聖濟總錄 [shèngjì zǒnglù]

Sheng Ji Zong Lu, "General Collection for Holy Relief" or "Imperial Encyclopaedia of Medicine", a monumental work consisting of 200 volumes (only 26 volumes exist today), which was compiled by a staff of physicians under imperial orders and completed around 1111-1117 A.D. It covers every branch of healing art, from internal medicine, surgery, gynecology, pediatrics, to acupuncture, charms, dieting, elixir of life, etc. About 20,000 recipes are recorded in it.

古今醫統　[gǔjīn yītǒng]

Gu Jin Yi Tong, "Ancient And Modern Medicine", or（古今醫統大全）Gu Jin Yi Tong Da Quan, "A Complete Work of Ancient and Modern Medicine", compiled by Xu Chun-fu（徐春甫）and completed in 1556 A.D. The book summed up and classified the contents of more than 100 medical and related works of the past generations.

證治準繩　[zhèngzhì zhǔnshéng]

Zheng Zhi Zhun Sheng, "Standards of Diagnosis and Treatments", also entitled（六科證治準繩）Liu Ke Zheng Zhi Zhun Sheng, written by Wang Ken-tang（王肯堂）in 1602 A.D., which gives a detailed and exhaustive description of symptoms and methods of treatment. The whole series consists of six branches, namely, febrile diseases, miscellaneous diseases of internal medicine, ulcers and boils, pediatrics, obstetrics and classified prescriptions. The work sums up the rich experiences of the doctors of the past generations and had the widest circultion in the 17th century.

景岳全書　[jǐngyuè quánshū]

Jing Yue Quan Shu, "Jing-yue's Complete Works", a book in 64 volumes, written by Zhang Jie-bin（張介賓）in 1624. The book includes studies of theories, pulse, febrile diseases, internal medicine, gynecology, pediatrics, surgery, materia medica, modern prescriptions, ancient prescriptions, etc. The author extracted the essence of various schools and made a systematical analysis of the diagnosis and treatment of diseases based on differentiation of their symptoms and signs. Advocating the theory "Yang is never in excess and Yin never sufficient", he recommended using warm, tonifying drugs and wrote 2 whole volumes of new prescriptions.

古今圖書集成醫部全集　[gǔjīn túshū jíchéng yībù quánjí]

Gu Jin Tu Shu Ji Cheng Yi Bu Quan Ji. "Collection of Ancient and Modern Books, The Part on Medicine", a book in 520 volumes, compiled by Jiang Ting-xi（蔣廷錫）et al. and published in 1723. This is a part of "Collection of Ancient and Modern Books", including "Internal Classic" and over 100 kinds of other medical works, with notes and commentaries on ancient medical works, diagnosis and treatment of various diseases, biography of physicians, etc.

390

醫宗金鑒 [yīzōng jīnjiàn]
Yi Zong Jin Jian, "The Golden Mirror of Medicine", in 90 volumes, one of the best treatises on general medicine, written by a staff of 80 persons headed by Wu Qian (吳謙) in compliance of an imperial order. A considerable part of the book is made up of extracts, revisions, and corrections of previous works. The book was issued in 1742 A.D.

中國醫學大辭典 [zhōngguó yīxué dàcídiǎn]
Zhong Guo Yi Xue Da Ci Dian, "A Dictionary of Chinese Medicine", compiled by Xie Guan (謝觀) et al. and published in 1921. The book collects more than 37,000 terms.

中國藥學大辭典 [zhōngguó yàoxué dàcídiǎn]
Zhong Guo Yao Xue Da Ci Dian, "A Dictionary of Chinese Pharmacy" published in 1935. The book includes all kinds of medicinal substances recorded in the medical literature of the past generations.

珍本醫書集成 [zhēnběn yīshū jíchéng]
Zhen Ben Yi Shu Ji Cheng, "Collection of Precious Medical Books", a collection of medical books compiled by Qiu Qing-yuan (裘慶元) and published in 1936. Of more than 3,000 kinds of books on medicine, the author chose 90 kinds, including editions de lure, the only extant books, copied editions, rarely extant ones and manuscripts. They were classified into 12 subjects, viz, medical classics, herbals, pulses, febrile diseases, general treatment, internal medicine, surgery, gynecology, pediatrics, prescriptions, medical case records and miscellaneous.

中國醫學大成 [zhōngguó yīxué dàchéng]
Zhong Guo Yi Xue Da Cheng, "A Great Collection of Chinese Medical Books", compiled by Cao Bing-zhang (曹炳章), published in 1936. A.D. Its compilation was based on 128 kinds of important medical works. The collection included 13 subjects, viz, medical classics, medical substances, diagnoses, prescriptions, general treatment, various clinical subjects, medical case records and miscellaneous topics, with abstracts and notes attached to each book.

Appendices

Appendix I Latin Names of Chinese Drugs in Common Use

Appendix II Chinese characters Strokes Index

Instruction:
1. The terms are arranged in the order of the number of brush strokes of Chinese characters;
2. Characters with the same number of strokes are arranged according the shape of strokes in the following order:
   — (horizontal bar), ｜ (vertical bar),
   丿 (slanting stroke), 丶 (dot), and → or 亅 (hook).

402

412

415

420